GLUCOSE TOLERANCE

Edited by **Sureka Chackrewarthy**

Glucose Tolerance
http://dx.doi.org/10.5772/2916
Edited by Sureka Chackrewarthy

Contributors

Paul Ernsberger, Richard J. Koletsky, Merita Emini Sadiku, Ayfer Colak, Gulden Diniz, Haifei Shi, Shiva Priya Dharshan Senthil Kumar, Ketut Suastika, Pande Dwipayana, Made Siswadi Semadi, R.A. Tuty Kuswardhani, Sylwia Dzięgielewska-Gęsiak, Ewa Wysocka, Soo-Jeong Kim, Dai-Jin Kim, Annadie Krygsman, Kia Halschou Hansen, Klaus Bukhave, Jens Rikardt Andersen, Nitsa Mirsky, Jackson Roberto Guedes da Silva Almeida, Grasielly Rocha Souza, Edigênia Cavalcante da Cruz Araújo, Fabrício Souza Silva, Julianeli Tolentino de Lima, Luciano Augusto de Araújo Ribeiro, Xirley Pereira Nunes, José Maria Barbosa Filho, Lucindo José Quintans Júnior, Márcio Roberto Viana dos Santos, Sureka Chackrewarthy, M.I. Thabrew, Yukihito Ishii, Takeshi Ohta, Tomohiko Sasase

Published by InTech

Janeza Trdine 9, 51000 Rijeka, Croatia

Publishing Process Manager Romina Skomersic
Technical Editor InTech Prepress, Novi Sad
Cover InTech Design team

Additional hard copies can be obtained from orders@intechopen.com

Glucose Tolerance, Edited by Sureka Chackrewarthy
p. cm.
ISBN 978-953-51-0891-7

For EU product safety concerns:
IN TECH d.o.o., Prolaz Marije Krucifikse Kozulić 3, 51000 Rijeka, Croatia,
info@intechopen.com or visit our website at intechopen.com.

Meet the editor

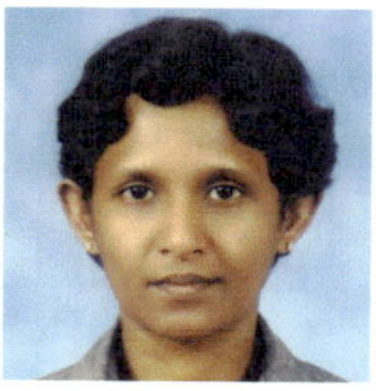

Dr. Sureka Chackrewarthy, graduated from University of Glasgow, UK with a PhD in Biochemistry. She is currently working as Head/ Senior Lecturer in Biochemistry and Clinical Chemistry at the Faculty of Medicine, University of Kelaniya, Sri Lanka.

Contents

Preface

With the rapidly rising rates of diabetes has come refreshed research efforts to understand the biological process impacting glucose tolerance. Glucose tolerance depends on a complex interaction among insulin secretion from the β-cells, clearance of the hormone, and the actions of insulin to accelerate glucose disappearance and inhibit endogenous glucose production. The research approaches the topic from several directions including insights into mechanisms of action, development of screening methods and novel therapeutic targets and the effectiveness of lifestyle and pharmacologic interventions in improving glucose tolerance. This book summarises the recent advances in research relating to glucose tolerance.

The book is divided into four sections and each section subdivided into individual chapters contributed by experts in that particular field. The progression from normal glucose tolerance to impaired glucose tolerance known as a prediabetic state, and then to overt diabetes is reviewed in the first section of this book. Usefulness of the oral glucose tolerance test in basic and clinical investigations and the effectiveness of interventions to prevent or delay the progression from a prediabetic to a diabetic state as demonstrated by findings of clinical trials are included in this section.

The second section reviews the potential mechanisms associated with insulin resistance leading to impaired glucose tolerance and type 2 diabetes. Our knowledge of the molecular basis of the signaling pathways mediating the various physiologic effects of insulin is steadily advancing. New substrates and signaling molecules have been identified and potential mechanisms involved in the pathophysiology of type II diabetes have been revealed. Each chapter in this section is an updated account of the advances in this field of research.

Third section reviews current evidence on the role of dietary constituents on insulin resistance and glycaemic control. Type of dietary fat and fatty acid composition in the modern diets contributing to the development of obesity and altered insulin action are reviewed. Further, research findings which demonstrate the effects of dietary sugars on postprandial glucose uptake and insulin secretion are included in this section.

Therapy of type 2 diabetes is also advancing and many new avenues of research have developed and established areas have taken new directions. The fourth section of this book includes several reviews on selected novel pharmacologic compounds with antidiabetic potential from natural sources. Their effectiveness in potentiating insulin action and improving glucose tolerance are discussed. In addition a review on experimental animal models extensively used in type 2 diabetes research and a mechanistic model of insulin dynamics with relevance to identifying new therapies is included to allow the reader to gain insights into potential new therapeutic targets.

This book is a team product, combining input from many individuals whose contributions are much appreciated. Each chapter is written as a focused review accompanied by extensive and updated reference lists providing a resource for further in-depth researching of the area of interest. All the contributing authors and co-authors are acknowledged for their scholarly approach and willingness to participate in this endeavor. Without their contributions this book could not have been successfully completed.

Sureka Chackrewarthy, PhD
Department of Biochemistry & Clinical Chemistry
Faculty of Medicine,
University of Kelaniya,
Sri Lanka

Section 1

Impaired Glucose Tolerance: Diagnosis, Prognosis and Treatment

Chapter 1

The Glucose Tolerance Test as a Laboratory Tool with Clinical Implications

Paul Ernsberger and Richard J. Koletsky

Additional information is available at the end of the chapter

http://dx.doi.org/10.5772/54785

1. Introduction

Metabolic syndrome is a cluster of abnormalities that are often associated with prediabetes, a condition present prior to the onset of diabetes (1). The hallmark of both metabolic syndrome and prediabetes is insulin resistance, an impairment of insulin action within tissues at the level of the insulin receptor and subsequent cellular events. Insulin resistance resides mainly within muscle, liver and adipose tissues (2). Type 2 diabetes arises from a combination of insulin resistance and a relative impairment of insulin secretion in response to meal ingestion. Type 2 diabetics differ in the relative contributions of insulin resistance and impaired insulin secretion to the development of hyperglycemia (3). Some diabetic patients predominantly have a secretory defect, while others may have normal or even excessive insulin secretion. The latter subgroup of diabetics has insulin resistance as the primary defect in their glucose homeostasis. Hyperglycemia by itself does not indicate whether there is an insufficiency of insulin secretion or a deficit in insulin action. Type 2 diabetics lie along a continuum between these two extremes, with a variable mix of secretory and cell signaling deficits. During the progression from normal glucose tolerance to impaired glucose tolerance to prediabetes to diabetes to severe diabetes over a number of years, individuals show a progressive decline in pancreatic insulin secretion in response to a glucose load(3). Insulin resistance may show progressive deterioration, but generally insulin resistance is the major defect early in the development of diabetes whereas late in the course of the disease pancreatic islet cell failure is more notable.

In Type 2 diabetes, determining the relative contribution of insulin secretion versus action has clinical implications. Knowledge of the predominant abnormalities in glucose homeostasis may well affect the choice of therapeutic agent for the treatment of diabetes. For example, metformin acts to reduce insulin resistance, particularly within the liver (4), and therefore is of considerable utility in early stages of Type 2 diabetes where insulin resistance is predominant. Sulfonylureas such as glyburide, in contrast, promote the secretion of endogenous insulin in response to a meal (5) and might therefore be more useful when insulin secretion is declining.

However, some have alleged that sulfonylureas may accelerate beta cell exhaustion over time and thereby accelerate the deterioration of diabetes (5). The incretin mimetic agents such as exendin and the DPP-IV inhibitors also promote insulin release from pancreatic islets but may also be cytoprotective within pancreatic islets and thereby delay the progression of diabetes (6). As shown in the Results section below, DPP-IV inhibitors are also effective in reversing metabolic syndrome prior to the onset of diabetes.

Diabetes typically manifests itself in the context of other abnormalities, especially the principal components of metabolic syndrome, namely hypertension and hyperlipidemia (2). The SHROB or Koletsky rat is a leading animal model of metabolic syndrome (7;8), as summarized in Table 1.

Trait	SHR(7)	SHROB(7)	Human Metabolic Syndrome(9)
Hypertension	SBP = 195	SBP = 185	SBP > 130
Insulin resistance	Absent	Profound	Present
Fasting glucose	Normal	Normal to slightly high	Normal to slightly high
Glucose tolerance	Normal	Impaired	Impaired
Triglycerides	Absent	>200 mg/dL	>150 mg/dL
Total Cholesterol	Normal	Slightly elevated	>200 mg/dL
Visceral obesity	Absent	Present	Present
Fasting insulin	Normal	Elevated 20-fold	Elevated
Fasting glucagon	Normal(10)	Elevated 2-fold(10)	Elevated(11;12)

Table 1. Characteristics of human metabolic syndrome compared with the SHROB model

Each of the primary abnormalities expressed in human metabolic syndrome are present in the SHROB rat. Other obese rodents fail to show these characteristics. In particular, the SHROB is only rodent model that incorporates hypertension and related cardiovascular changes together with insulin resistance and abnormal glucose homeostasis. The SHROB has marked hyperinsulinemia without hyperglycemia. Other rodent models show diabetes that ranges from mild (Zucker fatty rat) to fulminant Type 2 diabetes (db/db mouse) (8;13). In contrast, the SHROB is a model for the prediabetic state accompanied by hypertension and hyperlipidemia as well as obesity. Prediabetes can lead to secondary disease complications even in the absence of fasting hyperglycemia (14). The SHROB model can be used to understand the complex physiologic processes that contribute to metabolic syndrome. Dietary and pharmacologic interventions in this model may help identify the best prevention strategies and treatment combinations for metabolic syndrome as well.

Premise: The oral glucose tolerance test (OGTT) is vital for the characterization of metabolic syndrome, the natural progression from prediabetes to Type 2 diabetes, and characterization of the metabolic actions of cardiovascular and metabolic drugs. Although the OGTT is seldom used as a diagnostic test for Type 2 diabetes (15), it is extensively used as a sensitive indicator of gestational diabetes (16). As we demonstrate in the present work, the OGTT is an important laboratory tool in preclinical studies. In both humans and animals, the OGTT provides an indication of the relative roles of insulin secretion and insulin resistance in the progression of glucose intolerance. The impact of diet composition and pharmacologic interventions can be tested and possible target tissues identified. This in vivo, real time, whole body test can be used to identify the best treatments and possibly delay or prevent development of Type 2 diabetes.

Insulin release in response to a glucose load occurs in two phases in humans and in rodents. The early phase peaks within the first 15-30 min and is responsible for limiting the initial rise in glucose upon meal ingestion. The late phase of insulin secretion occurs later than 30 min after a meal, and may persist for several hours. This delayed burst of insulin secretion is responsible for returning glucose to baseline fasting levels. In the face of insulin resistance, the late phase of insulin secretion persists for an extended period and contributes to excessive insulin levels even after a return to the fasted state, resulting in fasting hyperinsulinemia (2).

Insulin and glucagon, derived from beta and alpha pancreatic islet cells, respectively, are the two most important hormones involved in glucose homeostasis. Together they determine whether food is utilized immediately for energy or put into storage for later use. Abnormalities in the release or actions of either or both of these hormones can be involved in the development of hyperglycemia and diabetes. Glucagon levels may influence glucose tolerance (11), although this hormone is seldom considered in the context of oral glucose tolerance. Glucagon raises glucose levels, and a higher level of insulin is needed to control glucose in the presence of glucagon (10).

The phases of insulin secretion in response to the oral ingestion of glucose are cephalic, gastric and intestinal. The cephalic phase begins with the sight of food and is strongly triggered by sweet taste receptors on the tongue (17). The cephalic and gastric phases are considered part of the early response, while the intestinal response is later. Interestingly, sweet taste receptors are also present in the small intestine and may shape the physiological response to carbohydrates (18;19). Sweet taste receptors in the small intestine not only regulate the rate of glucose absorption through glucose transporters (19), but also trigger the release of GLP-1 and cholecystokinin (18). GLP-1 and gastric inhibitory peptide (GIP) are incretins, gut hormones secreted from enteroendocrine cells into the blood in response to meal ingestion. Importantly, incretin secretion only occurs with oral ingestion of nutrients. Incretin secretion is not triggered in response to intravenous feeding, as the intestinal receptors are not activated when glucose is delivered through the circulation. Indeed, incretins were discovered as a result of the observation that the insulin stimulation and glucagon suppression by glucose was much greater when glucose was delivered orally or into the gut rather than by any other route (20). Thus, the normal physiological response to food ingestion can only be elicited through the oral route of administration.

Both incretins are rapidly deactivated by a degradative enzyme called dipeptidyl peptidase 4 (DPP4) (21). Since 2005, two new classes of drugs based on incretin action have been approved for Type 2 diabetes therapy: incretin analogs and incretin enhancers, which inhibit DPP4. DPP4 inhibitors act by slowing the breakdown of endogenous incretin peptides, thus extending their actions.

An OGTT is used clinically to diagnose impaired glucose tolerance and as a standardized test of carbohydrate metabolism and insulin secretion. The test is based on oral administration of glucose and subsequently following plasma glucose and insulin levels over time. A prolonged elevation (>120min) in both plasma glucose and insulin constitutes impaired glucose tolerance and insulin resistance and can be used in conjunction with fasting hyperglycemia in diagnosing Type 2 diabetes. A prolonged elevation in glucose with minimal changes in insulin secretion would be suggestive of impaired glucose stimulated insulin secretion. This procedure is directly applicable to rats and mice.

The OGTT was introduced first as a diagnostic tool for diabetes. Later studies focused on identifying patterns of the glucose curve during the OGTT that predicted the onset of diabetes years later. An OGTT profile during pregnancy can accurately predict which women will later develop Type 2 diabetes when they reach middle age (22). Clinically, the use of OGTT has fallen off because of the need for glucose loading, which many patients perceive as unpleasant. Furthermore, 4 to 6 separate blood samples are necessary. In the modern clinic, the OGTT has generally been supplanted by measuring fasting blood glucose, random post prandial blood glucose and glycosylated hemoglobin values.

The OGTT is influenced by many factors including age, diet, state of health, GI function, medications and emotional state. As age increases, the excursion of glucose during the OGTT progressively increases as a consequence of declining insulin sensitivity of target tissues, such as in muscle, fat and liver. The dose of glucose and standardization of measured responses including glucose levels and insulin have been debated over the years. When used in large population studies the OGTT test overestimates the prevalence of diabetes. In other words, it has a high false positive rate.

The intravenous glucose tolerance test is not sensitive for the diagnosis of diabetes and is used mainly as an assessment purely of glucose disposal i.e. the time required for glucose to clear circulation. It can be used as an index of residual beta cell function as well. The test bypasses the GI tract and eliminates the influence of intestinal hormones, especially incretins, on insulin and glucagon levels and subsequent glucose disposal. The endocrine system of the small intestine is important in the development of diabetes and has spawned new drugs to treat diabetes. The relative advantages of OGTT over other methods of assessing glucose homeostasis in the laboratory are summarized in Table 2.

The hyperinsulemic clamp has been described by some authors as "the gold standard" yet has a number of limitations. Indwelling catheters are required, necessitating some trauma.

Even with time for recovery, glucose homeostasis can be altered by ongoing wound healing and pain. For highly insulin resistant individuals, insulin must be elevated to very high levels. For example, insulin levels in SHROB rats must be raised to levels that would result in convulsions and death from hypoglycemia in a lean animal (results not shown). The OGTT allows all of the normal stages of insulin secretion and glucose processing to take place in sequence without causing stress or trauma to the subject.

	OGTT	IVGTT	Hyperinsulinemic Clamp
Incorporates cephalic phase	Yes	No	No
Incorporates gut-pancreatic axis	Yes	No	No
First pass through liver and portal circulation	Yes	No	No
Raises insulin to nonphysiologic levels	No	No	Yes
Requires surgery	No	Yes	Yes

Table 2. Advantages of OGTT over IVGTT and hyperinsulinemic clamps

2. Methods

Special diets are fed for 30 to 90d prior to the OGTT. Antihypertensive or antidiabetic medications are given in the drinking water or incorporated into the food and given for 42 to 90d. We carry out the OGTT by fasting animals for 18h, taking a baseline 200 μL blood sample from the tail under local anesthesia, and then gavaging with 12 mL/kg of a 50% glucose solution, which delivers 6g of glucose per kg of body weight. Blood samples are taken 30, 60, 120, 180, 240 and 360 minutes after the glucose meal and analyzed for blood glucose with a clinical meter. Plasma samples are frozen for later analysis of rat insulin by ELISA. The 240 and 360 minute time points are not typically used in OGTT, but the SHROB is so profoundly glucose intolerant that extended sampling is required to reliably establish the area under the curve. Area under the curve is determined for each subject using curve fitting software (Prism 5.0, GraphPad software, San Diego, CA).

Procedures:

1. Weigh the rats to the nearest 0.5g and place them into clean cages with new bedding. Rodents are copraphagic, so new cages will assure true fasting conditions over the next 18h.
2. Dextrose (D-glucose) solution: A 50% dextrose solution is made by weighing out the needed amount of dextrose and heating and stirring with water (be sure not to overheat solution or caramelization will take place). For example, if you need 50mL of workable solution, you would weigh out 25g of dextrose and add that to approximately 28mL of water then stir and heat until dextrose is in solution. Once in solution, pour into a graduated cylinder and dilute up to 50mL and allow cooling at room temperature prior to using.

3. Dose: We administer a 6g/kg body weight of a 50% dextrose solution for our studies to assure a significant challenge to glucose metabolism, but 2-4g/kg body weight is frequently reported by others.
4. Oral gavaging: Discharge rate should be slow so as not to cause a pressure induced "dumping syndrome". This will be apparent about 30-60min after gavaging with the presence of diarrhea.
5. Blood Collection: This is done by tail bleed. We recommend that blood be collected at least five times: 0, 30, 60, 120 and 180 min. However, we collect additional time points of 240 and 360 min in our SHROB rats, as this represents the delayed insulin peak response and allows an accurate estimate of the area under the curve for glucose, as glucose returns to fasting levels only very slowly. We also dip the cut tail tip into the local anesthetic, bupivacaine (Marcaine, 0.5%), after the first tail bleed and after each sample thereafter to minimize pain associated with the procedure.
6. Glucose measurement: A clinical glucose meter (One Touch Ultra, Lifescan) is used with 5 μL of whole blood.
7. Insulin and glucagon ELISA: Rodent-specific kits are available from several suppliers, including ALPCO (Salem, NH). The coefficient of variation is less than 10% in repeat measures and the sensitivity is 0.1 ng/mL. Plasma samples from our insulin resistant rats must be diluted 1:10 in assay buffer before addition to the assay plate.
8. Statistical analysis: Glucose and insulin data are processed through an analysis of variance with repeated measures to determine treatment effects, time effects, and treatment by time interaction terms by using the Prism 5.0 statistical and graphing program (GraphPad Software, Sand Diego, CA). Newman-Keuls post-hoc tests are used to determine significance of individual comparisons. Area under the curve measurement are also determined for each animal, expressed as mg*min/dL for glucose and ng*min/mL for insulin, and analyzed as a single datum.

3. Results

We review data from several contrasting interventions in SHROB rats, which includes diets and drug treatments with both beneficial and harmful effects on glucose tolerance. We contrast the use of OGTT with other measures such as fasting glucose and glucose to insulin ratios.

A relatively normal OGTT profile is illustrated by the data from lean SHR. Glucose starts at a low fasting level and rises only to a maximum of about 100 mg/dL at 60 min. Insulin levels are low in the fasted state and show a maximum 4-fold rise around 60 min and then return to baseline by 240 min. Not shown is the profile for normotensive Wistar or Sprague-Dawley control rats, which would show a similar profile but with even lower levels of insulin owing to a small amount of insulin resistance associated with hypertension (23).

SHROB on a control diet show a normal fasting level of glucose, but glucose ascends to a much higher peak around 60 min and takes much longer to return to baseline. Fasting insulin levels in the SHROB are 40-fold elevated compared to lean SHR littermates, and the further rise in insulin in response to a glucose load is delayed and prolonged. Dietary obese genetically lean SHR rats are only about 25% overweight compared to lean SHR on normal chow, in contrast to genetically obese SHROB which are about 100% overweight compared to lean SHR on normal chow (24). Despite the lesser degree of obesity, the dietary obese genetically lean SHR showed about the same degree of glucose intolerance as SHROB. Insulin levels at fasting and after the glucose load were unchanged relative to the SHR fed control diet. SHROB fed a high sucrose diet showed unchanged glucose tolerance. In contrast, the insulin response to a glucose load was greatly increased and prolonged beyond that observed for SHROB on a control diet. To our knowledge, the insulin levels in sucrose-fed SHROB during the OGTT, which exceed 100 ng/mL, are the highest ever recorded in a rodent. The data in Figure 1 illustrate the value of the OGTT. High sucrose input affected glucose levels in genetically lean animals without affecting insulin. In contrast, in genetically obese SHROB rats, high sucrose affected insulin without affecting glucose levels. None of this could be learned by obtaining fasting levels alone.

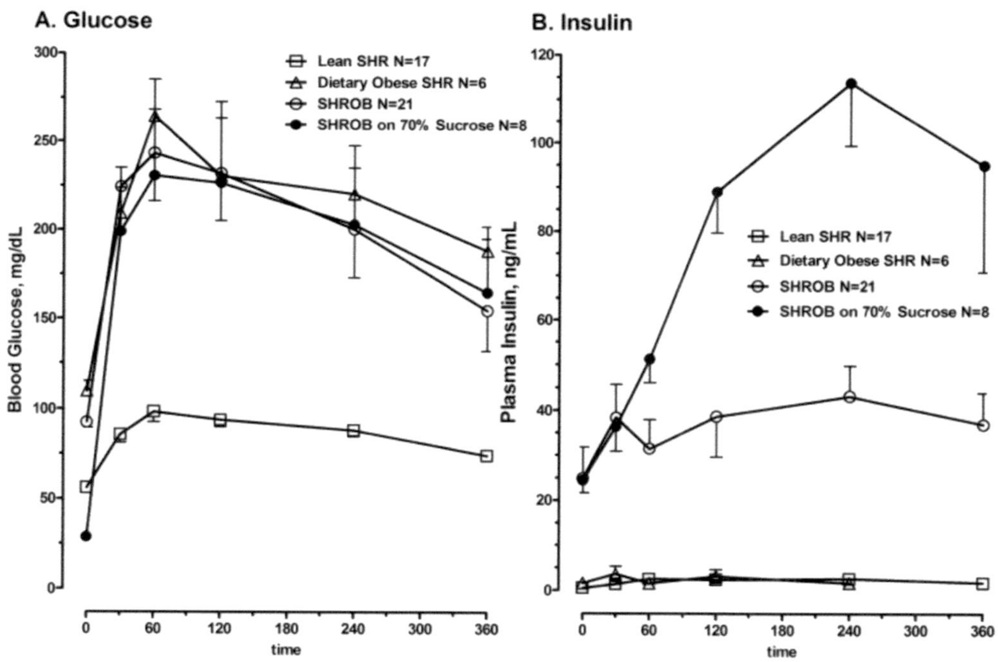

Figure 1. Glucose tolerance test: SHR versus SHROB on normal versus high sucrose diets. A: Glucose. B: Insulin. SHR were fed a supplementary sweet drink to induce dietary obesity in these genetically lean rats. SHROB were fed a high sucrose diet (70% sucrose by weight).

Figure 2 includes only the genetically obese SHROB fed a control diet, which were given vehicle or drug in their drinking water. Two oral antihyperglycemic agents, the insulin secretagogue glyburide (mg/kg) and the DPP4 inhibitor sitagliptin (mg/kg), were contrasted with the widely used antihypertensive hydrochlorothiazide (50 mg/kg). None of the agents had any effect on fasting glucose. The two antihyperglycemic agents, as expected, lowered the excursion of glucose in response to an oral load. The antihypertensive agent dramatically increased glucose levels following the oral load, with glucose rising to levels associated with frank diabetes (>400 mg/dL).

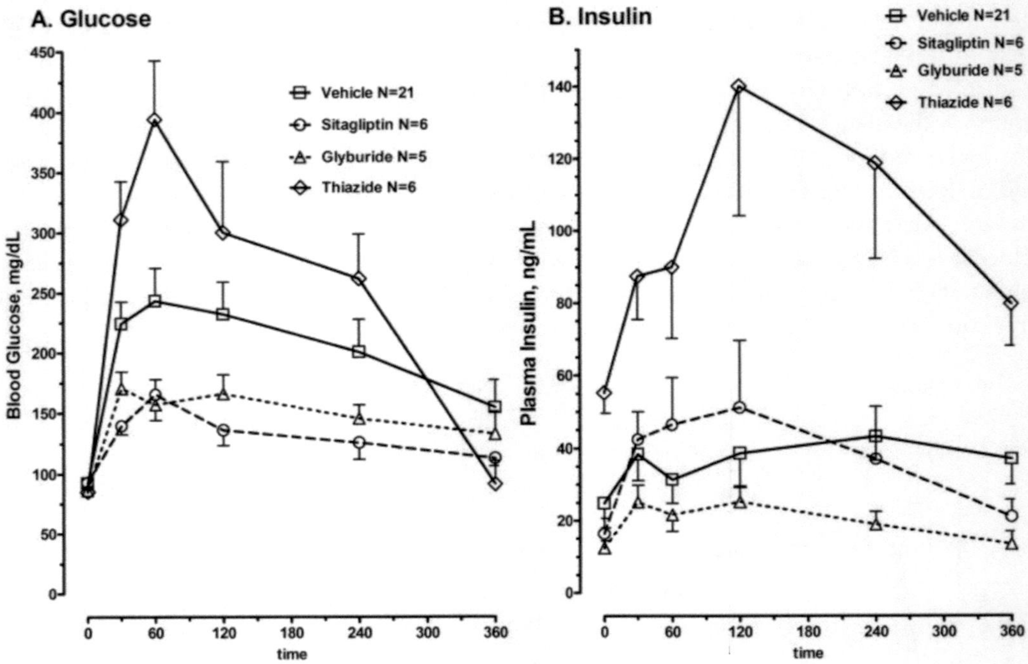

Figure 2. Glucose tolerance test: untreated SHROB versus SHROB treated with antihyperglycemic agents and one antihypertensive agent. A: Glucose. B: Insulin

Fasting insulin levels in vehicle controls (Figure 2) were very high, similar to those observed before in Figure 1. The oral antihyperglycemic drugs both reduced fasting insulin levels, although not to levels seen in lean SHR. Remarkably, hydrochlorothiazide further elevated fasting insulin. The post-load insulin curve in glyburide treated SHROB closely paralleled vehicle treated controls, but at a lower level. The insulin curve for the sitagliptin treated group showed a higher net response to the glucose load, especially at 30 min. This is consistent with the hypothesized role of incretin hormones in facilitating the insulin response to glucose. Hydrochlorothiazide greatly increased insulin levels, reminiscent of the effect of dietary sucrose in Figure 1.

Other hormones and metabolites can be measured during OGTT, not just glucose and insulin. Figure 3 illustrates changes in plasma glucagon during the first hour after an oral glucose load. Homeostasis predicts that glucagon would be high in the fasting state and decline when the fed state is restored. Glucagon levels are unchanged in SHR animals, possibly because the fall in glucagon is mainly mediated by gut hormones such as GLP-1 and GIP which are secreted later after the load has reached the distal small intestine where the L-cells that secrete these hormones reside. Remarkably, SHROB rats show a dramatic increase in glucagon from already high fasting levels. This paradoxical increase in glucagon in response to a glucose meal has been reported in humans with Type 2 diabetes (12).

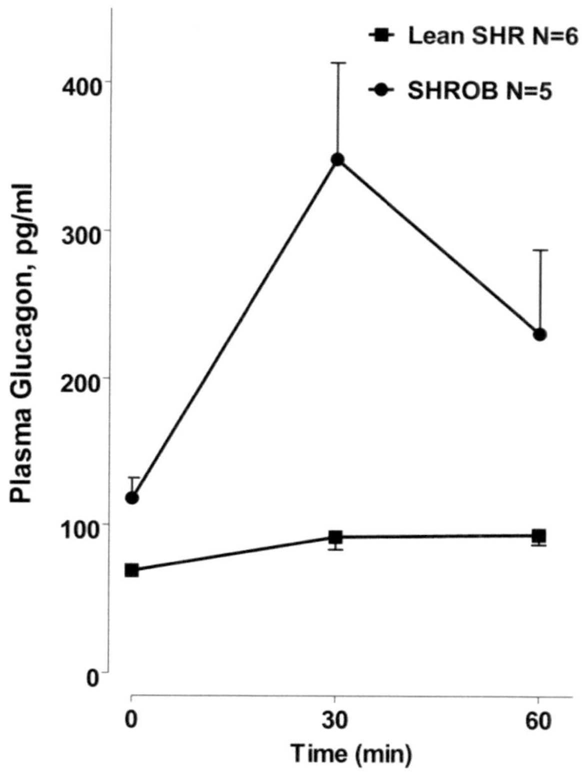

Figure 3. Changes in plasma glucagon level during an OGTT in SHROB and lean SHR littermates.

Besides glucose, another plasma substrate that can be assayed is the level of free fatty acids. We found that free fatty acids fall after glucose load in lean SHR, indicating reduced lipolysis when an abundant supply of glucose is present (10). Remarkably, the level of free fatty acids in SHROB rats stayed at the elevated level found in fasting (data not shown). This finding illustrates the multiple abnormalities in the whole body handling of metabolic fuels that can be uncovered in an OGTT.

4. Discussion

These data show that OGTT is much more sensitive than are other measures in identifying the loci of insulin resistance and its modulation by different interventions. Moreover, the results of OGTT testing in the SHROB model tracks closely with efficacy against metabolic syndrome and Type 2 diabetes in clinical trials. Thus, the OGTT yields laboratory data with greater relevance to the prevention and treatment of human disease.

The glucose tolerance test determines the rate at which glucose is cleared from blood. Glucose is administered either orally or intravenously and serial samples of glucose, insulin and glucagon are measured over time. Hypoglycemic medications used to treat diabetes have been developed that modify the actions of glucagon and insulin directly. Medications that are used to treat high blood pressure and lipid disturbances can also modify the responses to these hormones, sometimes improving the clearance of glucose and sometimes making it worse. Comparisons of the responses of glucose, insulin and glucagon levels during glucose tolerance testing with and without medications used to treat metabolic syndrome will lead to a better understanding of what combinations of these medications are the most beneficial and least toxic.

The current literature has many examples of inadequate assessments of glucose metabolism. Many authors report only on "random glucose" values, taken without regard to whether the animal had just eaten or had voluntarily fasted for several hours. If food is available ad libitum, then some animals may be postprandial and others will be fasted as a result of their sleep cycle. The glucose and insulin values obtained under these circumstances are highly variable and often irreproducible. A somewhat better approach is to determine fasting glucose and insulin levels. Various ratios between glucose and insulin can be calculated, with the most popular being the Homeostasis Model Assessment (HOMA). The mathematical derivation of the HOMA equation is sophisticated, but it is still based on only two numbers: fasting glucose and fasting insulin. The OGTT, by contrast, reflects the in vivo physiological response to a glucose meal and integrates the homeostatic response to a meal over time. Thus, the OGTT more accurately mirrors daily life.

The OGTT is useful as a research tool. It does allow for a more physiologic assessment of metabolism as it assesses a global response to the disposition of a meal. Neurologic and hormonal responses that influence the function of the gastric tract, absorption, transportation and processing of food in the liver and transport to and from storage tissue can be assessed. These include newly recognized hormones secreted from the GI tract in the presence of food known as incretins and previously recognized hormones such as insulin and glucagon. The OGTT is particularly useful in characterizing the actions of drugs which can be either beneficial or detrimental to glucose homeostasis.

Author details

Paul Ernsberger and Richard J. Koletsky
Department of Nutrition, Case Western Reserve University School of Medicine,
Cleveland, OH, USA

5. References

[1] Batsis JA, Nieto-Martinez RE, Lopez-Jimenez F. Metabolic syndrome: from global epidemiology to individualized medicine. Clin Pharmacol Ther 2007 Nov;82(5):509-24.

[2] Oda E. Metabolic syndrome: its history, mechanisms, and limitations. Acta Diabetol 2012 Apr;49(2):89-95.

[3] Haffner SM, Miettinen H, Gaskill SP, Stern MP. Decreased insulin action and insulin secretion predict the development of impaired glucose tolerance. Diabetologia 1996 Oct;39(10):1201-7.

[4] Cleasby ME, Dzamko N, Hegarty BD, Cooney GJ, Kraegen EW, Ye JM. Metformin prevents the development of acute lipid-induced insulin resistance in the rat through altered hepatic signaling mechanisms. Diabetes 2004 Dec;53(12):3258-66.

[5] Aston-Mourney K, Proietto J, Morahan G, Andrikopoulos S. Too much of a good thing: why it is bad to stimulate the beta cell to secrete insulin. Diabetologia 2008 Apr;51(4):540-5.

[6] Mu J, Petrov A, Eiermann GJ, Woods J, Zhou YP, Li Z, et al. Inhibition of DPP-4 with sitagliptin improves glycemic control and restores islet cell mass and function in a rodent model of type 2 diabetes. Eur J Pharmacol 2009 Nov 25;623(1-3):148-54.

[7] Ernsberger P, Koletsky RJ, Friedman JE. Molecular pathology in the obese spontaneous hypertensive Koletsky rat: a model of syndrome X. Ann N Y Acad Sci 1999 Nov 18;892:272-88.

[8] Koletsky RJ, Velliquette RA, Ernsberger P. The SHROB (Koletsky) rat as a model for metabolic syndrome. In: Shafrir E, editor. Animal Models of Diabetes: Frontiers in Research.Boca Raton, FL: CRC Press; 2007. p. 185-208.

[9] Hansen BC. The metabolic syndrome X. Ann N Y Acad Sci 1999 Nov 18;892:1-24.

[10] Velliquette RA, Koletsky RJ, Ernsberger P. Plasma glucagon and free fatty acid responses to a glucose load in the obese spontaneous hypertensive rat (SHROB) model of metabolic syndrome X. Exp Biol Med (Maywood) 2002 Mar;227(3):164-70.

[11] Unger RH. Glucagon and the insulin: glucagon ratio in diabetes and other catabolic illnesses. Diabetes 1971 Dec;20(12):834-8.

[12] Iannello S, Campione R, Belfiore F. Response of insulin, glucagon, lactate, and nonesterified fatty acids to glucose in visceral obesity with and without NIDDM: relationship to hypertension. Mol Genet Metab 1998 Mar;63(3):214-23.

[13] Rees DA, Alcolado JC. Animal models of diabetes mellitus. Diabet Med 2005 Apr;22(4):359-70.

[14] Reaven G. Insulin resistance and coronary heart disease in nondiabetic individuals. Arterioscler Thromb Vasc Biol 2012 Aug;32(8):1754-9.

[15] Inzucchi SE. Clinical practice. Diagnosis of diabetes. N Engl J Med 2012 Aug 9;367(6):542-50.

[16] Coustan DR, Carpenter MW. The diagnosis of gestational diabetes. Diabetes Care 1998;21 Suppl 2(Aug):B5-B8.

[17] Simon C, Schlienger JL, Sapin R, Imler M. Cephalic phase insulin secretion in relation to food presentation in normal and overweight subjects. Physiol Behav 1986;36(3):465-9.

[18] Gerspach AC, Steinert RE, Schonenberger L, Graber-Maier A, Beglinger C. The role of the gut sweet taste receptor in regulating GLP-1, PYY, and CCK release in humans. Am J Physiol Endocrinol Metab 2011 Aug;301(2):E317-E325.

[19] Mace OJ, Affleck J, Patel N, Kellett GL. Sweet taste receptors in rat small intestine stimulate glucose absorption through apical GLUT2. J Physiol 2007 Jul 1;582(Pt 1):379-92.

[20] Diakogiannaki E, Gribble FM, Reimann F. Nutrient detection by incretin hormone secreting cells. Physiol Behav 2012 Jun 6;106(3):387-93.

[21] Ahren B. GLP-1-based therapy of type 2 diabetes: GLP-1 mimetics and DPP-IV inhibitors. Curr Diab Rep 2007 Oct;7(5):340-7.

[22] Malcolm J. Through the looking glass: gestational diabetes as a predictor of maternal and offspring long-term health. Diabetes Metab Res Rev 2012 May;28(4):307-11.

[23] Reaven GM, Chang H, Hoffman BB, Azhar S. Resistance to insulin-stimulated glucose uptake in adipocytes isolated from spontaneously hypertensive rats. Diabetes 1989;38:1155-60.

[24] Johnson JL, Wan DP, Koletsky RJ, Ernsberger P. A new rat model of dietary obesity and hypertension. Obes.Res. 13, A113-A114. 2005.

Chapter 2

Can We Prevent or Delay Type 2 Diabetes?

Merita Emini Sadiku

Additional information is available at the end of the chapter

http://dx.doi.org/10.5772/54872

1. Introduction

Type 2 diabetes results from the interaction between genetic predisposition, behavioral and environmental risk factors (1). There is strong evidence that modifiable risk factors such as obesity and physical inactivity are the main non-genetic determinants of the disease(2). New figures indicate that the number of people living with diabetes is expected to rise from 366 million to 552 million by 2030, if no urgent action is taken (3).

Impaired glucose tolerance (IGT) is an intermediate category between normal glucose tolerance and overt diabetes, and it can be identified by glucose tolerance test. Subjects with IGT have an increased risk of type 2 diabetes (4), and consequently many trials of interventions for the prevention of type 2 diabetes have focused on such individuals. By 2025, the number of people with IGT is projected to increase to 418 million, or 8.1% of the adult population (5).

Interventions to delay or even to prevent type 2 diabetes have a potential to improve the health of the population and reduce the burden of healthcare costs. The interventions assessed have been diverse and include pharmacological and lifestyle changes.

Abnormal glucose tolerance is also a well-known risk factor of incident diabetes (6). The main known predictor of incident diabetes is the presence of insulin resistance. Direct measures of insulin sensitivity can be laborious, complicated, and expensive to be applicable for routine use in the general population as a screening tool. Markers like HOMA-IR index or 2-hour post-challenge glucose levels are being used to diagnose insulin resistance.

IGT when compared to impaired fasting glucose (IFG) is a stronger risk factor in predicting the onset of diabetes (7). Diagnosing of IGT requires oral glucose tolerance test (OGTT), a test of high specificity (92%) but low sensitivity (52%) in the prediction of diabetes (8). The World Health Organization (WHO) criteria including either IFG (≥6.1 mmol/L and <7.0 mmol/L and 2-h plasma glucose concentration <11.1 mmol/L during the oral glucose tolerance test) or IGT test (<7.0 mmol/L and 2-h plasma glucose concentration ≥7.8 mmol/L and <11.1mmol/L) are used to diagnose people with IGT (9).

The clinical characteristics associated with type 2 diabetes risk include obesity and overweight, age (the risk rises steadily from puberty into geriatric years), a history of gestational diabetes, polycystic ovary syndrome, a family history of type 2 diabetes, and membership in certain high-risk minority groups: African American, Hispanic, Native American, and Asian-Pacific Islanders (6). The ADA recommends screening youth and adults with multiple risk factors for type 2 diabetes; fasting plasma glucose is the preferred first-line test (10, 11).

People with metabolic syndrome are at a high risk to develop diabetes and ischemic atherosclerotic diseases (7). Several studies have shown that metabolic syndrome is a strong predictor of incident diabetes (12-14).

The Insulin Resistance Atherosclerosis Study (IRAS) assessed a series of risk factors and identified five significant risk factors for the development of type 2 diabetes including high plasminogen activator inhibitor 1 (PAI-1), hypertension (HTN), high triglycerides (TG), low high-density lipoprotein (HDL), and IGT. The incidence of type 2 diabetes increases with the increasing number of risk factors, 5% with 0 risk factors to 50% when all 5 risk factors are present (p<0.001) (15).

Every year about 5%-10% of people with IGT will develop diabetes and acquire the disease burden related to its diagnosis symptoms, need for surveillance for chronic consequences and associated costs, and increased risk of several chronic diseases (16).

The purpose of this article is to review available evidence on lifestyle and pharmacological intervention on the prevention or delay of the onset of type 2 diabetes and adapting these lessons from clinical trials to clinical practice.

2. How we can prevent type 2 diabetes?

The high economic and social costs of type 2 diabetes mellitus and its rising prevalence make a compelling case for its prevention (17). The most vulnerable groups to have diabetes are people with IFG and IGT and in the mean time they present the potent groups of preventing or delaying the progression to type 2 diabetes mellitus. These two groups are recognized as prediabetic states by the ADA (11).

3. Non pharmacological intervention

Four large prospective studies demonstrated that a treatment regimen using diet plus exercise reduces IGT progression to type 2 diabetes (18-21). Factor analysis showed that both insulin resistance and insulin secretion had a significant association with the development of diabetes, and lifestyle intervention was more effective in subjects with lower insulin resistance and higher insulin secretion (13).

3.1. Lifestyle trials - diet and physical activity

Overweight, obesity and physical inactivity are the major risk factors for developing type 2 diabetes mainly through insulin resistance. Therefore, interventions in weight reduction were shown to enhance insulin sensitivity and improve glucose tolerance in nondiabetic and diabetic subjects.

In the DaQing study, 577 subjects with IGT as defined by the WHO criteria were followed over 6 years. They were randomized into diet-only, exercise only, diet plus exercise groups, and a control group, which were associated with a 31% ($p \leq 0.03$), 46% ($p \leq 0.0005$) and 42% ($p \leq 0.005$) reduction in the risk of developing diabetes, respectively, when compared to the control group. Factor analysis showed that both insulin resistance and insulin secretion had a significant association with the development of diabetes, and lifestyle intervention was more effective in subjects with lower insulin resistance and higher insulin secretion (15,21,22).

The Swedish Diabetes Prevention Study was the first individually randomized clinical trial, where 522 middle-aged overweight subjects (body mass index/BMI >25) with IGT were randomized to the control group or intervention group and followed over a mean of 3.2 years. The intervention group received individual counseling regarding diet and exercise and lost 4.2±5.1 kg *versus* 0.8±3.7 kg in the control group, which translated to a 58% ($p \leq 0.001$) reduction in the risk of developing diabetes and was directly associated with changes in lifestyle (18,23).

The Diabetes Prevention Program (DPP) study was a double-blind randomized controlled trial (RCT) involving a larger number of subjects, 3234 with IGT or IFG with BMI >24 kg/m2 (>22 in Asian population) followed over 2.8 years. They were randomized to standard lifestyle recommendations with placebo or with metformin or to an intensive program of lifestyle modifications (19). The incidence of developing diabetes was 4.8 cases *versus* 11 cases *per* 100 person years for 3 years in the intensive lifestyle and placebo groups, respectively, which was a 58% lower incidence of developing diabetes in the intensive lifestyle group. In this study these changes were observed in all of the various ethnic and racial subgroups, and at least 50% of the lifestyle group had achieved the goal of >7% of weight reduction.

The Look AHEAD trial, which, like DPP, demonstrated impressive weight loss at year 1, was also followed by significant weight regain over the subsequent 3 years despite continued intensive intervention and follow-up (24).

In a recent community study in Finland, 2,797 high-risk individuals were enrolled in a diabetes prevention program designed to achieve 5–7% body weight loss. Only approximately one-third of participants were able to successfully decrease body weight by 2.5% (25).

From above mention studies it is obvious that successful weight reduction alone is not sufficient to prevent diabetes in a large percentage of individuals. The main issues is that it is difficult to maintain weight without an intervention program.

The key components of lifestyle interventions in clinical practice based on the studies analyzed by Burnet *et al.* (37) were as follows: the staff included were medical doctors, nurses, technicians, dietitians and physiotherapists. Trainings with patients were focused on nutrition, physical activity and behavioral self-management four times during the year in individualized sessions (in Diabetes Prevention Study) or small group counseling sessions weekly for one month, then monthly for three months (32). Physical activities were organized 2 times during the week as brisk walking (in Diabetes Prevention Program and Malmo Feasibility Study). Smokers were advised to stop or reduce smoking. It was a useful follow up session every 2 months with phone calls to patients between visits. In DPS study, if weight goal was not achieved in 6 to 12 months, a very low calorie diet was considered. As for social support, spouses were invited to join sessions.

The overall goal for diabetes prevention is to reach and maintain an active, healthy weight with a tendency toward a hypocaloric diet. Evidence supports limiting total calories and fat (25% of caloric intake) and increasing dietary fiber (20 to 30 g/day). Essential skills include understanding portion sizes and reading food labels (37).

4. Pharmacological interventions

Weight regain is a characteristic feature of most weight reduction programs, irrespective of the type of dietary intervention and similarly, weight loss achieved with pharmacological intervention is associated with major weight regain once medication is discontinued.

As shown above, lifestyle modification is the best strategy to prevent the progression of metabolic risk factors and to prevent cardiovascular events and the onset of diabetes. However, pharmacological trials have shown important results.

4.1. Metformin

Metformin (MF) 850 mg was used in one arm of the DPP study along with standard lifestyle recommendations. Subjects in this study had a decrease in their calorie intake by a mean of 296±23 kcal compared to 249±27 kcal in the placebo group; their average fat intake decreased by 0.8±0.2% in both the MF and the placebo group (*p*=NS).

The DPP demonstrated a 31% reduction in IGT conversion to type 2 diabetes in subjects receiving metformin, 850 mg twice daily (15,21).

4.2. α-Glucosidase inhibitors

Both acarbose (STOP-NIDDM) (26) and voglibose (27) have been shown to decrease conversion of IGT to type 2 diabetes. Although this preventive effect initially was believed to result from inhibition of carbohydrate absorption, α-glucosidases augment incretin hormone secretion; thus, enhanced b-cell function could, in part, explain their beneficial effects on glucose homeostasis (28). Subjects on acarbose were by 25% less likely to develop diabetes compared to placebo at the end of 1 year, and this continued to the end of the study. The reduced risk was present even after adjusting for change in weight, age, sex, or BMI (p=0.0063) (26).

4.3. Thiazolidinediones

Thiazolidinediones (TZD) are insulin sensitizers that act by facilitating glucose transport into the muscle and by acting on Perioxisome Proliferator Activated Receptor (PPAR)-γ receptors in the adipose cells to shift fat from visceral to less active subcutaneous fat compartment thus reducing insulin resistance. The TRIPOD was a single-center, placebo-controlled randomized controlled trials, which enrolled Mexican-American women with prior gestational diabetes mellitus (GDM) randomized to either placebo or troglitazone 400 mg/day. The mean annual incidence of diabetes was 5.4% in the troglitazone group *versus* 12.1% in the placebo group (p=0.009), which was a >50% reduction with troglitazone use (29). Analysis done 8 months after troglitazone had been stopped showed that the mean annual incidence of diabetes was 21.2% and 3.1% in the placebo and troglitazone group, respectively. This indicated that the protection by the drug persisted even after it had been stopped. The study was continued in the same group of women using pioglitazone called the Pioglitazone In the Prevention of Diabetes (PIPOD) study and the results published indicated that the benefit in terms of β-cell function achieved with troglitazone was maintained with the use of pioglitazone, indicating that it could be a class effect (30). Also, a report appeared on diabetes reduction assessment in the Ramipril and Rosiglitazone medication (DREAM) trial (16). This trial reported only combined results for individuals with either IGT or IFG. Briefly, it was found that the ACE inhibitor ramipril did not significantly reduce the incidence of diabetes (hazard ratio 0.91, 0.80 to 1.03) but rosiglitazone, an oral diabetes drug, did (0.38, 0.33 to 0.44).

In another study ACT NOW, pioglitazone (45 mg/day) decreased by 72% (P <0.00001) IGT conversion to type 2 diabetes (31).

4.4. Orlistat

Orlistat is another pharmacological agent used in the prevention of diabetes. Orlistat is a weight-reduction agent that inhibits the activity of intestinal lipase and thus decreases the amount of fat (triglycerides) absorbed. After 4 years' treatment, the cumulative incidence of diabetes was 9.0% with placebo and 6.2% with orlistat, corresponding to a risk reduction of 37.3% (P = 0.0032). Exploratory analyses indicated that the preventive effect was explained by the difference in subjects with IGT. Mean weight loss after 4 years was significantly greater with orlistat (5.8 vs. 3.0 kg with placebo; P < 0.001) and similar between orlistat recipients with impaired (5.7 kg) or normal glucose tolerance (NGT) (5.8 kg) at baseline. A second analysis in which the baseline weights of subjects who dropped out of the study was carried forward also demonstrated greater weight loss in the orlistat group (3.6 vs. 1.4 kg; P < 0.001)(32).

4.5. GLP-1 analogs

Liraglutide and exenatide are GLP-1 receptor agonists that mimic the actions of GLP-1 and are resistant to dipeptidyl peptidase-4 degradation. GLP-1 analogs represent a logical therapeutic intervention for treatment of IGT. Moreover, the stimulatory effect of GLP-1 and GLP-1 analogs on insulin secretion is glucose dependent, minimizing risk for hypoglycemia (33). Once-daily liraglutide also reduces body weight and decreases IGT conversion to type 2 diabetes in obese nondiabetic subjects (34).

4.6. Angiotensin converting enzyme inhibitor (ACEI)/angiotensinogen receptor blocker (ARB)

In addition to the beneficial effects on hypertension, the kidneys and the heart, both ACEI and ARBs have been shown to improve insulin sensitivity and glycemic control. Therapy with ACEI, like captopril and ramipril, and ARBs, like losartan and valsartan has been shown to reduce the incidence of new-onset diabetes anywhere by 14% to 34% (18). Although the exact mechanism how these agents reduce the incidence of diabetes is not known, it is well established that ACEI increases glucose uptake in skeletal muscle through increased synthesis of GLUT- 4 transporter protein secondary to up-regulation of insulin receptor substrate 1 (IRS 1) activity, enhanced bradykinin and nitric oxide (NO) activity (35).

4.7. Statins

The West of Scotland Coronary Prevention Study (WOSCOPS) examined the effect of pravastatin on cardiovascular (CV) events and observed that these pharmacological interventions were associated with a 30% reduction in the incidence of diabetes as secondary outcome (36). Therapeutic agents used to treat other coexisting conditions like hypertension and dyslipidemia with agents like ACEI/ARB/statins can also help with the prevention of diabetes and CV disease (15).

5. Conclusions and recommendations

From the trials discussed it was shown that both non pharmacological and pharmacological intervention can reduce the risk of type 2 diabetes in people with IGT, but lifestyle intervention seems to be more effective than pharmacological interventions. Lifestyle intervention, which aims to reduce obesity and increase physical activity, helps in addressing directly these risk factors. In the mean time lifestyle interventions incur fewer and less serious side effects than drug treatment. Like in pharmacological interventions, lifestyle interventions may not be permanent and advice on diet and exercise needs to be regularly reinforced by professional staff. For pharmacological interventions, adverse effects need to be fully understood to enable the potential harms and benefits to be assessed.

In lifestyle intervention, clinicians should recommend behavior changes for asymptomatic patients at a high risk of diabetes such as IGT. High-risk patients can be identified through clinical characteristics augmented with careful screening by fasting glucose. Although the diabetes prevention trials used intensive strategies for effecting lifestyle change, clinicians can translate key elements from those strategies into brief, office-based counseling on physical activity and dietary change. As it was proved by different trials in clinical practice, lifestyle changes should be made better through structured programs. These programs, proved to be successful in clinical practices from different countries, should emphasize goal setting, practice and motivational interviewing with patients, education and skills development, self-monitoring, behavior change (cognitive restructuring), physical activity, problem solving, stress and stimulus control, the importance of social support, and the utilization of community resources.

Multidisciplinary care teams consisting of nurses, clinicians, dietitians, psychologist physiotherapists and health educators may provide more intensive counseling and increase the motivation to continue and achieve the targets. Other forms of awareness rising as printed materials or if possible interactive computer programs in offices can reinforce counseling efforts. Implementing diabetes prevention will require significant changes for both patients and clinicians. Every health system that provide these special services need to educate clinicians in training and in practice about the potential benefits of diabetes prevention. Appropriate programs on the prevention or delay of type 2 diabetes have to be culturally adaptive for office-based counseling considering the better results planned to achieve. Besides office bases counseling with patients and family members, successful diabetes prevention efforts through lifestyle changes will likely require involvement broader societal entities such as schools, communities and workplaces.

Author details

Merita Emini Sadiku
University of Pristina, Kosovo

6. References

[1] Neel JV. Diabetes mellitus: a "thrifty" genotype rendered detrimental by "progress"? Am J Hum genet 1962;14:353-62.

[2] Manson JE, Rimm EB, Stampfer MJ, et al. Physical activity and incidence of non insulin dependent diabetes mellitus in women. Lancet 1991;338:774-8.

[3] International Diabetes Federation. Diabetes Atlas, 5rd ed. Brussels: International DiabetesFederation; 2011.

[4] The DECODE Study Group. Glucose tolerance and mortality: comparison of WHO and American Diabetes Association diagnostic criteria. Lancet 1999;354:617-21.

[5] International Diabetes Federation. Diabetes Atlas, 3rd ed. Brussels: International DiabetesFederation; 2006.

[6] Stern MP, Williams K, Haffner SM. Identification of persons at high risk for type 2 diabetes mellitus: do we need the oral glucose tolerance test? Ann Intern Med 2002;136:575-81.

[7] Emini-Sadiku M, Car N, Metelko Z, Bajraktari G, Morina N, Devolli D. Prevention or delay of type 2 diabetes by pharmacological or lifestyle interventions. Diabetologia Croatica 2008;37-1.

[8] Orio Jr, F Palomba S, Cascella T, et al. Improvement in endothelial structure and function after metformin treatment in young normal-weight women with polycystic ovary syndrome: results of a 6-month study. J Clin Endocrinol Metab 2005;90:6072-6.

[9] World Health Organization. Definition, diagnosis and classification of diabetes mellitus and its complications: report of a WHO consultation. Part1: diagnosis and classification of diabetes mellitus.Geneva: World Health Organization; 1999.

[10] American Diabetes Association. Type 2 diabetes in children and adolescents. Diabetes Care 2000;23:381-9.

[11] American Diabetes Association. Screening for type 2 diabetes. Diabetes Care 2004; 27:S11-3.

[12] Meigs JB, Williams K, Sullivan LM, et al. Using metabolic syndrome traits for efficient detection of impaired glucose tolerance. Diabetes Care 2004;27:1417-26.

[13] Hanley AJ, Festa A, D'Agostino Jr RB, et al. Metabolic and inflammation variable clusters and prediction of type 2 diabetes: factor analysis using directly measured insulin sensitivity. Diabetes 2004;53:1773-81.

[14] Grundy SM, Brewer Jr, HB Cleeman JI, et al.Definition of metabolic syndrome: Report of the National Heart, Lung, and Blood Institute/American Heart Association conference on scientific issues related to definition. Circulation 2004;109:433-8.

[15] Babu A, Fogelfeld L. Metabolic syndrome and prediabetes. Dis Mon 2006;52 (2-3):55-144.

[16] DREAM Trial Investigators. Effect of rosiglitazone on the frequency of diabetes in patients with impaired glucose tolerance or impaired fasting glucose: a randomised controlled trial. Lancet 2006; 368:1096-105.

[17] Zimmet P, Alberti KG, Shaw J. Global and societal implications of the diabetes epidemic. Nature 2001;414:782-7.

[18] Tuomilehto J, Lindstrom J, Eriksson JG, et al. Prevention of type 2 diabetes mellitus by changes in lifestyle among subjects with impaired glucose tolerance. N Engl J Med 2001;344:1343-50.

[19] Knowler WC, Barrett-Connor E, Fowler SE, et al. Reduction in the incidence of type 2 diabetes with lifestyle intervention or metformin. N Engl J Med 2002;346:393-403.

[20] Eriksson KF, Lindgärde F. Prevention of type 2 (non-insulin-dependent) diabetes mellitus by diet and physical exercise: the 6-year Malmö feasibility study. Diabetologia 1991;34:891–898

[21] Pan XR, Li GW, Hu YH, et al. Effects of diet and exercise in preventing NIDDM in people with impaired glucose tolerance: the Da Qing IGT and Diabetes Study. Diabetes Care 1997;20:537–544

[22] Li G, Hu Y, Yang W, et al. Effects of insulin resistance and insulin secretion on the efficacy of interventions to retard development of type 2 diabetes mellitus: the DA Qing IGT and Diabetes Study. Diabetes Res Clin Pract 2002;58:193-200.

[23] Lindstrom J, Eriksson JG, Valle TT, et al. Prevention of diabetes mellitus in subjects with impaired glucose tolerance in the Finnish Diabetes Prevention Study: results from a randomized clinical trial. J Am Soc Nephrol 2003;14:S108-13.

[24] Pi-Sunyer X, Blackburn G, Brancati FL, et al. Reduction in weight and cardiovascular disease risk factors in individuals with type 2 diabetes: one-year results of the Look AHEAD trial. Diabetes Care 2007;30:1374–1383

[25] Saaristo T, Moilanen L, Korpi-Hyövälti E, et al. Lifestyle intervention for prevention of type 2 diabetes in primary health care: one-year follow-up of the Finnish National Diabetes Prevention Program (FIN-D2D). Diabetes Care 2010; 33:2146–2151

[26] Chiasson JL, Josse RG, Gomis R, Hanefeld M, Karasik A, Laakso M; STOP-NIDDM Trial Research Group. Acarbose for prevention of type 2 diabetes mellitus: the STOP-NIDDM randomised trial. Lancet 2002;359:2072–2077

[27] Kawamori R, Tajima N, Iwamoto Y, Kashiwagi A, Shimamoto K, Kaku K; Voglibose Ph-3 Study Group. Voglibose for prevention of type 2 diabetes mellitus: a randomised, double-blind trial in Japanese individuals with impaired glucose tolerance. Lancet 2009;373:1607-1614.

[28] De Fronzo R, Abdul-Ghani M.Type 2 Diabetes Can Be Prevented With Early Pharmacological Intervention. Diabetes Care 34(Suppl. 2):S202–S209, 2011

[29] Buchanan TA, Xiang AH, Peters RK, et al. Preservation of pancreatic beta-cell function and prevention of type 2 diabetes by pharmacological treatment of insulin resistance in high-risk Hispanic women. Diabetes 2002;51:2796-803.

[30] Weiss R, Taksali SE, Tamborlane WV, et al. Predictors of changes in glucose tolerance status in obese youth. Diabetes Care 2005;28:902-9.

[31] De Fronzo RA, Tripathy D, Schwenke DC, et al. Pioglitazone for diabetes prevention in impaired glucose tolerance. N Engl J Med 2011;364:1104–1115

[32] Torgerson JS, Hauptman J, Boldrin MN, et al. XENical in the prevention of diabetes in obese subjects (XENDOS) study: a randomized study of orlistat as an adjunct to lifestyle changes for the prevention of type 2 diabetes in obese patients. Diabetes Care 2004;27:155-61.

[33] Triplitt C, DeFronzo RA. Exenatide: first in class incretin mimetic for the treatment of type 2 diabetes mellitus. Exp Rev Endocirnol Metab 2006;1:329–341

[34] Astrup A, Rössner S, Van Gaal L, et al. Effects of liraglutide in the treatment of obesity: a randomised, double-blind, placebo-controlled study. Lancet 2009; 374:1606–1616

[35] Kreutzfeldt J, Raasch W, Klein HH. Ramipril increases the protein level of skeletal muscle IRS- 1 and alters protein tyrosine phosphatase activity in spontaneously hypertensive rats. Naunyn Schmiedebergs Arch Pharmacol 2000;362:1-6.

[36] The WOSCOPS Study Group. West of Scotland Coronary Prevention Study: implications for clinical practice. The WOSCOPS Study Group. Eur Heart J 1996;17:163-4.

[37] Burnet DL, Elliott LD, Quinn MT, Plaut AJ, Schwartz MA, Chin MH. Preventing diabetes in the clinical setting. J Gen Intern Med 2006;21:84- 93.

Section 2

Insights into Potential Mechanisms of Insulin Resistance

Chapter 3

Impaired Glucose Tolerance, Obesity and Inflammatory Mediators

Ayfer Colak and Gulden Diniz

Additional information is available at the end of the chapter

http://dx.doi.org/10.5772/52378

1. Introduction

1.1. Plasma glucose levels and prediction of future type 2 diabetes

Prediabetes (PD) is a dysmetabolic state of glucose level between diabetes mellitus and normal glucose tolerance (NGT) which includes basically impaired fasting glucose (IFG) and impaired glucose tolerance (IGT). All these conditions are becoming a considerable public health problem worldwide [1]. Measurement of glucose in plasma of fasting subjects is widely accepted as a diagnostic criterion for diabetes. Oral glucose tolerance test (OGTT) evaluates the efficiency of the body to metabolize glucose. For many years, fasting plasma glucose (FPG) test and OGTT have been used as "gold standards" for diagnosis of glucose metabolism disorders [2]. In addition hemoglobin A1C (HbA1C) measurement has also become the focus of considerable attention for diagnosis of diabetes. HbA1C is formed by the nonenzymatic attachment of glucose to the N-terminal valin of the beta chain of hemoglobin and its normal range is between 4% and 6% [2-4]. Because of the long life span of erythrocytes, HbA1C reflects long-term glycemic exposure, representing the average glucose concentration over the preceding 8-12 weeks [2].

The hyperglycemic diagnostic criteria defined by American Diabetes Association (ADA) is widely used for the evaluation of glucose metabolism disorders [1]. Fasting plasma glucose (FPG) is less than 100 mg/dl and 2-hour postprandial plasma glucose (2hPG) [75g glucose OGTT) level is less than 140 mg/dl in normal glucose tolerance (NGT). If the FPG level is between 100 and 125 mg/ dl, but the 2hPG level is less than 140 mg/dl, this situation is defined as IFG. In IGT, the FPG level is between 100 and 125 mg/ dl, the 2hPG level is between 140 and 200 mg/dl. If 2hPG level is more than 200 mg/dl, it is termed as diabetes according to the ADA's criteria [1,2]. Similarly, the glycated hemoglobin (HbA1c) level is found more than 6.5% in type 2 diabetes [1,2].

There are some fundamental problems in using IGT and IFG to characterize abnormal glucose metabolism. These problems can be classified as; the best means of identifying at-risk populations, whether they characterize the same degree of risk, and whether IFG and IGT represent manifestations of the same process or fundamentally different mechanisms [5].

The results of recent studies demonstrate that, although both IFG and IGT are characterized by ß-cell dysfunction, the defects in insulin secretion in IFG and IGT are very distinct [6]. Subjects with IGT have impaired late-phase insulin secretion and increased insulin resistance (IR) in skeletal muscle. In contrasts, subjects with IFG have impaired early –phase insulin secretion and increased IR in liver [6-8]. Similarly there are some discrepancies between the clinical features of IFG and IGT. Subjects with isolated IFG are more insulin resistant, and subjects with isolated IGT exhibits a more severe deficit in insulin secretion [8]. IFG and IGT have been associated with other features of insulin resistance, including dyslipidaemia, hypertension, abdominal obesity, microalbuminuria, endothelial dysfunction, and markers of inflammation and hypercoagulability [5]. Combinations of these components have also been associated with progression to type 2 diabetes mellitus (T2DM), cardiovascular disease and increased mortality [10].

Impaired ß-cell function and increased IR in several peripheral tissues are both present in type 2 diabetes mellitus (T2DM) [9]. Currently it is understood that T2DM is also associated with obesity, hypertension and combined hyperlipidemia [10-12]. Populations at high risk for development of T2DM and atherosclerosis can be identified using markers of abnormal glucose metabolism, and recent studies have demonstrated that lifestyle modification and some pharmacological therapies have a favorable effect on reducing the risk for development of T2DM and increased mortality [5,10].

2. Relationship between obesity and glucose metabolism

Obesity is associated with an array of health problems including IR and T2DM, fatty liver disease, atherosclerosis, airway diseases, degenerative disorders, and various types of cancer [11,12]. IR is determined by impaired insulin sensitivity of its main target organs, such as adipose tissue, liver, and muscle. Insulin regulates glucose uptake and circulating free fatty acid (FFA) concentrations. Insulin decreases lipolysis in adipose tissue and inhibits gluconeogenesis in liver. Insulin resistance leads to increased circulating FFA concentrations and ectopic fat accumulation that impede insulin mediated glucose uptake in skeletal muscle and elevated glucose production in liver [13]. Finally, IR together with abnormalities in insulin secretion leads to T2DM [13].

Obesity is defined as abnormal or excessive fat accumulation and it is measured with body mass index (BMI) [10]. The conceptual transformation of adipose tissue from a passive organ to an active participant of homeostasis, has emerged relatively recently [12,14]. In 1994, adipose tissue was identified as the source of the hormone leptin, opening the door for a new area of research focused on adipocyte endocrinology [14]. Our understanding of the pathogenesis of obesity and its metabolic disturbances have advanced significantly over the past decades [11-14]. The growing evidence on obesity and associated pathologies has led to understand the role of adipose tissue as an active potential participant in controlling the physiological and pathological processes [11-15]. For many years, adipose tissue was regarded merely as a heat insulator and a store of excess FFAs that could be released when needed [14]. To date, the adipose tissue is considered as an endocrine organ able to mediate biological effects on metabolism and inflammation, contributing to the maintenance of energy homeostasis and, probably, pathogenesis of obesity-related metabolic and inflammatory complications [10-16]. Nowadays, worldwide increased obesity prevalence has been accompanied by a parallel rise in the glucose metabolism disorders [11,17]. There is evidence that IR and T2DM is also related to a chronic low-grade inflammatory state [17]. Therefore weight loss is associated both with an improvement of the inflammatory profile and a decreased risk of glucose metabolism disorders [9-11,13-15].

3. Effects of inflammatory mediators on glucose metabolism

Many complex signaling pathways regulate chronic low-grade inflammation associated with both the metabolism and immune systems [18]. Pro- inflammatory cytokines are mediators of these pathways and they enter the circulation as a result of lipolysis [10]. Recent data indicates that macrophages in adipose tissue are a major source of them [10-18]. Especially in obesity, adipose tissue is characterized by an increased production and secretion of a wide range of pro- inflammatory molecules which have been recognized as an active participant in numerous immunologic processes [13-16]. Cytokines play the crucial roles in many physiological and pathological processes such as hematopoiesis, angiogenesis, inflammation, atherosclerosis, allergy and autoimmunity [18]. The increased concentrations of circulatory cytokines are commonly determined in cardiovascular disease (CVD), the metabolic syndrome and T2DM. These cytokines are produced by different cell types and are secreted into circulation where they regulate different tissues through their local, central or peripheral action [19].

It is demonstrated that increases of these cytokines effect through intracellular signaling pathways which involve the nuclear factor kappa B (NF- κB) and c- Jun N-terminal kinase (JNK) systems [10]. Leptin also impairs glucose-stimulated insulin production of human β cells through activation of JNK. Moreover, hyperglycemia induces IL-1β production by pancreatic β-cells, which putatively contributes to glucotoxicity in human pancreatic islets [13].

The name of adipokine is nowadays generally given to any protein or cytokine that can be synthesized and secreted by adipocytes [11]. Several studies have shown that adipokine production is altered in obesity [11]. The first link between obesity and elevation of Tumor Necrosis Factor- Alpha (TNF-α) came from a study almost 20 years ago and this finding led to the concept of inflammation in obesity and demonstrated that adipocytes express TNF-α [17-23]. TNF-alpha is a pro- inflammatory cytokine, overproduced in adipose tissue of several rodent models of obesity and has an important role in the pathogenesis of IR in these species [21]. Interleukin-1 (IL-1) is one of the first identified cytokines and exert strong pro-inflammatory functions [10,20]. IL-1α has been demonstrated to be involved in the pathogenesis of glucose metabolism disorders in mice [18]. IL-1β is able to reduce IRS-1 expression at a transcriptional level through a mechanism that is ERK dependent and at a posttranscriptional level independent of ERK activation [18]. By targeting IRS-1, IL-1β is capable of impairing insulin signaling and action and could thus participate, in the development of IR, in concert with other cytokines [18-21]. IL-6 is also among the first identified cytokines and acts on the liver to stimulate the production of a number of acute-phase proteins [10]. It is implicated as a pathogenetic marker of IR and CVD. IL-1ß together with IL-6 concentration is suggested as a predictor for T2DM in humans better than either cytokine alone [9,19,23-28].

Similarly interleukin 8 (IL-8) is a pro- inflammatory cytokine, overproduced in adipose tissue of several rodent models of obesity and has an important role in the pathogenesis of IR in these species [12,21,29,30]. However, IL-8 is basically evaluated as a cytokine with atherogenic properties and its actual involvement in glucose metabolism disorders remains controversial in humans [29-31]. Through its multiple actions, IL-8 might promote intimal thickening and atherosclerosis. This cytokine is also able to increase the instability of atherosclerotic plaque [29-31]. Elevated circulating IL-8 levels were also reported in type 1 and type 2 diabetic patients. It was hypothesized that this cytokine could be involved in the pathogenesis of diabetic macroangiopathy. Especially T2DM is associated with accelerated atherogenesis and it is recognized as an independent risk factor for CVD. Precise mechanisms linking those conditions are not fully understood [18,19]. In recent years, theories about the role of chronic low-grade inflammation in the pathogenesis of both glucose metabolism disorders and atherosclerosis have been developed. Some investigations reported that elevated plasma IL-8 concentrations are related to obesity and hyperlipidemia [12].

C-reactive protein (CRP) is an acute-phase reactant, the elevation of which is indicative of acute or chronic inflammation [32,33]. CRP is produced solely by the liver [19]. An etiologic role for chronic inflammation in the development of IR has been hypothesized [32,33]. It has been recognized that elevation of CRP concentrations is an independent predictive parameter of T2DM, which is also associated with various components of the metabolic syndrome such as obesity, IR, and dyslipidemia [20-24]. A number of previous study have reported that high sensitivity (hs) CRP is also related to circulating IL-6 levels [24,32,33] and IL-6 is a powerful inducer of CRP production in the liver [18]. In addition, abdominal obesity is associated with elevated plasma hs-CRP concentration and it has shown that elevation of hs-CRP concentration is an independent predictive parameter of T2DM [32,33] Actually CRP is a most sensitive marker of inflammation and it is associated with features of IR [15,16].

More recently, hormone leptin has also been linked to inflammation in human. Leptin, is the product of the ob gene. It is involved in the regulation of energy homeostasis and is almost exclusively expressed and produced by white adipose tissue (WAT) and more particularly by differentiated mature adipocytes [11]. Circulating levels and adipose tissue mRNA expression of leptin are strongly associated with BMI and fat mass in obesity. Therefore, leptin appears as a real marker of adipose tissue mass in humans [11]. Leptin acts mainly at the level of the central nervous system to regulate food intake and energy expenditure. In addition, there is a relationship between leptin and the low-grade inflammatory state in obesity. It was suggested that leptin could exert peripheral biological effects as a function of its cytokine-like structure. It is similar to the IL-2 and receptors of leptin belong to the cytokine class I receptor family [14]. Some works have reported that there is an increased inflammatory response associated with the presence of hyperleptinemia without obesity. Leptin-deficient mice or humans display an altered immune status . The reduction in leptin levels could be responsible for fat-associated immunosuppression [11]. Leptin is able to control TNF-α production and activation by macrophages, however, the underlying mechanisms have not been clearly identified [11,14].

Adiponectin is an adipokine mainly produced by the adipose tissue and it is induced by activity of the nuclear peroxisome- proliferator–activated receptor (PPAR) γ. It exists both as a full-length protein as well as a proteolytic cleavage fragment, also known as globular adiponectin. Adiponectin circulates at high concentrations in human serum [5 to 10 μg/mL) and has a wide spectrum of biological activities. Adiponectin is unique that, unlike other adipokines, circulating concentrations are reduced with obesity. Serum levels of adiponectin are reduced in individuals with visceral obesity and states of IR. TNF-α suppresses the transcription of adiponectin in adipocytes, which might explain the lower adiponectin levels in serum in individuals who are obese. Weight loss induces adiponectin synthesis, as activation of PPARγ by its ligands thiazolidinediones (TZDs), which are used in the treatment of T2DM [19,21]

Data from epidemiological studies indicate that circulating adiponectin is reduced in patients with CVD and T2DM. Importantly, low adiponectin concentrations are strongly correlated with IR. In addition, adiponectin reduces glucose production in the liver by directly inhibiting the gluconeogenic enzymes phosphoenolpyruvate carboxykinase and glucose 6 phosphate , improving glycemic control and insulin sensitivity .The reduction in adiponectin with obesity and diabetes most likely arises from increased adipose tissue macrophage infiltration resulting in inflammation. In contrast, high concentrations of adiponectin are related to higher insulin sensitivity and decreased risk for CVD. The proinflammatory cytokines TNFα and IL-6 reduce adiponectin expression. Conversely, adiponectin has an antiinflammatory effect, inhibiting activation of NFκB by TNFα [19].

Resistin, also called FIZZ3 (found in inflammatory zones) or adipocyte secreted factor (ADSF) has been discovered in 2001 while looking for new molecular targets of TZDs in adipocytes [11,33]. It was shown that resistin levels were increased in obese rodents and resistin knock-out mice have lower fasting glycaemia, increased glucose tolerance and insulin sensitivity associated with a reduced liver glucose production [11]. Resistin is also expressed in the WAT, especially in the WAT of abdominal region and female gonadal adipose tissue [33]. Resistin has been linked with many facets of the metabolic syndrome, principally, obesity, insulin resistance and hyperlipidemia. The effect of resistin upon insulin resistance is mediated through increased expression of suppressor of cytokine signaling-3 (SOCS-3], which is a known inhibitor of insulin signaling [33]. Mice injected with resistin showed insulin resistance. Resistin was thus found to attend endocrine functions that led to insulin resistance. Increased expression of resistin was found to be associated with dyslipidemia and non-alcoholic fatty liver disease (NAFLD) in a few medical ranks. In patients with NAFLD, serum resistin levels were higher than those in control cases. The presence of metabolic syndrome with elevated levels of plasma resistin is associated with increased cardiovascular risk [33-35].

Osteopontin (OPN) actually is a secreted matrix glycoprotein and pro-inflammatory cytokine playing an important role in cell-mediated immunity. Its ability to interact with integrin surface molecules through an Arg-Gly-Asp sequence and with the CD44 receptor has established this mediator as an important signaling molecule [34]. Indeed, tissue infiltration of macrophages as observed in obesity is dependent on the expression of OPN, which promotes monocyte chemotaxis and motility. Obese mice lacking OPN showed improved insulin sensitivity and decreased macrophage infiltration into adipose tissue. These experiments add OPN to a long list of pro-inflammatory pathways involved in the development of IR [21]

However, actual involvement of all these mediators in glucose metabolism disorders in humans remains controversial. It is suggested that these mediators may alter insulin sensitivity by triggering different key steps in the insulin signaling pathway and overproduction of them is associated with the glucose metabolism disorders [36-40]. Many mediators contribute to the pathogenesis of impaired glucose homeostasis and most of them are overproduced during obesity. It now appears that obesity is associated with a low-grade inflammation of adipose tissue, resulting from activation of innate immune system. Especially in obesity, adipose tissue is characterized by an increased production and secretion of a wide range of pro- inflammatory molecules including IL-1ß, IL-6, IL-8, TNF-α, CRP, leptin, resistin and so on [23-35]. Recent data indicate that macrophages in obese adipose tissue are major source of most mediators. Therefore weight loss is associated with a reduction in the macrophage infiltration of adipose tissue and an improvement of the inflammatory profile [39-45].

4. Conclusion

During the last decades, understanding of the biology of adipose tissue and especially its secretory functions, have dramatically improved. This development has completely modified the understanding of the pathogenesis of obesity, glucose metabolism disorders and inflammation. Several cytokines attracted considerable attention as potential effectors in the pathology and physiology of insulin resistance associated with type 2 diabetes mellitus (T2DM) and obesity. Recent studies have implicated a number of inflammatory mediators including cytokines and adipokines in the inflammatory responses that accompany the glucose metabolism disorders. Therefore measurement of serum levels of inflammatory mediator is important in determining glucose regulation disorders and provides an improvement in therapeutic approaches to modulate the inflammatory responses and thereby alter disease progression. Elucidation of the mechanisms that link obesity with inflammation and glucose metabolism will contribute to the understanding of the physiopathology of obesity. As well as it will be probably provide the new strategies in the development of new therapeutic approaches.

Author details

Ayfer Colak
Izmir Tepecik Research Hospital, Biochemistry Department, Turkey

Gulden Diniz
Izmir Dr.Behcet Uz Children's Hospital, Pathology Department, Turkey

5. References

[1] Lu Q, Tong N, Liu Y, Li N, Tang X, Zhao J, et al. Community-based population data indicates the significant alterations of insulin resistance, chronic inflammation and urine ACR in IFG combined IGT group among prediabetic population.Diabetes Res Clin Pract 2009;84(3):319-24.
[2] Sacks DB. A1C versus glucose testing: a comparison. Diabetes Care 2011; 34(2):518-23.
[3] Kumar PR, Bhansali A, Ravikiran M, Bhansali S, Dutta P, Thakur JS, Sachdeva N, Bhadada SK, Walia R . Utility of glycated hemoglobin in diagnosing type 2 diabetes mellitus: a community-based study. J Clin Endocrinol Metab 2010;95(6):2832-5.
[4] Malkani S, DeSilva T. Controversies on how diabetes is diagnosed. Curr Opin Endocrinol Diabetes Obes 2012;19(2):97-103.
[5] Petersen JL, McGuire DK. Impaired glucose tolerance and impaired fasting glucose – a review of diagnosis, clinical implications and management Diabetes and Vascular Disease Research 2005 2: 9.
[6] Kanat M, Mari A, Norton L, Winnier D, DeFronzo RA, Jenkinson C, Abdul-Ghani MA. Distinct β-cell defects in impaired fasting glucose and impaired glucose tolerance. Diabetes 2012; 61(2):447-53.
[7] Abdul-Ghani MA, DeFronzo RA. Plasma glucose concentration and prediction of future risk of type 2 diabetes. Diabetes Care 2009;32 Suppl 2:S194-8.
[8] Oka R, Yagi K, Sakurai M, Nakamura K, Moriuchi T, Miyamoto S, Oka R, Yagi K, Sakurai M, Nakamura K, Moriuchi T, Miyamoto. Insulin secretion and insulin sensitivity on the oral glucose tolerance test (OGTT) in middle-aged Japanese. Endocr J 2012;59(1):55-64.
[9] Meyer C, Pimenta W, Woerle HJ, Van Haeften T, Szoke E, Mitrakou A, Gerich J. Different mechanisms for impaired fasting glucose and impaired postprandial glucose tolerance in humans. Diabetes Care 2006; 29(8):1909-14. A29.

[10] Colak A, Coker I, Diniz G, Karademirci I, Turkon H, Ergonen F, Hanci T, Bozkurt U et al. Interleukin 6 and Tumor Necrosis Factor-alpha Levels in Women with and without Glucose Metabolism Disorders. Turk J Biochem 2010; 35(3): 190- 194.

[11] Bastard JP, Maachi M, Lagathu C, Kim MJ, Caron M, Vidal H,et al. Recent advances in the relationship between obesity, inflammation, and insulin resistance. Eur Cytokine Netw 2006;17(1): 4-12.

[12] Gustafson B. Adipose tissue, inflammation and atherosclerosis. J Atheroscler Thromb 2010;17(4):332-41.

[13] Zeyda M, Stulnig TM. Obesity, inflammation, and insulin resistance. Gerontology 2009;55: 379-86.

[14] Wisse BE. The inflammatory syndrome: the role of adipose tissue cytokines in metabolic disorders linked to obesity. J Am Soc Nephrol 2004;15(11):2792-800.

[15] Chiang DJ, Pritchard MT, Nagy LE. Obesity, diabetes mellitus, and liver fibrosis. Am J Physiol Gastrointest Liver Physiol 2011;300(5):G697-702.

[16] Balistreri CR, Caruso C, Candore G. The role of adipose tissue and adipokines in obesity-related inflammatory diseases. Mediators Inflamm 2010; 2010:802078. 1.

[17] Rabe K, Lehrke M, Parhofer KG, Broedl UC. Adipokines and Insulin Resistance. Mol Med 2008; 14(11-12): 741–751.

[18] Rosa MS, Pinto AM. Cytokines. In: Tietz Textbook of Clinical Chemistry and Molecular Diagnostics. Burtis CA, Ashwood ER, Bruns MD DE (eds) 5th ed, Elsevier, Philadelphia 2005; Vol 1, p 645-723.

[19] Puglisi MJ, Fernandez ML. Modulation of C-reactive protein, tumor necrosis factor-alpha, and adiponectin by diet, exercise, and weight loss. J Nutr 2008;138(12):2293-6.

[20] Dogan Y, Akarsu S, Ustundag B, Yilmaz E, Gurgoze MK. Serum IL-1beta, IL-2, and IL-6 in insulin-dependent diabetic children. Mediators Inflamm 2006;2006(1):59206.

[21] Tilg H, Moschen AR. Inflammatory mechanisms in the regulation of insulin resistance. Mol Med 2008; 14(3-4):222-231.

[22] Popa C, Netea MG, van Riel PL, van der Meer JW, Stalenhoef AF. The role of TNF-alpha in chronic inflammatory conditions, intermediary metabolism, and cardiovascular risk. J Lipid Res 2007;48(4):751-62.

[23] Miyazaki Y, Pipek R, Mandarino LJ, DeFronzo RA. Tumor necrosis factor alpha and insulin resistance in obese type 2 diabetic patients. Int J Obes Relat Metab Disord 2003;27(1):88-94.

[24] Payette C, Blackburn P, Lamarche B, Tremblay A, Bergeron J, Lemieux I, Després JP, Couillard C. Sex differences in postprandial plasma tumor necrosis factor-alpha, interleukin-6, and C-reactive protein concentrations. Metabolism 2009;58(11):1593-601.

[25] Konukoglu D, Hatemi H, Bayer H, Bagriacik N. Relationship between serum concentrations of interleukin-6 and tumor necrosis factor alpha in female Turkish subjects with normal and impaired glucose tolerance. Horm Metab Res 2006, 38(1):34-37.

[26] Dinh W, Füth R, Nickl W, Krahn T, Ellinghaus P, Scheffold T, Bansemir L, Bufe A, Barroso MC, Lankisch M.. Elevated plasma levels of TNF-alpha and interleukin-6 in

patients with diastolic dysfunction and glucose metabolism disorders. Cardiovasc Diabetol 2009;8:58.
[27] Yeste D, Vendrell J, Tomasini R, Broch M, Gussinye M, Megia A, Carrascosa A. Interleukin-6 in obese children and adolescents with and without glucose intolerance. Diabetes Care 2007; 30(7):1892-1894.
[28] Cardellini M, Andreozzi F, Laratta E, Marini MA, Lauro R, Hribal ML, Perticone F, Sesti G.. Plasma interleukin-6 levels are increased in subjects with impaired glucose tolerance but not in those with impaired fasting glucose in a cohort of Italian Caucasians.Diabetes Metab Res Rev 2007;23(2):141-5. 1.
[29] Ruotsalainen E, Stancáková A, Vauhkonen I, Salmenniemi U, Pihlajamäki J, Punnonen K, Laakso M. Changes in cytokine levels during acute hyperinsulinemia in offspring of type 2 diabetic subjects. Atherosclerosis 2010;210(2):536-41.
[30] Kobashi C, Asamizu S, Ishiki M, Iwata M, Usui I, Yamazaki K, et al. Inhibitory effect of IL-8 on insulin action in human adipocytes via MAP kinase pathway. J Inflamm (Lond) 2009;6:25.
[31] Straczkowski M, Kowalska I, Nikolajuk A, Dzienis-Straczkowska S, Szelachowska M, Kinalska I. Plasma interleukin 8 concentrations in obese subjects with impaired glucose tolerance. Cardiovasc Diabetol 2003; 2: 5.
[32] Devaraj S, Singh U, Jialal I. Human C-reactive protein and the metabolic syndrome. Curr Opin Lipidol 2009;20(3):182-9.
[33] Gandhi H, Upaganlawar A, Balaraman R. Adipocytokines: The pied pipers. J Pharmacol Pharmacother 2010;1(1):9-17.
[34] Yuan G, Zhou L, Tang J, Yang Y, Gu W, Li F, Hong J, Gu Y, Li X, Ning G, Chen M. Serum CRP levels are equally elevated in newly diagnosed type 2 diabetes and impaired glucose tolerance and related to adiponectin levels and insulin sensitivity. Diabetes Res Clin Pract 2006;72(3):244-50.
[35] Ma K, Jin X, Liang X, Zhao Q, Zhang X. Inflammatory mediators involved in the progression of the metabolic syndrome. Diabetes Metab Res Rev 2012; 28(5):388-94.
[36] Fève B, Bastard JP .The role of interleukins in insulin resistance and type 2 diabetes mellitus. Nature Reviews Endocrinology 2009; 5, 305-311. |
[37] Wolowczuk I, Verwaerde C, Viltart O, Delanoye A, Delacre M, Pot B, Grangette C. Feeding our immune system: impact on metabolism. Clin Dev Immunol 2008:639803.
[38] Licastro F, Candore G, Lio D, Porcellini E, Colonna-Romano G, Franceschi C, Caruso C. Innate immunity and inflammation in ageing: a key for understanding age-related diseases. Immun Ageing 2005; 2:8.
[39] Kowalska I, Straczkowski M, Nikolajuk A, Adamska A, Karczewska-Kupczewska M, Otziomek E, et al. Insulin resistance, serum adiponectin, and proinflammatory markers in young subjects with the metabolic syndrome. Metabolism 2008; 57(11): 1539-1544.
[40] Flanagan AM, Brown JL, Santiago CA, Aad PY, Spicer LJ, Spicer MT. High-fat diets promote insulin resistance through cytokine gene expression in growing female rats. J Nutr Biochem 2008; 19(8):505-513.

[41] Goldberg RB.Cytokine and cytokine-like inflammation markers, endothelial dysfunction, and imbalanced coagulation in development of diabetes and its complications. J Clin Endocrinol Metab 2009;94(9):3171-82.

[42] Azar Sharabiani MT, Vermeulen R, Scoccianti C, Hosnijeh FS, Minelli L, Sacerdote C, Palli D, Krogh V, Tumino R, Chiodini P, Panico S, Vineis P . Immunologic profile of excessive body weight. Biomarkers 2011;16(3):243-51.

[43] Lamb RE, Goldstein BJ. Modulating an oxidative-inflammatory cascade: potential new treatment strategy for improving glucose metabolism, insulin resistance, and vascular function. Int J Clin Pract 2008;62(7):1087-95.

[44] de Rekeneire N, Peila R, Ding J, Colbert LH, Visser M, Shorr RI, Kritchevsky SB, Kuller LH, Strotmeyer ES, Schwartz AV, Vellas B, Harris TB. Diabetes, hyperglycemia, and inflammation in older individuals: the health, aging and body composition study. Diabetes Care 2006;29(8):1902-8.

[45] Kopp HP, Krzyzanowska K, Möhlig M, Spranger J, Pfeiffer AF, Schernthaner G. Effects of marked weight loss on plasma levels of adiponectin, markers of chronic subclinical inflammation and insulin resistance in morbidly obese women. Int J Obes (Lond) 2005;29(7):766-71.

Chapter 4

Sex Differences in Obesity-Related Glucose Intolerance and Insulin Resistance

Haifei Shi and Shiva Priya Dharshan Senthil Kumar

Additional information is available at the end of the chapter

http://dx.doi.org/10.5772/52972

1. Introduction

The prevalence of obesity has increased dramatically over the past decade (1) along with several health risks it encompasses, including non-insulin dependent type 2 diabetes, cardiovascular disease, fatty liver, dyslipidemia, and some types of cancer (2). The economic costs of caring for patients with obesity and diabetic complications are enormously high (3). There are important sex differences in the prevalence of these metabolic diseases. Premenopausal women have much less metabolic disorders than men; however, the prevalence of obesity and diabetes increases dramatically in postmenopausal women (4). Sex steroid hormone estrogen may be protective against the metabolic syndrome and may contribute to the maintenance of insulin sensitivity, and its deficiency leads to development of type 2 diabetes and insulin resistance. This has resulted in the use of estrogen hormone replacement therapy for the treatment of insulin resistance in postmenopausal women (5) and in men with congenital aromatase deficiency (6). Thus, estrogen has enormous potential as a therapeutic agent for use in the prevention or treatment of type 2 diabetes with glucose intolerance and insulin resistance.

1.1. Sex differences in genetic polymorphisms on the development of diabetes

The development and etiology of obesity and related diseases such as type 2 diabetes stems from a conflict between genes which allowed our ancestors to survive extended periods of famine and physiological responses to caloric excess and sedentary lifestyle of the modern world. Some studies have evaluated potential genetic components and reported sex differences in the effects of certain polymorphisms of several enzymes and genes on the development and etiology of diabetes. Several examples are listed below.

First example is protein tyrosine phosphatase, an enzyme involving signal transduction of T cell and insulin receptors. The activity of this enzyme, affected by certain genotypes, is related to age of onset of type 1 diabetes in a sex-specific manner (7). Specifically, genotypes associated with medium to high enzyme activity are correlated with younger age of onset in females but not in males, whereas low activity genotypes do not display sex differences. Second example is peroxisome proliferator-activated receptor γ_2 (PPARγ_2), whose polymorphism is correlated with increased insulin sensitivity and reduced risk for type 2 diabetes. Interestingly, in males, a more efficient shift from lipid oxidation in the basal state to carbohydrate oxidation during insulin stimulation has been observed in lean, glucose tolerant males with the polymorphism compared to wild-type males; whereas this difference has not been observed in females (8). Therefore, the PPARγ_2 polymorphism protects individuals from insulin insensitivity by promoting better suppression of lipid oxidation leading to more glucose disposal in males but not females. Another example is the 3′ untranslated region of the *PPP1R3A* gene, a gene involved in glycogen synthase activity and associated with development of type 2 diabetes (9). Males homozygous for the polymorphism of *PPP1R3A* gene are significantly younger at diagnosis than female carriers (10). Additionally, a polymorphism in the promoter region of uncoupling protein (UCP)-2, a mitochondrial inner membrane protein, may be involved in obesity and development of type 2 diabetes (11). In a study of 100 obese subjects, the genotype that causes increased transcription of UCP-2 mRNA is more prevalent in diabetic women than in nondiabetic women. However no difference in distribution of this genotype is detected in men (12). To summarize, sex differences in genetic polymorphisms exist in the development and etiology of diabetes.

1.2. Sex differences in physiologic mechanism on the development of diabetes

Obesity has been recognized as a major and an independent diabetes risk factor. The increase in type 2 diabetes is closely associated with the epidemic of obesity. Body composition is very closely associated with glucose tolerance and insulin sensitivity (13). Development of adverse metabolic complications has been attributed to increased body fat, not just body weight, and the fat distributed particularly in the abdominal visceral compartment, a source of bioactive mediators that directly contribute to insulin resistance (14). To be more specific, intra-abdominal visceral adipose tissue carries a stronger risk for the development of metabolic disorders, such as glucose intolerance and insulin resistance related type 2 diabetes, than subcutaneous adipose tissue. Therefore, risk for diabetes incidence is particularly high in individuals with large amounts of abdominal visceral fat.

Sex differences in the regional fat distribution exist. Males and females differ in terms of how and where they store body fat. In humans, premenopausal women usually have more subcutaneous fat, whereas men have more intra-abdominal visceral fat. Consequently, obesity-related metabolic disorders are much lower in premenopausal women than men (15). In addition, estrogens are responsible for body weight homeostasis in women. The prevalence of obesity is particularly high among middle-aged women. Symptoms of the metabolic syndrome, including increased visceral obesity and shifts in body fat distribution, as well as glucose intolerance and insulin resistance begin appearing in many women experiencing menopause and developing estrogen deficiency (16). Even in women who do not gain weight after menopause, fat shifts from a subcutaneous location into the abdomen. Women are at an increased risk to develop visceral obesity due to the loss of endogenous ovarian hormone production. The increased visceral obesity in menopausal women can be altered by exogenous hormone replacement therapy (17, 18). Researches using animal models have provided important insights into the pathogenesis of human diseases and new therapeutic approaches. Peripheral metabolic signals and hormones are not only involved in regulating adiposity and body fat distribution, but also involved in regulating glucose metabolism and glucose tolerance. In experimental rodent models, reductions in circulating estrogens, which occurs following removal of ovaries (i.e., ovariectomy), results in increased body adiposity. Such increase in body adiposity can be ameliorated by exogenous 17β – estradiol administration (19).

In addition, sex hormones are directly involved in the regulation of glucose tolerance (20, 21). In a prospective study that included over 500 women and men who did not have diabetes upon study entry, development of diabetes was associated with low levels of total testosterone in men and high levels of bioavailable testosterone in women (22). Therefore, differences in the regulation of glucose tolerance may be under the influence of sex hormones indirectly through their influence of body fat content and distribution or directly through their influence in the glucose metabolism and insulin signaling.

This chapter discusses the sex differences in regulation of glucose homeostasis, focusing on the roles of female sex hormone estrogens as determinants mediating body adiposity levels and body fat distribution as well as glucose metabolism and insulin sensitivity. We will use the term "sex difference" instead of "gender difference" throughout this chapter. The term "sex" refers to differences between males and females that result from the chromosomal complement and the effects of hormones; whereas the term "gender" refers to an individual's identity as a man or a woman, and the cultural and behavioral expectations associated with being a man or a woman. With regard to the regulation of glucose homeostasis and energy metabolism, little is known about gender differences, thus this chapter focuses primarily on sex differences.

2. Sex differences in body adiposity and fat distribution

The prevalence of obesity is higher in women than in men in many areas around the world (www.iaso.org). In addition there is a sex difference in body fat distribution. These sex differences in obesity incidence and fat distribution can be explained in part by the influence of gonadal steroids, as well as behavioral, socio-cultural and genetic factors. Several factors may play important roles to drive greater propensity for excess body fat in females than in males. It has been suggested that evolutionary pressures predispose females to store excess fat for reproduction and lactation. In contrast, evolutionary pressures predispose males to burn stored fuels in gathering and hunting. Adipose tissue plays a major role in the regulation of glucose homeostasis and insulin sensitivity, thus total body adiposity is closely associated with insulin sensitivity. Increased body fat is a risk factor for developing type 2 diabetes mellitus. A line of research has focused on behavioral and social differences between men and women that relate to eating or activity behaviors. Sex differences in body composition and insulin sensitivity are evident in humans throughout the lifespan. Pregnancy and menopause also have physiological and behavioral consequences on appetite and weight regulation that confer elevated obesity risk in many women. There is a sex difference in the regional fat distribution. Men and premenopausal women differ in their fat distribution. Females have "gynoid" or female-pattern fat distribution with more subcutaneous fat, whereas males have "android" or male-pattern body fat distribution with more abdominal visceral fat (15). Fat deposition in the subcutaneous depot is important for females during lactation. Despite the higher level of body fat, obesity-related metabolic disorders, such as type 2 diabetes, are much lower in premenopausal women and female animals than males. The role of estrogen in mediating body fat distribution and glucose homeostasis will be discussed in this chapter.

2.1. Difference between subcutaneous and abdominal adipose tissues

Body fat distribution is a more appropriate indicator than total adiposity for metabolic disorders, as obesity is not only a condition characterized by homogenous distribution of adipose tissue, but that the regional distribution of adipose tissue is more important in understanding the relationship between obesity and various metabolic diseases. Adipose tissue, which is distributed in the abdominal viscera, carries a greater risk for glucose intolerance and insulin resistance than adipose tissue subcutaneously. Specifically, abdominal adipose tissues contribute to the development of insulin resistance, glucose intolerance, hypertension, dyslipidemia, and atherosclerosis (23). Metabolites and secretions of visceral adipose tissue drain through the hepatic portal system, partially at least, to the liver. Insulin effect is lower and catecholamine effect is higher in visceral than subcutaneous adipose tissue. Specifically, visceral fat have higher rates of catecholamine-induced lipolysis (24, 25), express higher numbers of beta-1, -2 and -3 adrenergic receptors and are more sensitive to catecholamine-induced lipolysis (26, 27), and are less responsive to the cAMP-lowering effects of alpha-adrenergic agonists (28). In addition, visceral fat cells express higher levels of glucocorticoid receptor (29, 30) and have greater glucocorticoid response with lipoprotein lipase activation (31), produce more angiotensinogen (32, 33), and secrete more interleukin-6 and plasminogen activator inhibitor-1 (34) than subcutaneous adipose tissue. Accumulation of intra-abdominal/visceral adipose tissue carries a much greater risk for metabolic disorders than does adipose tissue distributed subcutaneously (35-37). In contrast, subcutaneous fat distribution is poorly correlated with risks for these metabolic disorders (23). Therefore, the elevated health risks in diabetes associated with obesity depend on the localization of the adipose tissue in the body, as the distribution of fat is more directly associated with glucose tolerance and insulin sensitivity than the total body adiposity. Consequently, there is a sex-based difference in the prevalence and incidence of metabolic complications associated with obesity. Males have an increased incidence of obesity-related metabolic diseases than females aged 12 to 18 years (38, 39). In premenopausal women, there is a lower incidence of metabolic disorders associated with obesity (38). The prevalence of the metabolic syndrome increases with age, and the prevalence of the metabolic syndrome is similar in middle-aged men and women (40).

There are noted functional differences between subcutaneous and abdominal adipose tissues. Subcutaneous tissue is poorly innervated compared to the abdominal adipose tissue (35). Consequently, subcutaneous adipose tissue takes up free fatty acids and stores the excess calories more readily than abdominal adipose tissue in both males and females. Lipoprotein lipase (LPL) is the major enzyme involved in the fatty acid uptake and is the key regulator of fat accumulation in adipose tissues. Estrogens decrease adipose tissue LPL activity (41-43), and thus males have a higher level of LPL activity and thus fat accumulation than females with higher levels of estrogens. The lipolytic pathway involves the breakdown of energy stored in the form of triglycerides and is initiated when the energy supply from the metabolic fuels is depleted. The lipolytic activity of the abdominal fat is higher compared to the lipolytic activity of the subcutaneous fat in premenopausal women; a phenomenon not observed in post-menopausal women lacking endogenous estrogen (24, 44, 45).

Recent evidence suggests that great subcutaneous fat accumulation may be protective against development of metabolic disorders. First, epidemiological studies indicate association of a high waist-to-hip ratio, instead of a large waist circumference alone, with the incidence of type 2 diabetes and other metabolic diseases (46-48). Indeed, a larger hip circumference has been shown to be protective against metabolic risk in multiple ethnic groups, independent of waist circumference or abdominal fat accumulation(49). Second, several animal studies reported that mice with transplantation of subcutaneous fat from the inguinal region of male donors into the intra-abdominal compartment of male recipient mice resulted in significantly protective effects on adiposity, insulin sensitivity and glucose tolerance (50-53). Since protective effect of a large hip circumference with regard to cardiovascular disease morbidity and mortality is significant in women but not in men (54), it would be expected that transplanting female subcutaneous adipose tissue might have greater protective effects.

2.2. Sex hormone estrogens and estrogen receptors regulate adiposity

Obesity development is accelerated after menopause in women; factors such as loss of estrogens, the ageing process and changes in lifestyle may all be contributors (Shi & Clegg 2009, Barton 2010). The effect of menopause is supported by animal models showing that a reduction in circulating estrogen levels following ovariectomy results in increased body adiposity (55). Body fat increases in several conditions associated with estrogen deficiency such as ovariectomy, polycystic ovary syndrome (PCOS), and the lack of a functional aromatase gene; all can be corrected and reversed by exogenous administration of 17β-estradiol, the active form of estrogens (56-61).

The classical nuclear estrogen receptors (ER) include estrogen receptor alpha (ERα) and estrogen receptor beta (ERβ).Genomic activation of ERs results from estrogens binding to estrogen response elements (EREs) in promoter regions of target genes (62, 63). Increased visceral adiposity is associated with the XbaI polymorphism of the human ERα gene when guanidine is substituted for adenine in exon one (64). Additionally, pre-menopausal women with increased of visceral adiposity, indicated by higher waist-hip ratios, have the XbaI polymorphism compared to the control cohort of women with the normal genotype (64).

Interestingly such polymorphism does not affect adiposity in postmenopausal women or in men(64). ERα gene expression in subcutaneous adipose tissue is reduced in obese pre-menopausal women, but increases after weight reduction (65). Furthermore several ERα single nucleotide polymorphisms have been associated with obesity phenotypes in women and men (64, 66, 67). Thus, polymorphisms of the human ERα gene may impair estrogen signaling and lead to increased visceral adiposity and its attendant health risks. In humans, polymorphisms in the ERβ gene have been associated with lower BMI although other investigators found no correlations (68, 69).

Utilizing targeted deletions in the ERα gene or both ERα and ERβ genes of male and female mice indicate increase in adiposity (70, 71). ERβ inhibits food intake and reduces body weight through effects in the central nervous system in rats (72). In addition, one study investigated the effect of estrogens on adipose tissue development using ERα knockout mice. Loss of estrogen following ovariectomy in ERα knockout mice resulted in decreased body fat and adipocyte size, which was reversed by 17β-estradiol treatment (73), suggesting that regulation of body adiposity is mediated by an ER other than ERα, possibly by ERβ. In contrast, mice lacking both ERα and ERβ develop obesity but increased adiposity is not observed in ERβ-knockout mice (71), questioning a role for ERβ and suggesting that the obesity-promoting effect of estrogen deficiency is mediated specifically through ERα. These findings support a substantial physiological role for ERα in mediating the effects of estrogens in the control of body adiposity. Replacement of 17β-estradiol prevents ovariectomized wild-type mice from developing obesity, such protective effects are not observed in ovariectomized ERα deficient mice (74). Therefore, estrogens, together with its ERα, play important roles to regulate total adiposity.

To summarize, the metabolic effects of estrogens appear to be largely mediated by ERα whereas the role of ERβ and possible cross-talk with other ERs is currently unclear. Indeed, ERβ inhibits ERα-mediated gene expression in certain cell types and often opposes the action of ERα (75), an interaction that might be also important for the regulation of body fat. Finally, it should be noted that compensatory developmental changes in both animal models and humans may alter hormone responsiveness in ways that are different from the inherent biology in healthy individuals or wild-type animals respectively.

2.3. Sex hormone estrogens regulate fat distribution

Because there are differential effects on health risk between subcutaneous and abdominal adipose tissues, it is important to understand mechanisms that determine not only total fat accumulation but also where fat is accumulated, and how fat distribution is regulated in males and females. Recent research using molecular approaches and animal models has provided greater understanding of the role of sex hormones and other molecules on fat partitioning.

The question of sex differences in fat distribution have been examined using animal models. Several animal species, including pigs and rodents, show sex-specific differences in fat distribution, with males having more abdominal fat and less subcutaneous fat than females.

Ovarian hormone estrogen appears to be a key regulator in mediating the sex-specific adipose tissue distribution pattern. Estrogens promote the accumulation of subcutaneous fat (76). In contrast, abdominal fat varies inversely with levels of estrogens (77). During the peri-menopausal period, depletion of ovarian follicles leads to a steady decline in 17β-estradiol production in post-menopausal women (78). Loss of estrogens with menopause is associated with an increase in abdominal fat accrual (36). Indeed, changes in body fat mass are positively correlated with serum 17β-estradiol concentration in post-menopausal women (79-81), although this association varies with time from the onset of menopause and may take up to 6 years to develop (81). In premenopausal women, there is a lower incidence of metabolic disorders associated with obesity. However, after menopause when there is a very low level of estrogen in the circulation, an increased risk of obesity-related metabolic disorders is reported (38). Therefore ovarian hormones might play a vital role in protecting the body against metabolic diseases via the sex-based differences seen in adipose tissue deposition.

The sexual dimorphism in adipose tissue distribution may partially explain the greater risk for the metabolic syndrome in men compared with premenopausal women. Estrogens are known to regulate body fat distribution in animals and humans. As being discussed earlier in this chapter, females tend to accumulate more fat in their subcutaneous depots whereas males tend to accumulate more fat in their visceral depots (82). Additionally, after the loss of endogenous estrogens as a result of menopause, a shift towards visceral adiposity occurs, which is sensitive to estrogen therapy (55).

Studies in ovariectomized rodent models have elucidated possible mechanisms by which changes in estrogen levels may impact fat distribution. Ovariectomized female rats gain fat, specifically visceral fat with a loss of subcutaneous fat (19, 83). Additionally peripheral or central administration of 17β-estradiol to OVX rats changes their body fat distribution to mirror that of intact females with normal estrous cycles. administration of exogenous estradiol reverses this increased visceral fat distribution pattern (19). Furthermore, altering the sex hormone milieu in males with exogenous 17β-estradiol administration to male rats decreases visceral fat and increases subcutaneous fat relative to males not given estrogen (19). An important implication from these findings is that estrogens are critical determinates of body fat distribution. Estrogen may influence fat distribution centrally by modulating leptin responsiveness, as leptin not only influences total body fat in rodents but also favors loss of visceral fat via Stat3 signaling in the hypothalamus (84). Female mice are more responsive than male mice to the effects of centrally administered leptin to decrease food intake and body weight and to increase c-fos and Stat3 expression in the arcuate nucleus (85). In addition, research has shown that both male and female aromatase-knockout mice, which are estrogen-deficient and have elevated testosterone, accumulate more abdominal adipose tissue with increased adipocyte size in the gonadal and intra-renal fat depots (57). Male aromatase-knockout mice also develop fatty liver, as do aromatase-deficient men, and this is reversible with estradiol treatment (86).

Sex hormones play important roles in adipose tissue lipolysis and fat uptake. Sex differences exist for regulation of lipolysis by alpha-2 adrenergic receptor(87). Estrogen treatment increases lipolysis in abdominal fat cells in mice(88). Lactation and menopausal status also impact the lipolytic responsiveness and lipoprotein lipase activity of fat cells. Higher adipose tissue lipoprotein lipase activity (promoting fat storage) occurs in subcutaneous femoral adipocytes compared with abdominal adipocytes in premenopausal women but not in postmenopausal, estrogen-deficient women(89). Additionally lipolysis increases in subcutaneous femoral fat during lactation but not in abdominal fat(89). Furthermore, estrogen treatment in postmenopausal women restores the lipoprotein lipase activity of the femoral adipocytes and attenuates lipolytic response in subcutaneous adipocytes but not in abdominal adipocytes (90). Subcutaneous gluteal adipocytes from premenopausal women are more sensitive to the antilipolytic effects of insulin than abdominal adipocytes (91).

Testosterone, male androgens also impact body fat distribution. Testosterone deficiency aggravates the development of obesity and hyperinsulinemia, which in turn will suppress testicular androgen synthesis even further and result in a vicious cycle (92). In 'andropause' men, gradual decline in circulating androgens with aging is accompanied by increased total and abdominal fat (93). Administration of aromatizable androgens such as testosterone (94, 95), but not nonaromatizable dihydrotestostone (94), reduces total and abdominal fat in older men. In contrast, androgen administration to ovariectomized female mice significantly increases body adiposity and abdominal fat (96). Such obesity development is associated with reduced fatty acid oxidation, indicated by decreased phosphorylation of adenosine monophosphate (AMP)-activated protein kinase and acetyl-CoA carboxylase in abdominal visceral fat (96). In humans, women with higher circulating androgen levels (97) or exogenous androgen administration (98, 99) increase abdominal fat. These findings raise significant clinical concern about the use of testosterone as a hormone replacement therapy in postmenopausal women.

In summary, sex differences in body fat distribution appear to be largely a result of differences in sex hormones between men and women. Estrogens reduce visceral fat in men and women, an effect that is likely mediated by both central and peripheral mechanisms. In contrast, opposite effects of androgens on fat distribution in men and women are seen, with aromatizable androgens decreasing visceral fat in men but increasing it in women.

2.4. Estrogen receptors regulate fat distribution

Gonadal hormones, including estrogen, progesterone and androgen, have their receptors expressed in the visceral and the subcutaneous adipose tissue depots (100). Subcutaneous adipose tissues have higher concentrations of estrogen receptors and progesterone receptors than androgen receptors in females, and estrogens down-regulates AR expression in subcutaneous fat (101). In contrast, visceral adipose tissue has higher concentrations of androgen receptors (102, 103). In visceral adipose tissue, there is an increase in the expression of androgen receptors in males relative to estrogen receptors. The development of knockout animals has provided a powerful tool to examine the role of individual receptors for estrogen, progesterone and androgen in the regulation of adipose tissue. Adipose tissue-specific androgen receptor knockout mice have increased intra-adipose tissue estradiol levels, which precedes increased subcutaneous obesity and hyperleptinemia (104). Additionally, androgens can be converted to estrogens through activation of the aromatase enzyme. Aromatase knockout mice have elevated testosterone and accumulate more abdominal adipose tissue with increased adipocyte size in the visceral fat depot. Hence, in adipose tissue, there is a counteracting effect between estrogen and androgen, which may lead to differences in fat distribution.

Estradiol regulates body fat distribution either directly at the level of the adipocyte or through augmenting the efficacy of the adiposity signals in the CNS. Subcutaneous and abdominal adipose tissues express both ERα and ERβ, but ERα is predominantly expressed in abdominal adipose tissue (105) and ERβ are higher in subcutaneous adipose tissue (106). ERα gene polymorphisms predict abdominal obesity in women, but not in men, suggesting a possible sexual dimorphism in the ERα effects (64). Female and male mice lacking ERα develop central obesity with increases in abdominal adipose tissue, which is reflected by increased adipocyte number and size (70). ERα is ubiquitously expressed in rodent brains, but the physiologically relevant sites of ERα in the regulation of food intake and energy expenditure have not been identified. ERα is expressed in the ventrolateral portion of the VMN, the ARC, the medial preoptic area (MPOA), and the paraventricular nuclei (PVN) (107-109). ERβ is found in the same hypothalamic nuclei as ERα, but ERβ expression is significantly reduced relative to ERα. Site-specific knock-down of ERα in bilateral ventromedial nucleus of the hypothalamus in mice using siRNA result in increased adiposity, no change in food intake, and suppression of energy expenditure, increased visceral adiposity, and decreased leptin sensitivity, implicating ventromedial hypothalamic ERα in energy homeostasis (110).

Both short-term and long-term castration in males resulted in increased insulin sensitivity and increased lipogenesis in both abdominal and subcutaneous adipose tissues, an event that is independent of changes in the fat pad weights (102). Thus, in contrast to the preferential effect of estrogen in females on the abdominal adipocytes, testosterone exerts an inhibitory effect on lipogenesis and insulin sensitivity in both abdominal and subcutaneous adipocytes.

3. Sex difference in glucose metabolism

Glucose challenge test is important in terms of understanding the pathophysiology of individuals at risk of progressing to type 2 diabetes. As recommended by the World Health Organization, the standardized, 75-g oral glucose tolerance test is used for diagnosis of impaired fasting glucose and impaired glucose tolerance. Plasma glucose at fasting and 2 hours after oral glucose tolerance test are measured to indicate glucose tolerance in individuals. Fasting glucose is the glucose concentration after an overnight fast and mostly reflects endogenous glucose production, whereas glucose level 2 hours after oral glucose tolerance test, *i.e.* post-load hyperglycemia, reflects the acute increase in blood glucose after a glucose challenge.

Several epidemiological investigations from European countries (111-113), Australia (114-116), Asian countries (117), and Mauritius (118) report that men have higher fasting plasma glucose levels and plasma glucose levels during the early course of the oral glucose tests than women, indicating that the prevalence of impaired fasting glycaemia is higher in men than in women; and women have higher plasma glucose levels 2 hours after oral glucose tolerance tests than men, suggesting that the prevalence of impaired glucose tolerance is higher in women than in men. The pre-diabetic condition of impaired fasting glycaemia is characterized by hepatic insulin resistance, elevated hepatic glucose production and beta cell dysfunction.

3.1. Sex difference in glucose tolerance

Men and women are given the same amount of glucose during a standard oral glucose tolerance test. In all ethnic groups throughout the world, women are on average shorter by approximately 15 cm and thus have smaller body sizes than men (119). Additionally, women generally have less absolute amount of fat-free muscle mass than men, which is the major metabolically active tissue involved in glucose uptake, and thus women are less able to metabolize the fixed amount of glucose (111, 115, 118). The higher prevalence of impaired glucose tolerance in women may be an artifact caused by the fact that individuals of different body sizes and lean muscle masses receive the same amount of glucose during glucose challenge test. This notion is supported by the observation that the increments of glucose, insulin and the incretin hormones glucagon-like peptide-1 and glucose-dependent insulinotropic polypeptide after an glucose challenge test are significantly higher in women than in men (120), indicating that the same amount of glucose represents a larger stimulus in women than in men when seen in relation to their body sizes.

Further analysis using anthropometric measures (*e.g.*, weights, heights and waist-hip circumferences) indicated that the differences in plasma glucose levels 2 hours after oral glucose tolerance tests, but not fasting plasma glucose levels, could be explained by differences in body size and/or body composition between men and women (113, 115, 118, 121). Consequently, women are more commonly diagnosed with diabetes on the basis of glucose level 2-hour post glucose tolerance test compared with fasting plasma glucose levels (112, 115).The risk of gestational diabetes is also higher in shorter compared with taller women (122). Women do not have higher glucose levels following glucose test than men when differences in height and high-waist circumference (113) or absolute amount of fat-free mass (121) are taken into account. This notion is supported by the observation that there is a higher risk of developing type 2 diabetes in men than in women with impaired glucose tolerance (123), suggesting that women with impaired glucose tolerance may be healthier than their male counterparts. In summary, sex difference in glucose tolerance without taking into account of body size is probably not related to sex-specific differences in the physiology of glucose regulation.

3.2. Sex difference in fasting plasma glucose

In contrast to the sex difference in glucose tolerance, sex difference in fasting plasma glucose levels is not related to differences in anthropometry and could not be explained by differences in body size and/or body composition between men and women. Indeed, higher fasting plasma glucose in men compared with women reflects differences in insulin sensitivity and pancreatic β cell function between men and women (113), suggesting that the sex difference in fasting plasma glucose has a true physiological basis.

During fasting females have decreased liver enzymes, lower creatinine and uric acid concentrations with a trend toward reduced triglycerides, but higher HDL cholesterol and body fat mass, which are generally seen as gender-related differences because of the direct effects by sex hormones (124, 125). There is an association between elevated FFA and increased endogenous glucose production (126). Interestingly, females displayed lower fasting endogenous glucose production than males, despite higher fasting plasma FFA concentrations (116). Study using laboratory rodent models indicate that there is no direct effect by FFA on hepatic glucose production in isolated perfused rat liver (127).

The possible physiological mechanism that is responsible for the higher fasting plasma glucose levels observed in men compared with women could be related to large waist circumference in men (128), suggesting that sex differences in body fat distribution contribute to the sex difference in fasting plasma glucose levels. Indeed, high waist circumference and hip circumference are associated with impaired glucose tolerance in both men and women (113), suggesting that obesity contributes and is related to disturbances of glucose metabolism. Visceral component of abdominal fat is strongly associated with insulin resistance (129). Abdominal adipose tissue has a reduced ability to metabolize the glucose load of a glucose challenge test (102). Homeostasis model assessment of insulin resistance (HOMA-IR), predominantly reflecting hepatic insulin resistance, is lower in men than in women in general (113). Homeostasis model assessment of β cell function (HOMA-β) is also slightly lower in men than in women.

In summary, sex differences in fasting plasma glucose levels are caused by underlying physiological differences in both insulin sensitivity and β cell function.

3.3. Sex difference in glucose absorption

Sex difference in carbohydrate metabolism may contribute to sex-specific glucose regulation. A glucose infusion at fasting and during hyperinsulinemia is used to measure whole-body insulin sensitivity and endogenous glucose production using hyperinsulinemic clamp technique. Healthy glucose-tolerant women have slower glucose absorption rates and slower liquid emptying from the stomach (130), and thus longer gut glucose half-life compared with glucose-tolerant men(116).Furthermore, there is an association between glucose absorption velocity and body size, with body tallness having strong influence on the glucose absorption velocity. This notion is supported by a recent study showing that, for both sexes, although people with different heights have similar fasting glucose levels, those in the shortest height quartile do have significantly higher 2 h glucose levels following oral glucose tolerance test compared with those in the tallest height quartile (115). As it is mentioned earlier in this section, women are on average shorter by approximately 15 cm than men (119). Consequently, women generally have lower glucose absorption rates and have higher plasma glucose levels 2 hours after oral glucose tolerance test than men (115).

Glucose absorption rates are higher in males in the initial phase and elevate in females in the end of the of the oral glucose tolerance tests three hours after oral glucose intake (116). The best-suited value to describe of glucose absorption velocity is glucose half-life in the gut. In all participants, glucose half-life is negatively related to body height and fat-free mass (116, 131), thus glucose half-life is prolonged in females in comparison with males. When adjusted for total fat-free body mass, females with similar gut absorption as males are slightly more insulin sensitive than males(116). The alterations of plasma glucose concentrations during glucose tolerance test in females and males are not only due to different glucose clearance rates but also due to different absorption rates from the gastrointestinal tract between sexes (116), which could serve to explain higher glucose concentrations at the end of the glucose challenge test in females. Additionally, postprandial insulin secretion affects glucose disappearance rate and glucose concentrations. One study has reported that females have greater peripheral insulin release and thus higher concentration during the first hour of oral glucose tolerance test (132). A separate study has reported that insulin secretion is comparable between young males and females following a high-carbohydrate mixed meal (133). Therefore, these available data from previous human studies suggest that the disturbance in insulin secretion does not contribute to the higher postprandial glucose concentrations in women. This notion is supported by animal studies using rodents, which have reported no sex associated difference in glucose-stimulated insulin secretion (134).

To summarize, sex difference in glucose absorption and concomitant effect of insulin release, but not insulin-induced glucose uptake or glucose metabolism, contributes to the higher prevalence of glucose intolerance in females diagnosed from oral glucose tolerance tests as observed in several epidemiological studies worldwide.

4. Sex differences in insulin sensitivity

Glucose homeostasis is maintained in a narrow range via glucose output by the liver and glucose uptake by tissues. Insulin, secreted by the pancreatic β cells in response to increased circulating levels of glucose, is the major anabolic hormone whose action is essential for maintenance of glucose homeostasis. Insulin regulates glucose homeostasis by reducing hepatic glucose production via decreased gluconeogenesis (de novo glucose synthesis) and glycogenolysis (glycogen breakdown), and increasing the rate of glucose uptake, primarily into skeletal muscle and adipose tissue (135). Insulin's actions are brought about by intracellular events following the binding of insulin to insulin receptor and the activation of its tyrosine kinase, which phosphorylates tyrosine residues of target proteins such as insulin receptor substrates (136). The phosphatidylinositol 3-kinase (PI3K)/Akt signaling cascade is activated by the IRS proteins to trigger the stimulation of glucose uptake (135). Insulin resistance, defined as a state of decreased responsiveness of target tissues to insulin, plays a major role in the development of type 2 diabetes. Increased plasma free fatty acid concentrations due to high-fat diet feeding are typically associated with many insulin-resistant states (135).Abnormalities in fatty acid metabolism result in inappropriate accumulation of lipids in myocytes and hepatocytes, thus impairing their function and leading to insulin resistance (135).

4.1. Female human and animals are more insulin sensitive

There is evidence indicating that insulin sensitivity differs between males and females (137). Premenopausal women have better glucose tolerance and insulin sensitivity compared with men in general. Despite having lower fat mass, the prevalence of diabetes and early abnormalities of glucose metabolism is three times higher in men than in women (138). Moreover, women have decreased susceptibility to fatty acid–induced peripheral insulin resistance (124, 139, 140). Female humans and rodents are more insulin-sensitive than their male counterparts.

In many different laboratory rodent models of glucose intolerance, insulin resistance, and diabetes, the different insulin sensitivity of female versus male mice can be detected by glucose tolerance tests and insulin tolerance tests. When various strains of mice are subjected to glucose tolerance tests, female mice have lower glucose levels than male mice at different time point throughout the tests (141-143). Additionally, female mice show a greater fall in blood glucose in response to insulin as compared with male mice during insulin tolerance tests (141-143). These data from our lab suggest that female animals are more insulin sensitive than males. Furthermore, female rodents are less prone to diet-induced insulin resistance, and many genetically induced forms of insulin resistance have a milder phenotype in females compared with males (141, 142, 144, 145).

4.2. Female fat cells are more insulin sensitive

Adipocytes in different fat depots appear to have a distinct impact in insulin sensitivity. As it is mentioned previously in this chapter, accumulation of visceral fat, but not subcutaneous fat, is linked to the development of metabolic complications. Fat accumulation in different depots is sexually dimorphic, i.e., men accumulate more visceral fat, whereas women accumulate more subcutaneous fat and have a higher percentage of body fat compared with men. These sex-related differences in insulin sensitivity and adipose tissue development and function could be attributable in part to actions of estrogen and testosterone. For example, decreases in estrogen and increases in testosterone levels that occur during menopause are associated with loss of subcutaneous and gain of visceral fat and increase in insulin resistance (146).

Female adipocytes have increased insulin sensitivity compared with male adipocytes, which is particularly true for abdominal adipocytes (102, 147). A recent study analyzed insulin sensitivity and glucose metabolism of adipocytes from abdominal and subcutaneous adipose tissue from normal, castrated, or steroid-implanted mice (102). The authors reported that both abdominal and subcutaneous adipocytes of females have greater lipogenic rates than those from males. Additionally, female abdominal adipocytes are more insulin sensitive than subcutaneous adipocytes and more insulin-sensitive than male adipocytes from either depot, with female abdominal adipocytes showing a robust increase in insulin-induced lipogenesis and insulin signaling, including downstream targets Akt and extracellular signal–related kinase phosphorylation, when stimulated by low physiological concentrations of insulin. In contrast, male adipocytes show activation only at much higher insulin concentrations (102). Furthermore, adipocytes from females have higher mRNA and protein levels of several genes involved in glucose and lipid metabolism, including glucose transporters and key lipogenic enzymes fatty acid synthase and acetyl CoA carboxylase (102), suggesting that the sex difference in insulin sensitivity at adipocyte level is attributable at least partially to increased glucose transporters and lipogenic enzyme levels. In summary, sex-specific differences in insulin action in adipocytes may contribute to the sexual dimorphism of insulin resistance.

Despite a higher lipogenic rates female adipocytes are smaller than male adipocytes, especially those from the abdominal adipose depot. This is because adipocytes of females also has a higher lipolytic capacity than those of males (148, 149), suggesting a higher metabolic turnover of female abdominal adipocytes leading to decreased fat accumulation in visceral depots in females compared with males. As a result, in humans, females have higher serum levels of free fatty acid than males (124, 139) but appear to be protected against insulin resistance induced by elevated free fatty acid (139).

Sex steroids are known to play a role in the regulation of adipose tissue development and function as well as whole body insulin sensitivity (146). These sex differences in insulin sensitivity in adipose tissue are regulated by physiological levels of sex steroids. Adipocytes of castrated male mice have increased insulin sensitivity and increased lipogenic rates, whereas adipocytes of ovariectomized females have lowered insulin sensitivity and reduced lipogenic capacity (102). The increased sensitivity to insulin and lipogenesis observed in adipocytes from females may account for their lower level of insulin resistance and diabetes risk despite similar or higher fat content than in male mice (102), indicating a positive role of estrogen in insulin sensitivity and lipogenesis in females. Therefore, gonadal hormones estrogen and testosterone contribute to the sexual dimorphism of lipogenesis and insulin sensitivity, lipogenic capacity of adipocytes.

4.3. Estrogens regulate insulin sensitivity

Gonadal hormones play critical roles in the regulation of glucose metabolism and maintenance of insulin sensitivity. Disturbances and changes in the relationship between estrogens and androgen metabolism seem to adversely affect fat metabolism and insulin sensitivity independent of sex (see below). Deficiency of estrogen leads to development of insulin resistance. Animals and humans lacking endogenous estrogen synthesis exhibit insulin resistance, which can be treated by estrogen supplementation (57, 61, 150). In humans, postmenopausal women with deficiency in endogenous estrogen have increased risk of insulin resistance and developing type 2 diabetes (4), while hormone replacement therapy or treatment with estradiol, the major bioactive form of estrogen, improves insulin sensitivity and lowers blood glucose levels (151, 152) and reduce incidence of diabetes (153,

154). Insulin resistance in a man with a homozygous inactivating mutation of the aromatase gene has been reported (60, 155). Estrogen deficiency also contributes to the development of insulin resistance and type 2 diabetes in rodent models (Louet et al 2004). Ovariectomized rodents with low level of endogenous estrogen have elevated basal glucose levels and impaired glucose tolerance (Bailey et al 1980). Aromatase knockout mice with a genetic impairment in endogenous estrogen synthesis exhibit decreased glucose tolerance and insulin resistance (Jones et al 2000; Takeda et al 2003).

The mechanism of regulation of estrogens on insulin sensitivity is not clear. Estrogens may increase hepatic insulin sensitivity by decreasing gluconeogenesis and glycogenolysis and increasing insulin release in islets of Langerhans (156). Estrogens also prevent β-cell apoptosis (157). Additionally, estrogens reduce pro-inflammatory adipokines and their signaling and therefore decrease inflammation (158, 159). Changes in the level of sex steroids had variable effects on levels of circulating adipokines, as ovariectomized females have lower level of adiponectin and females implanted with estradiol have higher adiponectin levels (102). It is increasingly evident that chronic activation of pro-inflammatory pathways may be at least partly responsible for obesity-induced insulin resistance and diabetes (25, 160). ERs are expressed in monocytes and macrophages, and estrogens activate these cells (161, 162). Female rats and mice are relatively protected from high-fat diet induced obesity, insulin resistance and inflammatory responses (141-143, 163-165). Recent studies have shown that 17β -estradiol may play a role in reducing the inflammatory response in adipose, cardiovascular, and neural systems (146). Suppression of pro-inflammatory responses with estrogens may represent a promising strategy to combat obesity and associated metabolic disorders. Furthermore estrogens may improve insulin action (166). Therefore, the greater amount of abdominal visceral adipose tissue in conjunction with lower endogenous estrogen levels found in men may be related to the higher insulin resistance when compared with pre-menopausal women.

4.4. Estrogen receptor regulates insulin sensitivity

Estrogen's action is via its classic nuclear receptors and non-classic membrane receptors (63, 167-172).Both ERα and ERβ are expressed in the liver, muscle, and adipose tissue, as well as in several key regions of the hypothalamus of the central nervous system that have been linked to the control of peripheral glucose homeostasis. In particular, recent evidence points to neurons in the arcuate nucleus as critical regulators of glucose homeostasis (173). ER subtype-specific ligands have been used to clarify the specific roles of ERα and ERβ, such as the selective ERα ligand propyl pyrazoletriol (PPT) and the selective ERβagonist (2,3-bis(4-hydroxyphenyl)-propionitrile (DPN). PPT has similar effects as estradiol, including increase of uterine weight, and prevention of increased body weight following ovariectomy (174). In addition, estrogen acts through other extranuclear pathways after ligands bind to the ERα or ERβ associated to the plasma membrane, as well as to ERs located at the plasma membrane, in the cytosol, or in the mitochondria (167, 171, 175) to regulate energy balance and glucose homeostasis (167). Estrogen may trigger its actions after binding to membrane ERs, such as GPR30 (176, 177), binding to receptors for other ligands, or binding to ion channels (167, 178,

179). The membrane ERs are characterized by a completely different pharmacological profile when compared to nuclear ERα and ERβ. They do not bind the antiestrogen ICI182,780 (167). These extranuclear actions of estrogen are the rapid activation of signaling cascades resulting in the activation of transcription factors and therefore in the regulation of gene expression.

Both animal and human studies suggest that ERα may play a critical role to regulate glucose tolerance and insulin sensitivity (see below). Impaired insulin sensitivity, glucose intolerance, and hyperinsulinemia in a man with a mutation of ERα and thus lacking functional ERα has been reported (180). Estrogen-dependent effects on glucose homeostasis through both ERα and ERβ, whereas glucose tolerance is normal in ERβ-knockout mice (70, 73, 181, 182). Additionally, ERα deficiency increases fasting insulin levels, impairs glucose tolerance, and results in skeletal muscle insulin resistance (182), suggesting that ERα may have a direct anti-diabetic role. Insulin sensitivity is preserved in mice lacking ERβ although these animals become obese following a high-fat diet (183). In addition, ERβ acts as an inhibitor of peroxisome proliferators-activated receptor gamma activity, a major inhibitory regulator of glucose and lipid metabolism (183). Therefore, previous studies argue in favor of an estrogen-dependent regulation of glucose tolerance and insulin sensitivity by ERα.

Several mechanisms of metabolic function of ERs involved in the regulation of estrogen-mediated insulin sensitivity have been suggested by animal studies.

First, estrogen's action helps to sustain insulin production. In the absence of ERα, 17β-estradiol only partially protects pancreatic β-cells from apoptosis in diabetic male and female mice (157), suggesting that this effect is at least in part ERα dependent. A recent study from the same group of investigators has demonstrated that estradiol stimulates islet insulin synthesis in an ERα independent manner, through interactions between non-classic extranuclear / membrane ERα and the tyrosine kinase Src, which activates ERK1/2 MAPK (184).

Second, estrogen's action facilitates insulin release. Glucose- and arginine-stimulated insulin release in pancreatic islets is similar in mice lacking either ERα or ERβ when compared with control animals (181).17β-estradiol does not increase insulin levels in isolated islets from ERαknockout animals compared to controls or to ERβ-knockout mice (156).

Third, estrogen's action regulates insulin sensitivity in liver and muscle. The development of ERα and ERβ knockout mice (185) has demonstrated the participation of these receptors in the regulation of many processes related to glucose metabolism, including insulin sensitivity in the liver and muscle. Impaired insulin sensitivity and glucose tolerance as determined by the hyperinsulinemic clamp technique in ERα deficient animals is attributed to either inadequate suppression of hepatic glucose production by insulin or impaired insulin action in skeletal muscle (181, 182).Furthermore, insulin-stimulated glucose uptake in skeletal muscle, mediated by the glucose transporter isoform GLUT4, is suppressed in the absence of ERα (181), however GLUT4 expression is not affected in mice lacking ERβ (186).

Fourth, estrogen's action mediates inflammation associated with insulin resistance. In both healthy and diabetic mice lacking ERβ, 17β-estradiol reduces inflammatory nitric oxide synthase expression in the aorta. This inhibitory effect is absent in ERα knockout animals

(187), indicating that the protective effects of estrogens on inflammatory responses in the vessel wall are mediated by ERα (187). In addition, adiponectin, an adipokine associated with suppression of insulin resistance and inflammation, is decreased in the absence of ERα whereas plasminogen activator inhibitor-1, a surrogate marker of systemic inflammation is increased (182). Increased inflammation-associated changes following streptozotocin-induced injury of pancreatic islets have been described in ERα-deficient mice (Le May et al. 2006). Moreover, enhanced inflammatory signaling and impaired fatty acid oxidation are found in the skeletal muscle of ERα-knockout mice (182), further indicating an ERα dependent regulation in inflammation which affects insulin resistance. In vitro studies have demonstrated 17β -estradiol-activated ERα decreases the number of pro-inflammatory cytokines (161). The anti-inflammatory properties of 17β-estradiol can be partially explained by the ability of ERs to act as transcriptional repressors by inhibiting the activity of nuclear factor kappa B (NFκB) through protein–protein interactions between agonist-bound ERs and activated NFκB subunits (188-190). Estrogens' inhibitory effect on NFκB function is not fully understood and may be target selective (189, 191). The PI3K pathway is also implicated in the anti-inflammatory effects of estrogens. For example, 17β-estradiol blocks LPS-induced NFκB nuclear translocation in macrophages, an effect that involves the activation of PI3K (188). Similarly, estradiol-17β decreases vascular leukocyte accumulation after an ischemia–reperfusion injury, and these effects are blocked by PI3K inhibitors (192)

In summary, previous studies not only support that estrogens and their cellular targets are important for the maintenance of glucose homeostasis, but also indicate an important role of ERα in the regulation of insulin sensitivity.

5. Conclusion

Sex differences and the role of gonadal hormones in modulating insulin sensitivity and glucose tolerance are of increasing interest and importance because of the increasing prevalence of type 2 diabetes mellitus and the metabolic abnormalities. Body composition is closely associated with insulin sensitivity, and increased body fat, particularly in the visceral compartment, is a risk factor for developing type 2 diabetes mellitus. Sex differences in body composition and/or insulin sensitivity are evident in humans and many non-human animal models.

Gonadal hormones estrogens and androgens are important, sex-independent regulators of body weight, body fat distribution, glucose metabolism and insulin resistance. When women enter menopause, they have a dramatically increased risk for developing obesity, type 2 diabetes and the metabolic syndrome. Although conventional hormone replacement therapy might beneficially to affect adiposity and to reduce diabetes risk, its previous use in women is associated with adverse effects including an increased risk for breast cancer and heart disease (i.e. thromboembolism). This increased risk may partly due to non-selective activation of ERs, which are ubiquitously expressed in the human body, especially in peripheral tissues, and due to complex intracellular events coupled to ERs genomic and non-genomic actions.

Future basic science investigations should therefore lead to a better understanding of the molecular mechanisms whereby different ERs regulate body weight, body fat, and insulin sensitivity in both females and males. Important gaps in the research need to be identified. In particular, potential interactions and cross-talk between ERα and G-protein-coupled estrogen receptor, which seem to mediate most beneficial effects, critical brain sites where ERs regulate glucose homeostasis, and intracellular signaling pathways that are required for estrogens' actions, need to be identified. Consequently only the ERs involved in energy homeostasis and glucose metabolism will be targeted. This identification would help to define novel pharmacological targets selectively associated with fat metabolism and glucose homeostasis and help to develop estrogen-like drugs that only initiate intracellular events that produce metabolically beneficial actions without deleterious side effects. Such an approach would also imply a therapeutic potential in men bypassing the unwanted effects of estrogens.

Author details

Haifei Shi and Shiva Priya Dharshan Senthil Kumar
Cellular, Molecular and Structural Biology, Miami University, Oxford, Ohio, USA

6. References

[1] James WPT 2008 The epidemiology of obesity: the size of the problem. J Intern Med 263:336-352
[2] Cummings DE, Schwartz MW 2003 Genetics and Pathophysiology of Human Obesity. Annual Review of Medicine 54:453-471
[3] Alberti K, Zimmet P, Shaw J 2005 IDF epidemiology task force consensus group: the metabolic syndrome - a worldwide definition. Lancet 366:1059 - 1062
[4] Ford ES 2005 Prevalence of the metabolic syndrome defined by the International Diabetes Federation among adults in the U.S. Diabetes Care 28:2745-2749
[5] Salpeter SR, Walsh JM, Ormiston TM, Greyber E, Buckley NS, Salpeter EE 2006 Meta-analysis: effect of hormone-replacement therapy on components of the metabolic syndrome in postmenopausal women. Diabetes Obes Metab 8:538-554
[6] Rochira V, Madeo B, Zirilli L, Caffagni G, Maffei L, Carani C 2007 Oestradiol replacement treatment and glucose homeostasis in two men with congenital aromatase deficiency: evidence for a role of oestradiol and sex steroids imbalance on insulin sensitivity in men. Diabetic Medicine 24:1491-1495
[7] Bottini N, Meloni GF, Borgiani P, Giorgini A, Buzzetti R, Pozzilli P, Lucarelli P, Gloria-Bottini F 2002 Genotypes of cytosolic low-molecular-weight protein-tyrosine-phosphatase correlate with age at onset of type 1 diabetes in a sex-specific manner. Metabolism 51:419-422
[8] Thamer C, Haap M, Volk A, Maerker E, Becker R, Bachmann O, Machicao F, Häring HU, Stumvoll M 2002 Evidence for Greater Oxidative Substrate Flexibility in Male Carriers of the Pro 12 Ala Polymorphism in PPARγ2. Horm Metab Res 34:132,136

[9] Delibegovic M, Armstrong CG, Dobbie L, Watt PW, Smith AJH, Cohen PTW 2003 Disruption of the striated muscle glycogen targeting subunit PPP1R3A of protein phosphatase 1 leads to increased weight gain, fat deposition, and development of insulin resistance. Diabetes 52:596-604
[10] Doney A, Fischer B, Cecil J, Cohen P, Boyle D, Leese G, Morris A, Palmer C 2003 Male preponderance in early diagnosed type 2 diabetes is associated with the ARE insertion/deletion polymorphism in the PPP1R3A locus. BMC Genet 4:11
[11] Wang H, Chu WS, Lu T, Hasstedt SJ, Kern PA, Elbein SC 2004 Uncoupling protein-2 polymorphisms in type 2 diabetes, obesity, and insulin secretion. Am J Physiol Endocrinol Metab 286:E1-E7
[12] D'Adamo M, Perego L, Cardellini M, Marini MA, Frontoni S, Andreozzi F, Sciacqua A, Lauro D, Sbraccia P, Federici M, Paganelli M, Pontiroli AE, Lauro R, Perticone F, Folli F, Sesti G 2004 The −866A/A Genotype in the Promoter of the Human Uncoupling Protein 2 Gene Is Associated With Insulin Resistance and Increased Risk of Type 2 Diabetes. Diabetes 53:1905-1910
[13] Björntorp P 1991 Metabolic implications of body fat distribution. Diabetes Care 14:1132-1143
[14] Xu H, Barnes GT, Yang Q, Tan G, Yang D, Chou CJ, Sole J, Nichols A, Ross JS, Tartaglia LA, Chen H 2003 Chronic inflammation in fat plays a crucial role in the development of obesity-related insulin resistance. J Clin Invest 112:1821-1830
[15] Shi H, Seeley RJ, Clegg DJ 2009 Sexual differences in the control of energy homeostasis. Front Neuroendocrinol 30:396-404
[16] Pokrywka GS 2007 Diagnosis and Treatment of Metabolic Syndrome in Menopausal Women. Menopause Management 16:16-25
[17] Ryan AS, Nicklas BJ, Berman DM 2002 Hormone replacement therapy, insulin sensitivity, and abdominal obesity in postmenopausal women. Diabetes Care 25:127-133
[18] Samaras K, Hayward CS, Sullivan D, Kelly RP, Campbell LV 1999 Effects of postmenopausal hormone replacement therapy on central abdominal fat, glycemic control, lipid metabolism, and vascular factors in type 2 diabetes: a prospective study. Diabetes Care 22:1401-1407
[19] Clegg DJ, Brown LM, Woods SC, Benoit SC 2006 Gonadal hormones determine sensitivity to central leptin and insulin. Diabetes 55:978-987
[20] Livingstone C, Collison M 2002 Sex steroids and insulin resistance. Clin Sci (Lond) 102:151-166
[21] Bruns CM, Kemnitz JW 2004 Sex hormones, insulin sensitivity, and diabetes mellitus. ILAR J 45:160-169
[22] Oh J-Y, Barrett-Connor E, Wedick NM, Wingard DL 2002 Endogenous Sex Hormones and the Development of Type 2 Diabetes in Older Men and Women: the Rancho Bernardo Study. Diabetes Care 25:55-60
[23] Björntorp P 1992 Abdominal obesity and the metabolic syndrome. Ann Med 24:465-468
[24] Rebuffé-Scrive M, Andersson B, Olbe L, Björntorp P 1989 Metabolism of adipose tissue in intraabdominal depots of nonobese men and women. Metabolism 38:453-458
[25] Kahn BB, Flier JS 2000 Obesity and insulin resistance. The Journal of Clinical Investigation 106:473-481

[26] Hellmer J, Marcus C, Sonnenfeld T, Arner P 1992 Mechanisms for differences in lipolysis between human subcutaneous and omental fat cells. J Clin Endocrinol Metab 75:15-20

[27] Arner P, Hellström L, Wahrenberg H, Brönnegård M 1990 Beta-adrenoceptor expression in human fat cells from different regions. J Clin Invest 86:1595-1600

[28] Vikman HL, Savola JM, Raasmaja A, Ohisalo JJ 1996 Alpha 2A-adrenergic regulation of cyclic AMP accumulation and lipolysis in human omental and subcutaneous adipocytes. Int J Obes Relat Metab Disord 20:185-189

[29] Rebuffé-Scrive M, Brönnegard M, Nilsson A, Eldh J, Gustafsson J-A, Björntorp P 1990 Steroid hormone receptors in human adipose tissues. J Clin Endocrinol Metab 71:1215-1219

[30] Lundholm K, Rebuffe-Scrive M, Bjc-Rntorp P 1985 Glucocorticoid hormone binding to human adipose tissue. Eur J Clin Invest 15:267-271

[31] Fried SK, Russell CD, Grauso NL, Brolin RE 1993 Lipoprotein lipase regulation by insulin and glucocorticoid in subcutaneous and omental adipose tissues of obese women and men. J Clin Invest 92:2191-2198

[32] Karlsson C, Lindell K, Ottosson M, Sjöström L, Carlsson B, Carlsson LMS 1998 Human adipose tissue expresses angiotensinogen and enzymes required for its conversion to angiotensin II. J Clin Endocrinol Metab 83:3925-3929

[33] Dusserre E, Moulin P, Vidal H 2000 Differences in mRNA expression of the proteins secreted by the adipocytes in human subcutaneous and visceral adipose tissues. Biochim Biophys Acta 1500:88-96

[34] Weisberg SP, McCann D, Desai M, Rosenbaum M, Leibel RL, Ferrante AW 2003 Obesity is associated with macrophage accumulation in adipose tissue. The Journal of Clinical Investigation 112:1796-1808

[35] Wajchenberg BL 2000 Subcutaneous and visceral adipose tissue: Their relation to the metabolic syndrome. Endocr Rev 21:697-738

[36] Lee CG, Carr MC, Murdoch SJ, Mitchell E, Woods NF, Wener MH, Chandler WL, Boyko EJ, Brunzell JD 2009 Adipokines, Inflammation, and Visceral Adiposity across the Menopausal Transition: A Prospective Study. J Clin Endocrinol Metab 94:1104-1110

[37] Björntorp P 1997 Body fat distribution, insulin resistance, and metabolic diseases. Nutrition 13:795-803

[38] Ford ES, Li C, Zhao G, Pearson WS, Mokdad AH 2008 Prevalence of the metabolic syndrome among U.S. adolescents using the definition from the International Diabetes Federation. Diabetes Care 31:587-589

[39] O'Dea JA 2008 Gender, ethnicity, culture and social class influences on childhood obesity among Australian schoolchildren: implications for treatment, prevention and community education. Health Soc Care Community 16:282-290

[40] Villegas R, Perry IJ, Creagh D, Hinchion R, O'Halloran D 2003 Prevalence of the metabolic syndrome in middle-aged men and women. Diabetes Care 26:3198-3199

[41] Dark J, Wade GN, Zucker I 1984 Ovarian modulation of lipoprotein lipase activity in white adipose tissue of ground squirrels. Physiol Behav 32:75-78

[42] Gray JM, Greenwood MR 1983 Uterine and adipose lipoprotein lipase activity in hormone-treated and pregnant rats. Am J Physiol 245:E132-E137

[43] Ramirez I 1981 Estradiol-induced changes in lipoprotein lipase, eating, and body weight in rats. Am J Physiol 240:E533-E538

[44] Llado I, Rodriguez-Cuenca S, Pujol E, Monjo M, Estrany ME, Roca P, Palou A 2002 Gender effects on adrenergic receptor expression and lipolysis in white adipose tissue of rats. Obesity 10:296-305

[45] Rebuffé-Scrive M, Enk L, Crona N, Lönnroth P, Abrahamsson L, Smith U, Björntorp P 1985 Fat cell metabolism in different regions in women. Effect of menstrual cycle, pregnancy, and lactation. J Clin Invest 75:1973-1976

[46] Canoy D, Boekholdt SM, Wareham N, Luben R, Welch A, Bingham S, Buchan I, Day N, Khaw K-T 2007 Body fat distribution and risk of coronary heart disease in men and women in the European Prospective Investigation Into Cancer and Nutrition in Norfolk cohort: : a population-based prospective study. Circulation 116:2933-2943

[47] Yusuf S, Hawken S, Ôunpuu S, Bautista L, Franzosi MG, Commerford P, Lang CC, Rumboldt Z, Onen CL, Lisheng L, Tanomsup S, Wangai Jr P, Razak F, Sharma AM, Anand SS 2005 Obesity and the risk of myocardial infarction in 27 000 participants from 52 countries: a case-control study. The Lancet 366:1640-1649

[48] Snijder MB, Dekker JM, Visser M, Bouter LM, Stehouwer CD, Kostense PJ, Yudkin JS, Heine RJ, Nijpels G, Seidell JC 2003 Associations of hip and thigh circumferences independent of waist circumference with the incidence of type 2 diabetes: the Hoorn Study. Am J Clin Nutr 77:1192-1197

[49] Snijder MB, Zimmet PZ, Visser M, Dekker JM, Seidell JC, Shaw JE 2004 Independent association of hip circumference with metabolic profile in different ethnic groups. Obesity 12:1370-1374

[50] Foster M, Shi H, Softic S, Kohli R, Seeley R, Woods S 2011 Transplantation of non-visceral fat to the visceral cavity improves glucose tolerance in mice: investigation of hepatic lipids and insulin sensitivity. Diabetologia 54:2890-2899

[51] Foster MT, Shi H, Seeley RJ, Woods SC 2010 Transplantation or removal of intra-abdominal adipose tissue prevents age-induced glucose insensitivity. Physiol Behav 101:282-288

[52] Hocking S, Chisholm D, James D 2008 Studies of regional adipose transplantation reveal a unique and beneficial interaction between subcutaneous adipose tissue and the intra-abdominal compartment. Diabetologia 51:900-902

[53] Tran TT, Yamamoto Y, Gesta S, Kahn CR 2008 Beneficial effects of subcutaneous fat transplantation on metabolism. Cell Metabolism 7:410-420

[54] Heitmann BL, Frederiksen P, Lissner L 2004 Hip circumference and cardiovascular morbidity and mortality in men and women. Obesity 12:482-487

[55] Shi H, Clegg DJ 2009 Sex differences in the regulation of body weight. Physiol Behav 97:199-204

[56] Asarian L, Geary N 1999 Cyclic estradiol treatment phasically potentiates endogenous cholecystokinin's satiating action in ovariectomized rats. Peptides 20:445-450

[57] Jones MEE, Thorburn AW, Britt KL, Hewitt KN, Wreford NG, Proietto J, Oz OK, Leury BJ, Robertson KM, Yao S, Simpson ER 2000 Aromatase-deficient (ArKO) mice have a phenotype of increased adiposity. Proc Natl Acad Sci U S A 97:12735-12740

[58] Gambineri A, Pelusi C, Vicennati V, Pagotto U, Pasquali R 2002 Obesity and the polycystic ovary syndrome. Int J Obes Relat Metab Disord 26:883-896

[59] Misso ML, Murata Y, Boon WC, Jones MEE, Britt KL, Simpson ER 2003 Cellular and molecular characterization of the adipose phenotype of the aromatase-deficient mouse. Endocrinology 144:1474-1480

[60] Maffei L, Rochira V, Zirilli L, Antunez P, Aranda C, Fabre B, Simone ML, Pignatti E, Simpson ER, Houssami S, Clyne CD, Carani C 2007 A novel compound heterozygous mutation of the aromatase gene in an adult man: reinforced evidence on the relationship between congenital oestrogen deficiency, adiposity and the metabolic syndrome. Clin Endocrinol (Oxf) 67:218-224

[61] Takeda K, Toda K, Saibara T, Nakagawa M, Saika K, Onishi T, Sugiura T, Shizuta Y 2003 Progressive development of insulin resistance phenotype in male mice with complete aromatase (CYP19) deficiency. J Endocrinol 176:237-246

[62] Razandi M, Pedram A, Greene GL, Levin ER 1999 Cell membrane and nuclear estrogen receptors (ERs) originate from a single transcript: studies of ERα and ERβ expressed in Chinese hamster ovary cells. Mol Endocrinol 13:307-319

[63] Pappas T, Gametchu B, Watson C 1995 Membrane estrogen receptors identified by multiple antibody labeling and impeded-ligand binding. FASEB J 9:404-410

[64] Okura T, Koda M, Ando F, Niino N, Ohta S, Shimokata H 2003 Association of polymorphisms in the estrogen receptor [alpha] gene with body fat distribution. Int J Obes Relat Metab Disord 27:1020-1027

[65] Nilsson M, Dahlman I, Ryden M, Nordstrom EA, Gustafsson JA, Arner P, Dahlman-Wright K 2007 Oestrogen receptor alpha gene expression levels are reduced in obese compared to normal weight females. Int J Obes 31:900-907

[66] Deng H-W, Li J, Li J-L, Dowd R, Davies KM, Johnson M, Gong G, Deng H, Recker RR 2000 Association of estrogen receptor-alpha genotypes with body mass index in normal healthy postmenopausal Caucasian women. J Clin Endocrinol Metab 85:2748-2751

[67] Fox CS, Yang Q, Cupples LA, Guo C-Y, Atwood LD, Murabito JM, Levy D, Mendelsohn ME, Housman DE, Shearman AM 2005 Sex-specific association between estrogen receptor-alpha gene variation and measures of adiposity: the Framingham Heart Study. J Clini Endocrinol Metab 90:6257-6262

[68] Goulart AC, Zee RYL, Rexrode KM 2009 Association of estrogen receptor 2 gene polymorphisms with obesity in women (obesity and estrogen receptor 2 gene). Maturitas 62:179-183

[69] Saltiki K, Mantzou E, Doukas C, Kanakakis I, Zotos P, Lazaros L, Georgiou I, Alevizaki M 2009 Estrogen receptor beta gene variants may be associated with more favorable metabolic profile in postmenopausal women undergoing coronary angiography. Exp Clin Endocrinol Diabetes 117:610-615

[70] Heine PA, Taylor JA, Iwamoto GA, Lubahn DB, Cooke PS 2000 Increased adipose tissue in male and female estrogen receptor-α knockout mice. Proc Natl Acad Sci U S A 97:12729-12734

[71] Ohlsson C, Hellberg N, Parini P, Vidal O, Bohlooly M, Rudling M, Lindberg MK, Warner M, Angelin B, Gustafsson J-Å 2000 Obesity and disturbed lipoprotein profile in estrogen receptor-α-deficient male mice. Biochem Biophys Res Commun 278:640-645

[72] Liang YQ, Akishita M, Kim S, Ako J, Hashimoto M, Iijima K, Ohike Y, Watanabe T, Sudoh N, Toba K, Yoshizumi M, Ouchi Y 2002 Estrogen receptor beta is involved in the anorectic action of estrogen. Int J Obes Relat Metab Disord 26:1103-1109

[73] Naaz A, Zakroczymski M, Heine P, Taylor J, Saunders P, Lubahn D, Cooke PS 2002 Effect of ovariectomy on adipose tissue of mice in the absence of estrogen receptor alpha (ERα): a potential role for estrogen receptor beta (ERβ). Horm Metab Res 34:758,763

[74] Geary N, Asarian L, Korach KS, Pfaff DW, Ogawa S 2001 Deficits in E2-dependent control of feeding, weight gain, and cholecystokinin satiation in ER-α null mice. Endocrinology 142:4751-4757

[75] Matthews J, Gustafsson J-Å 2003 Estrogen signaling: a subtle balance between ER alpha and ER beta. Mol Interv 3:281-292

[76] Krotkiewski M, Björntorp P, Sjöström L, Smith U 1983 Impact of obesity on metabolism in men and women. Importance of regional adipose tissue distribution. J Clin Invest 72:1150-1162

[77] Bouchard C, Despres, JEAN-PIERRE, Mauriege P 1993 Genetic and nongenetic determinants of regional fat distribution. Endocr Rev 14:72-93

[78] Gruber CJ, Tschugguel W, Schneeberger C, Huber JC 2002 Production and actions of estrogens. N Engl J Med 346:340-352

[79] Haffner SM, Katz MS, Dunn JF 1991 Increased upper body and overall adiposity is associated with decreased sex hormone binding globulin in postmenopausal women. Int J Obes 15:471-478

[80] Kaye SA, Folsom AR, Soler JT, Prineas RJ, Potter JD 1991 Associations of body mass and fat distribution with sex hormone concentrations in postmenopausal women. Int J Epidemiol 20:151-156

[81] Baglietto L, English D, Hopper J, MacInnis R, Morris H, Tilley W, Krishnan K, Giles G 2009 Circulating steroid hormone concentrations in postmenopausal women in relation to body size and composition. Breast Cancer Res Treat 115:171-179

[82] Enzi G, Gasparo M, Biondetti P, Fiore D, Semisa M, Zurlo F 1986 Subcutaneous and visceral fat distribution according to sex, age, and overweight, evaluated by computed tomography. Am J Clin Nutr 44:739-746

[83] Asarian L, Geary N 2006 Modulation of appetite by gonadal steroid hormones. Philos T Roy Soc B 361:1251-1263

[84] Barzilai N, Wang J, Massilon D, Vuguin P, Hawkins M, Rossetti L 1997 Leptin selectively decreases visceral adiposity and enhances insulin action. J Clin Invest 100:3105-3110

[85] Clegg DJ, Riedy CA, Smith KAB, Benoit SC, Woods SC 2003 Differential sensitivity to central leptin and insulin in male and female rats. Diabetes 52:682-687

[86] Simpson ER, Jones ME 2007 Of mice and men: the many guises of estrogens. In: Korach KS, Wintermantel T eds. Tissue-specific estrogen action: Springer Berlin Heidelberg; 45-68

[87] Wahrenberg H, Lönnqvist F, Arner P 1989 Mechanisms underlying regional differences in lipolysis in human adipose tissue. The Journal of Clinical Investigation 84:458-467

[88] D'Eon TM, Souza SC, Aronovitz M, Obin MS, Fried SK, Greenberg AS 2005 Estrogen regulation of adiposity and fuel partitioning. Evidence of genomic and non-genomic regulation of lipogenic and oxidative pathways. J Biol Chem 280:35983-35991

[89] Rebuffé-Scrive M, Eldh J, Hafström L-O, Björntorp P 1986 Metabolism of mammary, abdominal, and femoral adipocytes in women before and after menopause. Metabolism 35:792-797

[90] Lindberg U-B, Crona N, Silfverstolpe G, Björntorp P, Rebuffé-Scrive M 1990 Regional adipose tissue metabolism in postmenopausal women after treatment with exogenous sex steroids. Horm Metab Res 22:345,351

[91] Johnson JA, Fried SK, Pi-Sunyer FX, Albu JB 2001 Impaired insulin action in subcutaneous adipocytes from women with visceral obesity. Am J Physiol Endocrinol Metab 280:E40-E49

[92] Zitzmann M 2009 Testosterone deficiency, insulin resistance and the metabolic syndrome. Nat Rev Endocrinol 5:673-681

[93] Blouin K, Després J-P, Couillard C, Tremblay A, Prud'homme D, Bouchard C, Tchernof A 2005 Contribution of age and declining androgen levels to features of the metabolic syndrome in men. Metabolism 54:1034-1040

[94] Marin P, Holmang S, Gustafsson C, Jonsson L, Kvist H, Elander A, Eldh J, Sjostrom L, Holm G, Bjorntorp P 1993 Androgen treatment of abdominally obese men. Obes Res 1:245-251

[95] Lovejoy JC, Bray GA, Greeson CS, Klemperer M, Morris J, Partington C, Tulley R 1995 Oral anabolic steroid treatment, but not parenteral androgen treatment, decreases abdominal fat in obese, older men. Int J Obes Relat Metab Disord 19:614-624

[96] McInnes KJ, Corbould A, Simpson ER, Jones ME 2006 Regulation of adenosine 5',monophosphate-activated protein kinase and lipogenesis by androgens contributes to visceral obesity in an estrogen-deficient state. Endocrinology 147:5907-5913

[97] Pasquali R, Casimirri F, Cantobelli S, Morselli Labate AM, Venturoli S, Paradisi R, Zannarini L 1993 Insulin and androgen relationships with abdominal body fat distribution in women with and without hyperandrogenism. Horm Res 39:179-187

[98] Lovejoy JC, Bray GA, Bourgeois MO, Macchiavelli R, Rood JC, Greeson C, Partington C 1996 Exogenous androgens influence body composition and regional body fat distribution in obese postmenopausal women--a clinical research center study. J Clin Endocrinol Metab 81:2198-2203

[99] Elbers JMH, Asscheman H, Seidell JC, Megens JAJ, Gooren LJG 1997 Long-term testosterone administration increases visceral fat in female to male transsexuals. J Clin Endocrinol Metab 82:2044-2047

[100] Crandall DL, Busler DE, Novak TJ, Weber RV, Kral JG 1998 Identification of estrogen receptor β RNA in human breast and abdominal subcutaneous adipose tissue. Biochem Biophys Res Commun 248:523-526

[101] Björntorp P 1997 Hormonal control of regional fat distribution. Hum Reprod 12:21-25

[102] Macotela Y, Boucher J, Tran TT, Kahn CR 2009 Sex and depot differences in adipocyte insulin sensitivity and glucose metabolism. Diabetes 58:803-812

[103] Lu S-f, McKenna SE, Cologer-Clifford A, Nau EA, Simon NG 1998 Androgen receptor in mouse brain: sex differences and similarities in autoregulation. Endocrinology 139:1594-1601

[104] Yu I-C, Lin H-Y, Liu N-C, Wang R-S, Sparks JD, Yeh S, Chang C 2008 Hyperleptinemia without obesity in male mice lacking androgen receptor in adipose tissue. Endocrinology 149:2361-2368

[105] Dieudonné MN, Leneveu MC, Giudicelli Y, Pecquery R 2004 Evidence for functional estrogen receptors α and β in human adipose cells: regional specificities and regulation by estrogens. Am J Physiol Cell Physiol 286:C655-C661

[106] Mayes JS, Watson GH 2004 Direct effects of sex steroid hormones on adipose tissues and obesity. Obes Rev 5:197-216

[107] Österlund M, G.J.M. Kuiper G, Gustafsson J-Å, Hurd YL 1998 Differential distribution and regulation of estrogen receptor-α and -β mRNA within the female rat brain. Mol Brain Res 54:175-180

[108] Merchenthaler I, Lane MV, Numan S, Dellovade TL 2004 Distribution of estrogen receptor α and β in the mouse central nervous system: In vivo autoradiographic and immunocytochemical analyses. J Comp Neurol 473:270-291

[109] Simerly RB, Swanson LW, Chang C, Muramatsu M 1990 Distribution of androgen and estrogen receptor mRNA-containing cells in the rat brain: An in situ hybridization study. J Comp Neurol 294:76-95

[110] Musatov S, Chen W, Pfaff DW, Mobbs CV, Yang X-J, Clegg DJ, Kaplitt MG, Ogawa S 2007 Silencing of estrogen receptor α in the ventromedial nucleus of hypothalamus leads to metabolic syndrome. Proc Natl Acad Sci U S A 104:2501-2506

[111] Glümer C, Jørgensen T, Borch-Johnsen K 2003 Prevalences of diabetes and impaired glucose regulation in a Danish population: the Inter99 study. Diabetes Care 26:2335-2340

[112] Group tDS 2003 Age- and sex-specific prevalences of diabetes and impaired glucose regulation in 13 European cohorts. Diabetes Care 26:61-69

[113] Færch K, Borch-Johnsen K, Vaag A, Jørgensen T, Witte D 2010 Sex differences in glucose levels: a consequence of physiology or methodological convenience? The Inter99 study. Diabetologia 53:858-865

[114] Dunstan DW, Zimmet PZ, Welborn TA, de Courten MP, Cameron AJ, Sicree RA, Dwyer T, Colagiuri S, Jolley D, Knuiman M, Atkins R, Shaw JE 2002 The rising prevalence of diabetes and impaired glucose tolerance: the Australian Diabetes, Obesity and Lifestyle Study. Diabetes Care 25:829-834

[115] Sicree RA, Zimmet PZ, Dunstan DW, Cameron AJ, Welborn TA, Shaw JE 2008 Differences in height explain gender differences in the response to the oral glucose tolerance test— the AusDiab study. Diabet Med 25:296-302

[116] Anderwald C, Gastaldelli A, Tura A, Krebs M, Promintzer-Schifferl M, Kautzky-Willer A, Stadler M, DeFronzo RA, Pacini G, Bischof MG 2011 Mechanism and effects of glucose absorption during an oral glucose tolerance test among females and males. J Clini Endocrinol Metab 96:515-524

[117] Group EHBCC 2003 Body Mass Index, Serum Sex Hormones, and Breast Cancer Risk in Postmenopausal Women. J Natl Cancer Inst 95:1218-1226

[118] Williams JW, Zimmet PZ, Shaw JE, De Courten MP, Cameron AJ, Chitson P, Tuomilehto J, Alberti KGMM 2003 Gender differences in the prevalence of impaired fasting glycaemia and impaired glucose tolerance in Mauritius. Does sex matter? Diabet Med 20:915-920

[119] Nettle D 2002 Women's height, reproductive success and the evolution of sexual dimorphism in modern humans. Proc Biol Sci 269:1919-1923

[120] Vaag AA, Holst JJ, Vølund A, Beck-Nielsen H 1996 Gut incretin hormones in identical twins discordant for non-insulin-dependent diabetes mellitus (NIDDM)—evidence for decreased glucagon-like peptide 1 secretion during oral glucose ingestion in NIDDM twins. Eur J Endocrinol 135:425-432

[121] Rathmann W, Strassburger K, Giani G, Döring A, Meisinger C 2008 Differences in height explain gender differences in the response to the oral glucose tolerance test. Diabet Med 25:1374-1375

[122] Anastasiou E, Alevizaki M, Grigorakis SJ, Philippou G, Kyprianou M, Souvatzoglou A 1998 Decreased stature in gestational diabetes mellitus. Diabetologia 41:997-1001

[123] Magliano DJ, Barr ELM, Zimmet PZ, Cameron AJ, Dunstan DW, Colagiuri S, Jolley D, Owen N, Phillips P, Tapp RJ, Welborn TA, Shaw JE 2008 Glucose indices, health behaviors, and incidence of diabetes in Australia: the Australian Diabetes, Obesity and Lifestyle Study. Diabetes Care 31:267-272

[124] Soeters MR, Sauerwein HP, Groener JE, Aerts JM, Ackermans MT, Glatz JFC, Fliers E, Serlie MJ 2007 Gender-related differences in the metabolic response to fasting. J Clin Endocrinol Metab 92:3646-3652

[125] Li Z, McNamara JR, Fruchart JC, Luc G, Bard JM, Ordovas JM, Wilson PW, Schaefer EJ 1996 Effects of gender and menopausal status on plasma lipoprotein subspecies and particle sizes. J Lipid Res 37:1886-1896

[126] Bogardus C, Lillioja S, Howard BV, Reaven G, Mott D 1984 Relationships between insulin secretion, insulin action, and fasting plasma glucose concentration in nondiabetic and noninsulin-dependent diabetic subjects. J Clin Invest 74:1238-1246

[127] Anderwald C, Brunmair B, Stadlbauer K, Krebs M, Fürnsinn C, Roden M 2007 Effects of free fatty acids on carbohydrate metabolism and insulin signalling in perfused rat liver. Eur J Clin Invest 37:774-782

[128] Færch K, Vaag A, Witte DR, Jørgensen T, Pedersen O, Borch-Johnsen K 2009 Predictors of future fasting and 2-h post-OGTT plasma glucose levels in middle-aged men and women—the Inter99 study. Diabet Med 26:377-383

[129] Wagenknecht LE, Langefeld CD, Scherzinger AL, Norris JM, Haffner SM, Saad MF, Bergman RN 2003 Insulin sensitivity, insulin secretion, and abdominal fat: the Insulin Resistance Atherosclerosis Study (IRAS) Family Study. Diabetes 52:2490-2496

[130] Datz FL, Christian PE, Moore J 1987 Gender-related differences in gastric emptying. J Nucl Med 28:1204-1207

[131] Anderwald C, Tura A, Winhofer Y, Krebs M, Winzer C, Bischof MG, Luger A, Pacini G, Kautzky-Willer A 2011 Glucose absorption in gestational diabetes mellitus during an oral glucose tolerance test. Diabetes Care 34:1475-1480

[132] Flanagan DE, Holt RIG, Owens PC, Cockington RJ, Moore VM, Robinson JS, Godsland IF, Phillips DIW 2006 Gender differences in the insulin-like growth factor axis response to a glucose load. Acta Physiol (Oxf) 187:371-378

[133] Basu R, Dalla Man C, Campioni M, Basu A, Klee G, Toffolo G, Cobelli C, Rizza RA 2006 Effects of age and sex on postprandial glucose metabolism: differences in glucose turnover, insulin secretion, insulin action, and hepatic insulin extraction. Diabetes 55:2001-2014

[134] Sugden M, Holness M 2002 Gender-specific programming of insulin secretion and action. J Endocrinol 175:757-767

[135] Shulman GI 2000 Cellular mechanisms of insulin resistance. J Clin Invest 106:171-176
[136] Saltiel AR, Kahn CR 2001 Insulin signalling and the regulation of glucose and lipid metabolism. Nature 414:799-806
[137] Mittendorfer B 2005 Insulin resistance: sex matters. Current Opinion in Clinical Nutrition & Metabolic Care 8:367-372
[138] Kuhl J, Hilding A, Östenson CG, Grill V, Efendic S, Båvenholm P 2005 Characterisation of subjects with early abnormalities of glucose tolerance in the Stockholm Diabetes Prevention Programme: the impact of sex and type 2 diabetes heredity. Diabetologia 48:35-40
[139] Frias JP, Macaraeg GB, Ofrecio J, Yu JG, Olefsky JM, Kruszynska YT 2001 Decreased susceptibility to fatty acid-induced peripheral tissue insulin resistance in women. Diabetes 50:1344-1350
[140] Hevener A, Reichart D, Janez A, Olefsky J 2002 Female rats do not exhibit free fatty acid-induced insulin resistance. Diabetes 51:1907-1912
[141] Shi H, Sorrell JE, Clegg DJ, Woods SC, Seeley RJ 2010 The roles of leptin receptors on POMC neurons in the regulation of sex-specific energy homeostasis. Physiol Behav 100:165-172
[142] Shi H, Strader AD, Sorrell JE, Chambers JB, Woods SC, Seeley RJ 2008 Sexually different actions of leptin in proopiomelanocortin neurons to regulate glucose homeostasis. Am J Physiol Endocrinol Metab 294:E630-639
[143] Shi H, Strader AD, Woods SC, Seeley RJ 2007 The effect of fat removal on glucose tolerance is depot specific in male and female mice. Am J Physiol Endocrinol Metab 293:E1012-1020
[144] Trevaskis JL, Meyer EA, Galgani JE, Butler AA 2008 Counterintuitive effects of double-heterozygous null melanocortin-4 receptor and leptin genes on diet-induced obesity and insulin resistance in C57BL/6J mice. Endocrinology 149:174-184
[145] Li AC, Brown KK, Silvestre MJ, Willson TM, Palinski W, Glass CK 2000 Peroxisome proliferator–activated receptor γ ligands inhibit development of atherosclerosis in LDL receptor–deficient mice. J Clin Invest 106:523-531
[146] Turgeon JL, Carr MC, Maki PM, Mendelsohn ME, Wise PM 2006 Complex actions of sex steroids in adipose tissue, the cardiovascular system, and train: Insights from basic science and clinical studies. Endocr Rev 27:575-605
[147] Guerre-Millo M, Leturque A, Girard J, Lavau M 1985 Increased insulin sensitivity and responsiveness of glucose metabolism in adipocytes from female versus male rats. J Clin Invest 76:109-116
[148] Pujol E, Rodríguez-Cuenca S, Frontera M, Justo R, Lladó I, Kraemer FB, Gianotti M, Roca P 2003 Gender- and site-related effects on lipolytic capacity of rat white adipose tissue. Cellular and Molecular Life Sciences 60:1982-1989
[149] Mittendorfer B, Horowitz JF, Klein S 2001 Gender differences in lipid and glucose kinetics during short-term fasting. Am J Physiol Endocrinol Metab 281:E1333-1339
[150] Morishima A, Grumbach MM, Simpson ER, Fisher C, Qin K 1995 Aromatase deficiency in male and female siblings caused by a novel mutation and the physiological role of estrogens. J Clin Endocrinol Metab 80:3689-3698
[151] Crespo CJ, Smit E, Snelling A, Sempos CT, Andersen RE 2002 Hormone replacement therapy and its relationship to lipid and glucose metabolism in diabetic and nondiabetic

postmenopausal women: results from the Third National Health and Nutrition Examination Survey (NHANES III). Diabetes Care 25:1675-1680

[152] Saglam K, Polat Z, Yilmaz M, Gulec M, Akinci S 2002 Effects of postmenopausal hormone replacement therapy on insulin resistance. Endocrine 18:211-214

[153] Bonds DE, Larson JC, Schwartz AV, Strotmeyer ES, Robbins J, Rodriguez BL, Johnson KC, Margolis KL 2006 Risk of fracture in women with type 2 diabetes: the Women's Health Initiative Observational Study. J Clin Endocrinol Metab 91:3404-3410

[154] Margolis KL, Bonds DE, Rodabough RJ, Tinker L, Phillips LS, Allen C, Bassford T, Burke G, Torrens J, Howard BV, for the Women's Health Initiative I 2004 Effect of oestrogen plus progestin on the incidence of diabetes in postmenopausal women: results from the Women's Health Initiative Hormone Trial. Diabetologia 47:1175-1187

[155] Maffei L, Murata Y, Rochira V, Tubert G, Aranda C, Vazquez M, Clyne CD, Davis S, Simpson ER, Carani C 2004 Dysmetabolic syndrome in a man with a novel mutation of the aromatase gene: effects of testosterone, alendronate, and estradiol treatment. J Clin Endocrinol Metab 89:61-70

[156] Alonso-Magdalena P, Ropero AB, Carrera MP, Cederroth CR, Baquié M, Gauthier BR, Nef S, Stefani E, Nadal A 2008 Pancreatic insulin content regulation by the estrogen receptor ER alpha. PLoS One 3:e2069

[157] Le May C, Chu K, Hu M, Ortega CS, Simpson ER, Korach KS, Tsai M-J, Mauvais-Jarvis F 2006 Estrogens protect pancreatic β-cells from apoptosis and prevent insulin-deficient diabetes mellitus in mice. Proc Natl Acad Sci U S A 103:9232-9237

[158] Evans MJ, Eckert A, Lai K, Adelman SJ, Harnish DC 2001 Reciprocal antagonism between estrogen receptor and NF-kappaB activity in vivo. Circ Res 89:823-830

[159] Evans MJ, Lai K, Shaw LJ, Harnish DC, Chadwick CC 2002 Estrogen receptor alpha inhibits IL-1beta induction of gene expression in the mouse liver. Endocrinology 143:2559-2570

[160] Wellen KE, Hotamisligil GS 2005 Inflammation, stress, and diabetes. J Clin Invest 115:1111-1119

[161] Vegeto E, Belcredito S, Etteri S, Ghisletti S, Brusadelli A, Meda C, Krust A, Dupont S, Ciana P, Chambon P, Maggi A 2003 Estrogen receptor-α mediates the brain antiinflammatory activity of estradiol. Proc Natl Acad Sci U S A 100:9614-9619

[162] Pozzi S, Benedusi V, Maggi A, Vegeto E 2006 Estrogen action in neuroprotection and brain inflammation. Ann N Y Acad Sci 1089:302-323

[163] Payette C, Blackburn P, Lamarche B, Tremblay A, Bergeron J, Lemieux I, Després J-P, Couillard C 2009 Sex differences in postprandial plasma tumor necrosis factor–α, interleukin-6, and C-reactive protein concentrations. Metabolism 58:1593-1601

[164] Gallou-Kabani C, Vigé A, Gross M-S, Boileau C, Rabes J-P, Fruchart-Najib J, Jais J-P, Junien C 2007 Resistance to high-fat diet in the female progeny of obese mice fed a control diet during the periconceptual, gestation, and lactation periods. Am J Physiol Endocrinol Metab 292:E1095-E1100

[165] Dhar MS, Sommardahl CS, Kirkland T, Nelson S, Donnell R, Johnson DK, Castellani LW 2004 Mice heterozygous for Atp10c, a putative amphipath, represent a novel model of obesity and type 2 diabetes. J Nutr 134:799-805

[166] Brussaard HE, Leuven JAG, Frölich M, Kluft C, Krans HMJ 1997 Short-term oestrogen replacement therapy improves insulin resistance, lipids and fibrinolysis in postmenopausal women with NIDDM. Diabetologia 40:843-849
[167] Nadal A, Ropero AB, Laribi O, Maillet M, Fuentes E, Soria B 2000 Nongenomic actions of estrogens and xenoestrogens by binding at a plasma membrane receptor unrelated to estrogen receptor α and estrogen receptor β. Proc Natl Acad Sci U S A 97:11603-11608
[168] Beato M, Klug J 2000 Steroid hormone receptors: an update. Hum Reprod Update 6:225-236
[169] Monje P, Boland R 2001 Subcellular distribution of native estrogen receptor α and β isoforms in rabbit uterus and ovary. J Cell Biochem 82:467-479
[170] Yang S-H, Liu R, Perez EJ, Wen Y, Stevens SM, Valencia T, Brun-Zinkernagel A-M, Prokai L, Will Y, Dykens J, Koulen P, Simpkins JW 2004 Mitochondrial localization of estrogen receptor β. Proc Natl Acad Sci U S A 101:4130-4135
[171] Pedram A, Razandi M, Wallace DC, Levin ER 2006 Functional estrogen receptors in the mitochondria of breast cancer cells. Mol Biol Cell 17:2125-2137
[172] Ropero AB, Eghbali M, Minosyan TY, Tang G, Toro L, Stefani E 2006 Heart estrogen receptor alpha: distinct membrane and nuclear distribution patterns and regulation by estrogen. J Mol Cell Cardiol 41:496-510
[173] Sandoval DA, Bagnol D, Woods SC, D'Alessio DA, Seeley RJ 2008 Arcuate glucagon-like peptide 1 receptors regulate glucose homeostasis but not food intake. Diabetes 57:2046-2054
[174] Harris HA, Katzenellenbogen JA, Katzenellenbogen BS 2002 Characterization of the biological roles of the estrogen receptors, ERalpha and ERbeta, in estrogen target tissues in vivo through the use of an ERalpha-selective ligand. Endocrinology 143:4172-4177
[175] Kelly MJ, Levin ER 2001 Rapid actions of plasma membrane estrogen receptors. Trends Endocrinol Metab 12:152-156
[176] Revankar CM, Cimino DF, Sklar LA, Arterburn JB, Prossnitz ER 2005 A transmembrane intracellular estrogen receptor mediates rapid cell signaling. Science 307:1625-1630
[177] Filardo E, Quinn J, Pang Y, Graeber C, Shaw S, Dong J, Thomas P 2007 Activation of the novel estrogen receptor G protein-coupled receptor 30 (GPR30) at the plasma membrane. Endocrinology 148:3236-3245
[178] Ropero AB, Soria B, Nadal A 2002 A Nonclassical Estrogen Membrane Receptor Triggers Rapid Differential Actions in the Endocrine Pancreas. Molecular Endocrinology 16:497-505
[179] Valverde MA, Rojas P, Amigo J, Cosmelli D, Orio P, Bahamonde MI, Mann GE, Vergara C, Latorre R 1999 Acute activation of Maxi-K channels (hSlo) by estradiol binding to the beta subunit. Science 285:1929-1931
[180] Smith EP, Boyd J, Frank GR, Takahashi H, Cohen RM, Specker B, Williams TC, Lubahn DB, Korach KS 1994 Estrogen resistance caused by a mutation in the estrogen-receptor gene in a man. N Engl J Med 331:1056-1061
[181] Bryzgalova G, Gao H, Ahren B, Zierath JR, Galuska D, Steiler TL, Dahlman-Wright K, Nilsson S, Gustafsson JÅ, Efendic S, Khan A 2006 Evidence that oestrogen receptor-α plays an important role in the regulation of glucose homeostasis in mice: insulin sensitivity in the liver. Diabetologia 49:588-597

[182] Ribas V, Nguyen MTA, Henstridge DC, Nguyen A-K, Beaven SW, Watt MJ, Hevener AL 2010 Impaired oxidative metabolism and inflammation are associated with insulin resistance in ERα-deficient mice. Am J Physiol Endocrinol Metab 298:E304-E319

[183] Foryst-Ludwig A, Clemenz M, Hohmann S, Hartge M, Sprang C, Frost N, Krikov M, Bhanot S, Barros R, Morani A, Gustafsson J-Å, Unger T, Kintscher U 2008 Metabolic actions of estrogen receptor beta (ERβ) are mediated by a negative cross-talk with PPARγ. PLoS Genet 4:e1000108

[184] Wong WPS, Tiano JP, Liu S, Hewitt SC, Le May C, Dalle S, Katzenellenbogen JA, Katzenellenbogen BS, Korach KS, Mauvais-Jarvis F 2010 Extranuclear estrogen receptor-α stimulates NeuroD1 binding to the insulin promoter and favors insulin synthesis. Proc Natl Acad Sci U S A 107:13057-13062

[185] Dupont S, Krust A, Gansmuller A, Dierich A, Chambon P, Mark M 2000 Effect of single and compound knockouts of estrogen receptors alpha (ERalpha) and beta (ERbeta) on mouse reproductive phenotypes. Development 127:4277-4291

[186] Barros RPA, Machado UF, Warner M, Gustafsson J-Å 2006 Muscle GLUT4 regulation by estrogen receptors ERβ and ERα. Proc Natl Acad Sci U S A 103:1605-1608

[187] Cignarella A, Bolego C, Pelosi V, Meda C, Krust A, Pinna C, Gaion RM, Vegeto E, Maggi A 2009 Distinct roles of estrogen receptor-alpha and beta in the modulation of vascular inducible nitric-oxide synthase in diabetes. J Pharmacol Exp Ther 328:174-182

[188] Ghisletti S, Meda C, Maggi A, Vegeto E 2005 17beta-estradiol inhibits inflammatory gene expression by controlling NF-kappaB intracellular localization. Mol Cell Biol 25:2957-2968

[189] Kalaitzidis D, Gilmore TD 2005 Transcription factor cross-talk: the estrogen receptor and NF-κB. Trends Endocrinol Metab 16:46-52

[190] Stein B, Yang MX 1995 Repression of the interleukin-6 promoter by estrogen receptor is mediated by NF-kappa B and C/EBP beta. Mol Cell Biol 15:4971-4979

[191] Chadwick CC, Chippari S, Matelan E, Borges-Marcucci L, Eckert AM, Keith JC, Albert LM, Leathurby Y, Harris HA, Bhat RA, Ashwell M, Trybulski E, Winneker RC, Adelman SJ, Steffan RJ, Harnish DC 2005 Identification of pathway-selective estrogen receptor ligands that inhibit NF-κB transcriptional activity. Proc Natl Acad Sci U S A 102:2543-2548

[192] Simoncini T, Hafezi-Moghadam A, Brazil DP, Ley K, Chin WW, Liao JK 2000 Interaction of oestrogen receptor with the regulatory subunit of phosphatidylinositol-3-OH kinase. Nature 407:538-541

Age is an Important Risk Factor for Type 2 Diabetes Mellitus and Cardiovascular Diseases

Ketut Suastika, Pande Dwipayana,
Made Siswadi Semadi and R.A. Tuty Kuswardhani

Additional information is available at the end of the chapter

http://dx.doi.org/10.5772/52397

1. Introduction

A field study by World Health Organization (WHO), World Bank and Harvard University in 1990 found a changing pattern of diseases caused by unhealthy lifestyle changes that may eventually lead to metabolic syndrome, type 2 diabetes mellitus, coronary arterial diseases, depression, and traffic accidents (Kinsella and Phillips, 2005). The study also predicted that cerebrovascular diseases would become the most prevalent disease, whereas human HIV infection would sharply increase in the year 2020 (Kinsella and Phillips, 2005). The lifestyle-related and degenerative diseases are significant problems in the old aged population group.

The number of elderly population has increased worldwide, and recently it has been increasing sharply in the developing countries. The projection of the number of elderly population in Indonesia by the year 2010 is 23,992. The Indonesian Central Bureau for Statistics (*Badan Pusat Statistik*) has reported that Indonesia is the world's fourth in the number of elderly population after China, India, and USA (Komala *et al.*, 2005). US Bureau of Census predicted that from 1990 to 2020, the Indonesian elderly population would increase to 41.4%. The predicted increased number of elderly was ascribed to the success of health promotion and improvement of social and economic status (Kinsella and Taeuber, 1993).

Metabolic disorders including type 2 diabetes mellitus (T2DM) and cardiovascular diseases are closely related with the aging process. Central obesity and insulin resistance as the initial preconditions and its consequences related to metabolic diseases and cardiovascular diseases are frequently found among the elderly. Decline in lean body mass and increase in body fat, particularly visceral adiposity that often accompanies aging, may contribute to the development of insulin resistance. As for the mechanism of T2DM, it is known that aging induces a decrease of insulin sensitivity and alteration or insufficient compensation of beta cell functional mass in the face of increasing insulin resistance (Meneilly and Elliot, 1999). Related to beta cell functions, aging correlates with a decrease of beta cell proliferation capacity and enhances sensitivity to apoptosis (Maedler *et al.*, 2006). It has recently been proposed that an age-associated decline in mitochondrial function contributes to insulin resistance in the elderly (Petersen *et al.*, 2003). Other metabolic diseases are also frequently related with aging such as coronary arterial disease, malignancies, cognitive disorders, and vitamin D deficiency (Yaffe *et al.*, 200; Lu *et al.*, 2009).

2. Age and related risk factors for type 2 diabetes mellitus and cardiovascular diseases

2.1. Age, mitochondrial dysfunction and inflammation

Mitochondria, a membrane-enclosed organelle found in most eukaryotic cells, generate most of the cell's supply of adenosine triphosphate (ATP), are used as a source of chemical energy, and are involved in a range of other processes such as signaling, cellular differentiation, cell death, as well as the control of the cell cycle and cell growth. Mitochondria have been implicated in several human diseases, including mitochondrial disorders, aging process and cardiac dysfunction. Mitochondrial dysfunction is central to the theories of aging because age-related changes of mitochondria are likely to impair a host of cellular physiological functions in parallel and thus contribute to the development of all the common age-related diseases (Dai *et al.*, 2012). Rising cellular oxidative stress due to any cause induces mtDNA and mitochondria damage and culminates in a mitochondria function crisis, cell death and aging. Otherwise, aging itself causes abnormal mitochondrial morphology and cell death or apoptosis (Seo *et al.*, 2010). Judge *et al.* (2005) in their study on rats found that accumulation of oxidant-induced damage in interfibrillar mitochondria might be a major contributing factor to the age-related alterations in myocardial function. How old age can be a major risk factor for CVD via mitochondrial dysfunction has been completely reviewed by Dai *et al.* (2012).

Chronic inflammation is a characteristic feature of aging. A study by Sarkar et al. (2004) showed that human polynuleotide phosphrylase might play a significant role in producing pathological changes associated with aging by generating proinflammatory cytokines via reactive oxidative stress (reactive oxygen species(ROS) and NF-κB. The role of NF-κB in bridging the explanation of how aging is associated with inflammation and endothelial dysfunction is reviewed well by Csiszar *et al.* (2008). Another study has shown that depletion of cellular (GSH) during aging plays an important role in regulating the hepatic response to IL-1β (Rutkute *et al.*, 2007). At rest, skeletal muscles of elderly people showed a lower number of macrophages, higher gene expression of several cytokines, and activation of stress signaling proteins, compared with skeletal muscles of young people (Peake et al., 2010). Human aging is associated with the development of insulin resistance, β-cell dysfunction and glucose intolerance. The level of suppression of the TNF-α production was observed and found to be significantly correlated with insulin action. Reduced suppression of TNF-α production in the elderly may in part contribute to the decline in insulin sensitivity (Kirwan et al., 2001). Hyperglycemia in patients with prediabetes and diabetes is associated with inflammation (de Rekeneire *et al.*, 2006).

2.2. Age and lipid metabolism

Aging and age are often associated with lipid metabolism disorders. Lipid metabolism disorders that are associated with aging process constitute the early stage in the emergence of a constellation of risk factors for metabolic disorders (Sawabe *et al.*, 2009; Gobal and Metha, 2010). After the age of 20 years, low-density lipoprotein cholesterol (LDL-C) increases significantly in both men and women. LDL-C does not increase or is in a flat state between the age of 50-60 years (male) and 60-70 years (female) (Gobal and Mehta, 2010). On the other hand, high–density lipoprotein cholesterol (HDL-C) levels decrease during puberty to young adulthood (in males). Throughout their lives women have lower total cholesterol compared to men, but the levels will rise sharply after menopause and will be higher in the age >60 years as compared to men. Concentrations of triglyceride (TG) increase sharply in males, reaching a peak at the age 40-50 years and decline gradually thereafter. TG levels increase in women throughout their lives, especially in women taking estrogen replacement therapy (Gobal and Mehta, 2010).

With the increase of age the composition of body fat also increases, which especially accumulates in the abdomen triggering the incidence of central obesity. TG composition in the muscle and liver are higher in older age compared with younger age groups (Cree *et al.*, 2004). Increased body fat composition is associated with reduced fat oxidation both at rest and in activity (Nagy *et al.*, 1996). Aging (age) affects the release of fatty acids (FFA),from fat tissue (adipose), and the capacity of peripheral tissues such as muscles, to oxidize fat. These are some of the changes in lipid metabolism influenced by age and aging, which decreases lipolysis response and capacity of fat oxidation.

Lipolysis is modulated by various hormones such as catecholamines, glucagon, adrenocorticotropic hormone, growth hormone, prostaglandin, and thyroid hormone (Toth and Tchernof, 2000). Lipolysis response regulated by these hormones will decrease with aging. Decreased ability of catecholamines to stimulate lipolysis in the elderly is caused by decreased fat tissue response to adrenergic stimulation (Dillon *et al.*, 1984). This response involves reduced role of protein kinase A, G-protein complex adenylil cyclase, or the stages in the cyclic AMP signaling cascade (Toth and Tchernof, 2000). Effects of insulin on plasma FFA was different between in the elderly compared with in younger subjects. Insulin infusions showed that plasma FFA, turnover and oxidation, and total lipid oxidation were higher significantly in the elderly than in the younger group (Bonadonna *et al.*, 1994). Aging is also associated with decreased sensitivity to antilipolysis effects of insulin (Toth and Tchernof, 2000). Hence this will also increase the release of free fatty acids to the blood in the elderly.

Age is associated with decline in fat oxidation during activity, after meal and in resting condition (Robert *et al.*, 1996). In principle, the capacity of metabolically active tissues such as the muscles to oxidize fat represents a combination of the tissue mass and oxidative capacity of the tissue. Fat free mass decreases with age (Poehlman *et al.*, 1992) and in resting condition fat oxidation tends to be influenced by the size of fat free mass itself. Changes in lipid metabolism in the aging process are associated with dysfunction of endothelial cells pseudocapillarization of the liver sinusoid. This change causes decreased endocytosis, increased leukocyte adhesion, decreased hepatic perfusion and will potentially reduce the passage of chylomicron remnants into hepatocytes (Denke and Grundy, 1990). After activity or after meal, fat oxidation rate is more influenced by the oxidative capacity of muscle tissue. Decreased muscle oxidative capacity with aging is associated with reduced activity of enzymes involved in oxidative metabolic processes (such as succinate dehydrogenase; citrate synthase; cytrochrome c oxidase) and β-oxidation of fatty acids (such as H-3-CoA dehydrogenase Hydroacyl) (Coggan *et al.*, 1992; Rooyackers *et al.*, 1996).

Changes in lipid metabolism due to aging will lead to increased accumulation of body fat, resulting in increased concentrations of free fatty acids in the blood/plasma, and disposal of non-oxidative or free fatty acids. Increased concentrations of free fatty acids in blood increases glucose production, and this will inhibit insulin-stimulated glucose uptake and decrease hepatic insulin extraction (Fanelli *et al.*, 1993; Toth and Tchernof, 2000). The changes will be followed by insulin resistance and hyperinsulinemia. Disposal of non-oxidative free fatty acids into the liver will increase the formation of triglyceride-rich very low-density lipoprotein (VLDL) that plays a role in the formation of atherogenic dyslipidemia. Increased levels of TG and decrease HDL-C are features of atherogenic dyslipidemia in people with central obesity, hypertension and insulin resistance (Linblad et al, 2001). In relation to BMI, although older age correlates with lower BMI and higher fat mass, dramatically decreased insulin sensitivity and lack of physical activity are the most important risk factors for metabolic disorders in the elderly (Gobal and Metha, 2010; Linbald *et al.*, 2001). Insulin resistance itself is associated with decreased glucose carrier protein in the muscle (Sawabe *et al.*, 2009).

The incidence of heart attacks is higher in the elderly compared to middle age group with high cholesterol levels. Van der Meer *et al.* (2008) studied the association of myocardial TG content with diastolic function. They found that myocardial TG content was significantly associated with age ($r = 0.57$, $p < 0.05$) and TG was negatively related to left ventricular diastolic function ($r = 0.68$, $p < 0.05$). Multivariate analysis showed that myocardial TG content was an independent predictor ($p < 0.05$) for decreased diastolic function associated with age. Lower HDL cholesterol is an important risk factor for not only ischemic heart disease but also for cerebrovascular disease, especially in diabetic elderly individuals (Hayashi *et al.*, 2009).

2.3. Age, insulin resistance and metabolic syndrome

Metabolic syndrome is a group of metabolic abnormalities of which central obesity and insulin resistance are believed to be the primary backgrounds. The diagnostic criteria for metabolic syndrome have been proposed by several organizations and associations, all of which are based on five parameters i.e. central obesity, high blood pressure, high fasting blood glucose levels, high TG levels and low levels of HDL-C. The pathogenesis of how central obesity causes insulin resistance and metabolic syndrome has been explained in many publications. Decreased insulin sensitivity, reduced muscle mass, and increased body fat mass, especially visceral fat that accompanies aging contribute to insulin resistance in the elderly. Aging process is also associated with reduced compensatory beta cell mass function of the pancreas and to insulin resistance (Maneilly and Elliott, 1999) as well as with decreased mitochondrial function that contributes to insulin resistance (Petersen *et al.*, 2003). A study by Gupta *et al.* (2000) showed that hepatic insulin resistant was related to body fat and its distribution, and hepatic insulin action could be preserved by caloric restriction in aging caloric restriction rat.

A study conducted in the metropolitan area of St. Louis on 100 women aged ≥ 65 years found higher fasting blood sugar levels in subjects with insulin resistance (94.1 ± 8.1 *vs.* 87.9 ± 8.2 mg/dl, $p < 0.05$) (Banks *et al.*, 2007). A study by Kuusisto *et al.* (2001) showed that the insulin resistance syndrome is a risk factor for coronary heart disease (CHD) in the elderly with a hazard ratio of 1.71. Insulin resistance as risk factor for cardiovascular disease (CVD) is associated with increase of acute phase protein response and inflammatory markers. The Rotterdam study that enrolled 574 non-diabetic elderly population showed that insulin correlated strongly and significantly with C-reactive protein (CRP), α-1-antichymotrypsin, interleukin (IL)-6 and soluble intercellular adhesion molecule-1, indicating that insulin resistance is an integral part of inflammation (Hak *et al.*, 2001). A study by Suastika *et al.* (2011) on the population of Bali, Indonesia, has showed a tendency of increasing frequency of metabolic syndrome and its components with increasing age (Table 1). A study on the elderly by Zambon *et al.* (2009) found that metabolic syndrome was associated with increased mortality by various causes (HR 1:41) and mortality from CVD (HR 1.60). The association of metabolic syndrome and increased frequency of carotid plaque and thickening of the carotid artery intima media in elderly subjects (aged 65-85 years) was noted in a study by Empana *et al.* (2007). Subjects with metabolic syndrome have two-fold higher levels of oxidized LDL-C than those without Metabolic syndrome, and they are associated with increased risk of myocardial infarction with relative risk of 2.25 (Holvoet *et al.*, 2004). Metabolic syndrome in the elderly was associated with two-times increase of CRP levels (3.1 *vs.* 1.5 mg/l), compared with the elderly without metabolic syndrome (Hassinen, 2006).

Decreased physical activity/less exercise in the elderly has also contributed to the occurrence of obesity and metabolic syndrome. A study by Hahn *et al.* (2009) on subjects aged 55-74 years found that regular exercise at least ≤1 hour per week reduced the risk of metabolic syndrome. Sports activities >2 hours per week would be effective in lowering the risk of metabolic syndrome.

3. Age and type 2 diabetes mellitus

Similar to metabolic syndrome, the prevalence of impaired fasting glycemia (IFG) and T2DM increase with rising age. In the United States, the estimated percentage of people aged 20 years or older having diagnosed or undiagnosed diabetes in 2005-2008 was increasing with age. In the age group of 20-44 years, it was estimated about 3.7% people had diabetes; while in the age group 45-64 years the number increased to 13.7%; and the highest percentage of 26.9% was found in the age group of ≥ 65 years (Centers for Disease Control and Prevention, 2011). Similar feature was also observed n England, where the prevalence of diabetes was increasing with age. The peak prevalence of diabetes can be found in the age group of 65-74 years with 15.7% in men and 10.4% in women (Shelton, 2006). The study by Suastika *et al.* (2011) on Bali population showed that the prevalences of IFG and T2DM were higher in the elderly than in the younger age group, i.e. nearly two-fold and more than two fold, respectively (Figure 2). There was a tendency of increasing frequency of IFG and T2DM with increasing age (Table 2). Data from rural Taiwan showed that prevalence of DM was 16.9% and that of IFG was 25.5% among elderly Chinese in 2000. During a 5 year follow up, cumulative prevalences of DM and IFG were 23.7% and 27.9%, respectively. The 5-years cumulative incidence of newly onset diabetes was 6.8%. Hypertension, overt proteinuria, IFG and high total cholesterol were independent risk factors for new onset diabetes (Peng *et al.*, 2006).

Metabolic syndrome and its components	~19 (%)	20-29 (%)	30-39 (%)	40-49 (%)	50-59 (%)	60-69 (%)	≥70 (%)
Metabolic syndrome	5.5	4.8	15.9	17.6	29.6	26.0	17.3
Increased waist circumference	12.5	24.6	37.9	40.1	43.6	29.7	13.8
Elevated triglyceride	1.7	10.3	24.6	26.1	31.3	25.9	18.3
Reduced HDL-cholesterol	25.9	31.3	34.2	27.6	30.2	33.5	31.4
Elevated blood pressure	12.5	15.1	19.2	31.5	45.8	55.1	60.0
Elevated fasting blood glucose	6.9	9.5	12.9	17.3	27.4	34.9	29.9

Suastika et al. J Clin Gerontol Geriatrics 2011; 2: 47-52.

Table 1. Frequency of metabolic syndrome and its components, by age (years)

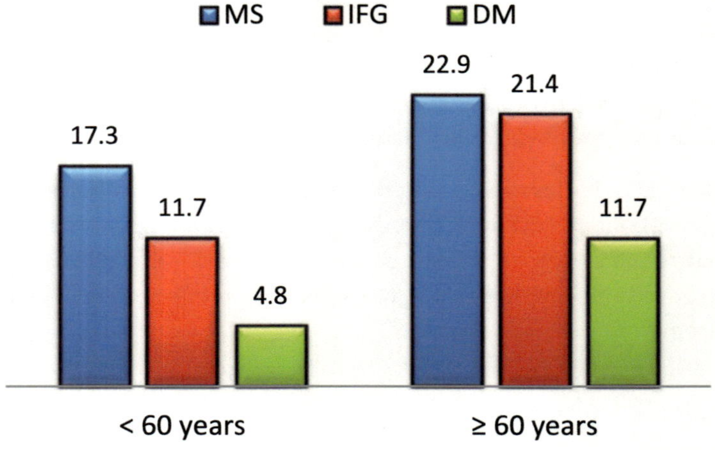

Figure 1. Frequency of metabolic syndrome (MS), impaired fasting glycemia (IFG), and diabetes mellitus (DM) in the younger-aged and elderly. Suastika et al. J Clin Gerontol Geriatrics 2011; 2: 47-52.

The prevalence of glucose intolerance (pre-diabetes and T2DM) increases with advancing age. Some factors involve in the pathophysiology of glucose intolerance in the elderly. The main factors are that aging induces decrease insulin sensitivity and alteration or insufficient compensation of beta cell functional in the face of increasing insulin resistance (Chang and Halter, 2003). Decrease in beta cell proliferation capacity and enhanced sensitivity to apoptosis are the states related with aging (Maedler *et al.*, 2006). A study by Szoke *et al.* (2008) showed that the first and second phase of insulin secretion normally decreases at the rate of approximately 0.7% per year with aging, this decrease in β cell function is accelerated about two-fold in people with impaired glucose tolerance. But aging per se has no effect on insulin sensitivity independent of change in body composition. Decline in lean body mass and the increase in body fat particularly visceral adipocytes ("central obesity") that accompanies aging may contribute to insulin resistance. It has recently been proposed that an age-associated decline in mitochondrial function contributes to insulin resistance in elderly. Mitochondrial oxidative and phosphorylation function was reduced about 40% in association with increased intramyocellular and intrahepatocellular lipid content and decreased insulin-stimulated glucose uptake (Petersen *et al.*, 2003). The pathophysiological basis of sarcopenia (loss of muscle mass with age) has a relationship with oxidative stress, reduced neuronal stimulation, subclinical inflammatory and insulin resistant state. Those conditions contribute to the development of glucose intolerance and type 2 diabetes (Khamseh *et al.*, 2011).

Minamino *et al.* (2009) in their study on mice proposed a model in which aging and inflammation was initiated in adipose tissue and subsequently induced insulin resistance in adipose tissue, liver and muscle. They also proposed that adipose tissue p53 tumor suppressor mediated the lipid abnormalities and cardiovascular morbidity associated with obesity. The study found that excessive calorie intake caused accumulation of oxidative stress in the adipose tissue of mice with type 2 diabetes–like disease and promoted senescence-like changes, such as increased activity of senescence-associated β-galactosidase, increased expression of p53 and increased production of proinflammatory cytokines. Inhibition of p53 activity in adipose tissue decreased the expression of proinflammatory cytokines and improved insulin resistance. Conversely, up-regulation of p53 in adipose tissue caused an inflammatory response that led to insulin resistance.

Classification	~19 (N=59)	20-29 (N=201)	30-39 (N=454)	40-49 (N=490)	50-59 (N=304)	60-69 (N=199)	≥70 (N=111)
Normoglycemia	93.1	90.5	87.1	82.7	72.6	65.1	70.1
Impaired fasting glycemia	6.9	7.0	10.9	11.7	16.9	23.4	17.8
Diabetes mellitus	0	2.5	2.0	5.6	10.5	11.5	12.1

Suastika et al. J Clin Gerontol Geriatrics 2011; 2: 47-52.

Table 2. Frequency of glycaemic status (), by age (years)

4. Age and cardiovascular diseases

Cardiovascular disease remains to be the most important cause of death in all countries over the world. Although certain reports from some developed countries indicate the incidence tends to decrease, from many countries there are reports mentioning that its incidence tends to increase. Cardiovascular disease is a complex disease; too many risk factors are involved in its pathogenesis. In general, risk factors for CVD can be divided into two main groups, namely traditional and non-traditional risk factors. Traditional risk factors include age (older than 40 years for men, 45 years for women), male sex, family history of coronary heart disease, smoking, hypertension, diabetes, central obesity, unhealthy cholesterol levels (high total cholesterol, low high-density lipoprotein [HDL] cholesterol, high low-density lipoprotein [LDL] cholesterol, high triglycerides), and low physical activity (Fonseca *et al.*, 2004; Torpy *et al.*, 2009). In addition, some non-traditional risk factors for CVD are reported elsewhere (Fonseca *et al.*, 2004; Vasan, 2006; Helfland *et al.*, 2009).

Several reviews have stressed that age is the strongest risk factor for CVD (Ref). Age itself may be an independent risk factor or may have other risk factors related to aging or exposure to risk factors during their lifetime. In the United States, CVD was the leading cause of death for persons 65 years of age and over in 2007, which accounted for 28% of deaths in this age group (National Center for Health Statistics, 2011). In Asian population, age is also one of the most important determinants of CVD. The studies by Suastika *et al.* in a remote area of Ceningan Island found that coronary heart disease (CHD) prevalence was relatively high (11.5%), and older age (male ≥45 years and female ≥55 years) had higher risk for CHD than younger age group (OR, 27.0). By logistic regression analysis of all variables of the risk factors, age (β=3.937) consistently appeared to be the risk factor for CHD (Suastika *et al.*, 2012a). Age in the group with CHD (old myocardial infarction and myocardial ischemia) was significantly higher than those without CHD (65.0 *vs.* 58.5 *vs.* 40.5 years) (Suastika *et al.*, 2012b).

Several changes in cardiovascular system related with aging include changes in vascular function (increase wall thickening and arterial stiffening, endothelial dysfunction) and cardiac function (heart rate and cardiac output, left ventricular wall function and myocardial contraction). The stiffness of arterial walls increase with age. This increase includes luminal enlargement with wall thickening and a reduction of elastic properties at the level of large elastic arteries. Long standing arterial pulsation in the central artery has a direct effect on the structural matrix proteins, collagen and elastin in the arterial wall, disrupting muscular attachments and causing elastin fibers to fatigue and fracture. Increased vascular calcification and endothelial dysfunction is also characteristic of arterial aging. These changes lead to increased pulse wave velocity, especially along central elastic arteries, and increase in systolic blood pressure and pulse pressure (Lee and Oh, 2010). Aging cardiovascular tissues are exemplified by pathological alterations including hypertrophy, altered left ventricular (LV) diastolic function, and diminished LV systolic reverse capacity, increased arterial stiffness, and impaired endothelial function. Study by Cheng *et al.* (2009) revealed that age was associated with a phenotype of LV remodeling marked by increased mass-to-volume ratio and accompanied by systolic as well as diastolic myocardial dysfunction that is not reflected by preserved ejection fraction. This pattern of ventricular remodeling confers significant cardiovascular risk, particularly when present earlier in life.

Peripheral artery disease (PAD), a marker of systemic atherosclerosis, is frequently related with age. It mostly starts at 40 and increases after the age 70 years. PAD is the independent risk factor for mortality caused by CVD (Norman *et al.*, 2004). A study by Kuswardhani and Suastika (2010) on elderly patients who visited the Geriatric Outpatient Clinic, Sanglah Hospital showed that diabetic patients with PAD had higher age (70.7 *vs.* 65 years, $p<0.001$) and higher homocystein levels (13.4 *vs.* 11.5 mmol/L, $p = 0.023$), compared with those without PAD. High age (70-80 years) had 7.4 times risk than those with lower age (60-69 years) and high homocystein levels (≥ 11 mmol/L) had 2.5 times risk than those with lower homocystein levels, to develop PAD. By multivariate analysis (logistic regression), it was found that only age played a role in PAD event.

How the age/aging relates to T2DM and CVD based on above review is summarised in Figure 2.

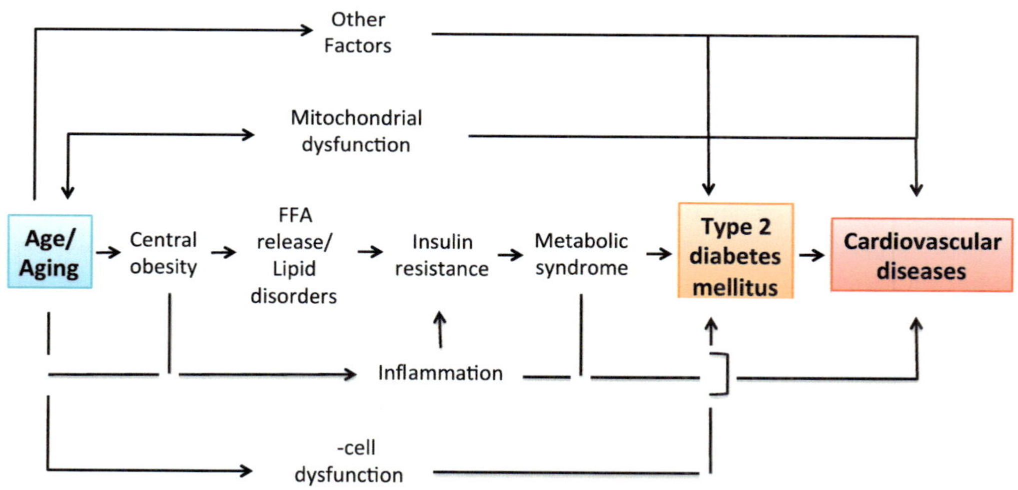

Figure 2. Summary of the relationship between age/aging and type 2 diabetes mellitus and cardiovascular diseases. .

5. Conclusion

The number of elderly population has increased worldwide, and recently it has been increasing sharply in the developing countries. Prolong survival in the elderly creates an impact on the appearance of metabolic diseases and CVD. Increase in the prevalence of metabolic diseases (such as T2DM and CVD) in old age may be related directly with age or aging process itself or indirectly through several other age-related risk factors of T2DM and CVD such as central obesity, mitochondrial dysfunction, FFA and lipid metabolisms disorders, inflammation, β-cell dysfunction, insulin resistance, metabolic syndrome, and other factors which are not discussed in this review.

Author details

Ketut Suastika, Pande Dwipayana and Made Siswadi Semadi
Division of Endocrinology and Metabolism, Internal Medicine, Faculty of Medicine, Udayana University, Sanglah Hospital, Denpasar, Indonesia

RA Tuty Kuswardhani
Division of Geriatrics; Department of Internal Medicine, Faculty of Medicine, Udayana University, Sanglah Hospital, Denpasar, Indonesia

6. References

Akbaraly TN, Kivimaki M, Ancelin ML, Barberger-Gateau P, Mura T, Tzourio C, Touchon J, Ritchie K, Berr C. Metabolic syndrome, its components, and mortality in the elderly. J Clin Endocrinol Metab 2010, 95: E327-E332.

Banks WA, Willoughby LM, Thomas DR, Morley JE. Insulin resistance syndrome in the elderly. Diabetes Care 2007, 30: 2369-2373.

Bonadonna RC, Groop LC, Simonson DC, DeFronzo RA. Free faty acid and glucose metabolism in human aging: evidence for operation of the randle cycle. Am J Physiol Endocrinol Metab 1994, 266: E501-E509.

Centers for Disease Control and Prevention. National diabetes fact sheet: national estimates and general information on diabetes and prediabetes in the United States, 2011. Atlanta: U.S. Department of Health and Human Services, Centers for Disease Control and Prevention.

Chang AM and Halter JB. Aging and insulin secretion. Am J Physiol Endocrinol metab 2003, 248: E7-E12.

Cheng S, Fernandes VRS, Bluemke DA, McClelland RL, Kronmal RA, Lima JAC. Age-related left ventricular remodeling and associated risk for cardiovascular outcomes. The multi-ethnic study of atherosclerosis. Circ Cardiovascular Imaging 2009, 2: 191-198.

Coggan AR, King OS, Rogers MA, Brown M, Nemeth PM. Histochemical and enzymatic comparison of the gastrocnemius muscle of young and elderly men and women. J. Gerontol 1992, 47: B71-B76.

Cree MG, Newcomer BR, Katsanos CS, Moore MS, Chinkes D, Aarsland A, Urban R, & Wolfe RR. Intramuscular and liver triglycerides are increased in the elderly. J Clin Endocrinol Metab 2004, 89: 3864-3871.

Csiszar A, Wang M, Lakatta EG, Ungvari Z. Inflammation and endothelial dysfunction during aging: role of NF- κB. J Appl Physiol 2008, 105:1333-1341.

Dai DF, Rabinovitch PS, Ungvari Z. Mitochondria and cardiovascular aging. Circ Res 2012, 110:1109-1124.

Denke MA, and Grudy SM. Hypercholesterolemia in elderly persons: resolving the treatment dilemma. Ann Intern Med 1990, 112: 780-792.

De Rekeire N, Piela R, Ding J, Colbert LH, Visser M, Shorr RI. Kristchevsky SB, Kuller LH, Stropmeyer ES, Schwartz AV, Vellas B, Harris TB. Diabetes, Hyperglycemia, and Inflammation in Older Individuals. The Health, Aging and Body Composition study. Diabetes Care 2006, 29: 1902-1908.

Dillon N, Chung S, Kelly J. & Malley K. Age and beta adrenoceptor-mediated function. Clin Pharmac Ther 1984, 24: 769-772.

Empana JP, Zureik M, Gariepy J, Courbon D, Dartigues JF, Ritchie K, Tzourio C, Alperovitch A, Ducimetiere P. The metabolic syndrome and the carotid artery structure in non-institutionalized elderly subjects. The Three-City Study. Stroke 2007, 38: 893-899.

Fanelli C, Epifano L, DeVincenzo A, Modarelli F, Pampanelli and DeFeo P, Brunetti P, Gerich JE & Bolli GB. Demonstration of a critical role for free fatty acids in mediating counter regulatory stimulation of gluconeogenesis and suppression of glucoseutilization in humans. J Clin Invest 1993, 92: 1617-1622.

Fonseca V, Desouza C, Asnani S, Jialal I. Nontraditional risk factors for cardiovascular disease in diabetes. Endocr Rev 2004, 25: 153–175.

Gobal FA, and Metha FL. Management of dyslipidemia in the elderly population. Ther Adv Cardiovasc Dis 2010, 4: 375-383.

Gupta G, Cases JA, She LI, Hui MA, Man Yang X, Hu M, Wu J, Rossetti L, Barzilai N. Ability of Insulin to modulate hepatic glucose production in aging rats is impaired by fat accumulation. Am J Physiol Endocrinol Metab 2000, 278: E985-E991.

Hahn V, Halle M, Schmidt-Truckass A, Rathmann W, Meisinger C, Mielck A. Physical activity and metabolic syndrome in elderly German men and women. Diabetes Care 2009, 32: 511-513.

Hak AE, Pols HAP, Stehouwer CDA, Meijer J, Kiliaan AJ, Hofman A, Breteler MMB, Witteman JCM. Markers of inflammation and cellular adhesion molecules in relation to insulin resistance in nondiabetic elderly: The Rotterdam Study. J Clin Endocrinol Metab 2001, 86: 4398-4405.

Hassinen M, Lakka TA, Komulainen P, Gylling H, Nissinen A, Rauramaa R. C-reactive protein and metabolic syndrome in elderly women. Diabetes Care 2006, 29: 931-932.

Hayashi T, Kawashima S, Itoh H, Yamada N, Sone H, Watanabe H, Hattori Y, Ohrui T, Yokote K, Nomura H, Umegaki H, Iguchi A; Japan CDM Group. Low HDL cholesterol is associated with the risk of stroke in elderly diabetic individuals: changes in the risk for atherosclerotic diseases at various ages. Diabetes Care 2009, 32: 1221-1223.

Helfand M, Buckley DI, Freeman M, Fu R, Rogers K, Flemming C, Humphrey LL. Emerging risk factors for coronary heart disease: A summary of systematic reviews conducted for the U.S. Preventive Services Task Force. Ann Intern Med 2009, 151: 496-507.

Holvoet P, Kritchevsky SB, Tracy RP, Mertens A, Rubin SM, Butler J, Goodpaster B, Harris TB. The metabolic syndrome, circulating oxidized LDL, and risk of myocardial infarction in well-functioning elderly people in the health, aging, and body composition cohort. Diabetes 2004, 53: 1068-1073.

Judge S, jang YM, Smith A, Hagen T, Leeuwenburg C. FASEB J 2005, 19: 419-421.

Khamseh ME, Malek M, Aghili R, Emami Z. Sarcopenia and diabetes: pathogenesis and consequences. Br J Diabetes Vasc Dis 2011, 11: 230-234.

Kinsella K and Taeuber CM. An Aging World II, International population reports. Washington DC: US Bureau of the Census; 1993, Pp. 92-93.

Kinsella K and Phillips DR. Global Aging: The challenge of success. Popul Bull 2005, 60: 3-40.

Kirwan JP, Khrisnan RK, Weaver JA, Del Aguila LF, Evans WJ. Human aging is associated with altered TNF-a production during hyperglycemia and hyperinsulinemia. Am J Physiol Endocrinol Metab 2001, 281: E1137-E1143.

Komala LR, Heriawan R, Coquelin B. Proyeksi penduduk Indonesia (Indonesia population projection) 2000–2025. Jakarta, Indonesia: Badan Perencanaan dan Pengembangan Nasional (BAPPENAS), Badan Pusat Statistik (BPS), United Nations Population Fund (UNPF); 2005.

Kuswardhani RAT and Suastika K. Age and homocystein were risk factor for peripheral arterial disease in elderly with type 2 diabetes mellitus. Indonesian J Intern Med 2010, 42: 94-99.

Kuusisto J, Lempiainen P, Mykkanen L, Laakso M. Insulin resistance syndrome predicts coronary heart disease events in elderly type 2 diabetic men. Diabetes Care 2001, 24: 1629-1633.

Lee HY and Oh BH. Aging and arterial stiffness. Circ J 2010, 74: 2257–2262.

Linbald U, Langer RD, Wingard DL, Thomas RG, and Barret-Connor EL. Metabolic syndrome and ischemic heart diseases in elderly men and women. Am J Epidemiol 2001, 153: 481-489.

Lu L, Yu Z, Pan A, Hu FB, Franco OH, Li H, Li X, Yang X, Chen Y, Lin X. Plasma 25-hydroxyvitamin d concentration and metabolic syndrome among middle-aged and elderly Chinese individuals. Diabetes Care 2009, 32: 1278-1283.

Maedler K, Schumann DM, Schulthess F, Oberholzer J, Bosco D, Berney T, Donath MY. Aging correlates with decreased β-cell proliferative capacity and enhanced sensitivity to apoptosis. A potential role for FAS and pancreatic duodenal homeobox-1. Diabetes 2006, 55: 2455-2462.

Meneilly GS and Elliott T. Metabolic alterations in middle-aged and elderly obese patients with type 2 diabetes. Diabetes Care 1999, 22:112-118.

Minamino T, Orimo M, Shimizu I, Kunieda T, Yokoyama M, Ito T, Nojima A, Nabetani A, Oike Y, Matsubara H, Ishikawa F, Komuro I. A crucial role for adipose tissue p53 in the regulation of insulin resistance. Nature Med 2009, 15: 1082-1088.

Nagy TR, Goran MI, Weinsier RL, Toth J, Schutz Y, Poehlman ET. Determinant of basal fat oxidation in healthy Caucasians. J Appl Physiol 1996, 80: 1743-1748

National Center for Health Statistics. Health, United States, 2010: with special feature on death and dying. Washington DC: US Government Printing Office. Available from: http://www.cdc.gov/nchs/data/hus/hus10.pdf. 2011

Norman PE, Eikelboom JW, Hankey GJ. Peripheral arterial disease: prognostic significance and prevention of atherothrombotic complications. Med J Aust 2004, 181: 150-154.

Peake J, Gatta PD, Cameron-Smith D. Aging and its effects on inflammation in skeletal muscle at rest and following exercise-induced muscle injury. Am J Physiol Regul Comp Physiol 2010, 298: R1485-R1495.

Peng LN, Lin MH, Lai HY, Hwang SJ, Chen LK, Chiou ST. Risk factors of new onset diabetes mellitus among elderly Chinese in rural Taiwan. Age Ageing 2010, 39: 125-128.

Petersen KF, Befroy D, Dufour S, Dziura J, Ariyan C, Rothman DL, DiPietro L, Cline GW, Shulman GI. Mitochondrial dysfunction in the elderly: possible role in insulin resistance. Science 2003, 300: 1140-1142.

Poehlman ET, Berke EM, MI Joseph JR, Gardner AW, Ades PA, Katzan-Rook SR, Goran MI. Influence of aerobic capacity, body composition, and thyroid hormone on age-related decline in resting metabolic rate. Metabolism 1992, 41: 915-921.

Robert SB, Fuss P, Dallal GE, Atknson A, Evans WJ, Joseph L, Fiatarone MA, Greenberg AS, Young VR. Effect of age on energy expenditure and substrate oxidation during experimental overfeeding in healthy men. J Gerontol A Biol Sci Med Sci 1996, 51A: B148-B157.

Rooyakers OE, Adey DB, Ades PA, Nair KS. Effect of age on in vivo rates of mitochondrial protein synthesis in human skeletal muscle Proc Natl Acad Sci 1996, 93: 15364–15369.

Sarkar D, Lebedeva IV, Emdad L, Kang D, Baldwin Jr AS, Fisher PB. Human polynucleotide phosphorylase (hPNPaseold-35): A potential link between aging and inflammation. Cancer Res 2004, 64: 7473-7478.

Sawabe M, Tanaka N, Nakahara K, Hamamatsu A, Chida K, Arai T. High liporotein (a) level promotes both coronary atherosclerosis and myocardial infarction: a path analysis using a large number of autosy cases. Heart 2009, 95: 1997-2002.

Seo AY, Joseph AM, Dutta D, Hwang JCY, Aris JP, Leeuwenburg C. New insight into the role of mitochondria in aging: mitochondrial dynamics and more. J Cell Sc 2010, 123: 2533-2542.

Shelton N. Diabetes. In: Ali A, et al. Health survey for England 2006: Volume 1 Cardiovascular disease and risk factors in adults. United Kingdom: The Information Center, 2008.

Suastika K, Dwipayana P, Saraswati IMR, Kuswardhani T, Astika N, Putrawan IB, Matsumoto K, Kajiwara N, Taniguchi H. Relationship between age and metabolic disorder in the population of Bali. J Clin Ge rontol Geriatrics 2011, 30: 1-6.

Suastika K, Dwipayana P, Saraswati MR, Gotera W, Budhiarta AAG, Sutanegara ND, Gunadi GNP, Nadha KB, Wita W, Rina K, Santoso A, Soegondo S, Kajiwara N, Taniguchi H.. Underweight is an important risk factor for coronary heart disease in the population of Ceningan Island, Bali. Diabetes Vasc Dis Res 2012a, 9: 75-77.

Suastika K, Dwipayana P, Saraswati MR, Gotera W, Budhiarta AAG, Gunadi GNP, Nadha KB, Wita W, Rina K, Santoso A, Malik S, Sudoyo H, Kajiwara N, Taniguchi H. Coronary Heart Disease in a Remote Area. J Clin Exp Cardiol 2012b, S:6. http://dx.doi.org/10.4172/2155-9880.S6-002

Szoke E, Shrayyef MZ, Messing S, Woerle HJ, Van Haeften TW, Meyer C, Mitrakou A, Pimenta W, Gerich JE. Effect of aging on glucose homeostasis: Accelerated deterioration of β-cell function in individuals with impaired glucose tolerance. Diabetes Care 2008, 31: 539-543.

Torpy JM, Burke AE, Glass RM. Coronary heart disease risk factors. J Am Med Assoc 2009, 302: 2388.

Toth MJ and Tchernof A. Lipid metabolism in the elderly. Eur J Clin Nutrition 2000, 54 (Suppl. 3): S121-125.

van der Meer RW, Rijzewijk LJ, Diamant M, Hammer S, Schär M, Bax JJ, Smit JW, Romijn JA, de Roos A, Lamb HJ. The ageing male heart: myocardial triglyceride content as independent predictor of diastolic function. Eur Heart J 2008, 29: 1516-1522.

Vasan RS. Biomarkers of cardiovascular disease molecular basis and practical considerations. Circulation 2006, 113: 2335-2362.

Yaffe K, Weston AL, Blackwell T, Krueger KA. The metabolic syndrome and development of cognitive impairment among older women. Arch Neurol 2009, 66: 324-328.

Zambon S, Zanoni S, Romanato G, Corti MC, Noale M, Sartori L, Musacchio E, Baggio G, Crepaldi G, Manzato E. Metabolic syndrome and all-cause and cardiovascular mortality in an Italian elderly population. Diabetes Care 2009, 32: 153-159.

Chapter 6

Glucose Tolerance and Elders – Lessons We Have Learned and Challenges for the Future

Sylwia Dzięgielewska-Gęsiak and Ewa Wysocka

Additional information is available at the end of the chapter

http://dx.doi.org/10.5772/46247

1. Introduction

The worsening of glucose metabolism as well as increasing risk for cardiovascular disease while aging is documented (Wild S. et al., 2004; Okereke OI. et al., 2008). According to gold standard research in diabetes - the United Kingdom Prospective Diabetes Study (UKPDS) (Matthews D.R 1999; Turner R.C. et al., 1998) - about 40% of patients with type 2 diabetes mellitus (T2DM) suffer from late diabetic complications, including atherosclerosis, hypertension and dyslipidemia and microangiopathies (nephropathy, retinopathy). From epidemiological point of view, 40% of dysglycemic patients are 65 years old or over (Barnett T. 1998; Harris M. 19962).

An impaired fasting glycemia (IFG) and an impaired glucose tolerance (IGT) are categories of increased risk for type 2 diabetes mellitus (prediabetes) (ADA 2012). There is no separate algorithm for dysglycaemia in elders, however glucose concentrations in plasma increases with aging (from 30 years old, fasting glycemia about 1-2 mg/dl for the every decade and postprandial glycaemia about 2-4 mg/dl for the every decade), and is caused by insulin-resistance (Winger JM & Hornick T. 1996). Paralleled to glucose concentration glycated hemoglobin - HbA_{1c} rise with age – round 0,11 to 0,15 % of HbA_{1c} per decade (Nuttal F.Q. 1999).

Aging is a universal process that can be determined by genetic, the environment or diseases. Biological theories are the most promising in relation to finding answers about aging.

1.1. Aging theories

There are many aging theories. From the very easy one, like programmed death theories, to the more complicated as concerning mistake accumulation theories (Table 1).

THEORIES OF PROGRAMED DEATH	THEORIES OF MISTAKE ACCUMULATION
programmed cellular aging theory clock theory	autoimmune theory random mistake theory free radical theory cross-links theory calories restriction theory glycation theory

Table 1. Theories of aging (examples)

The gerontological theories try to explain aging from the biological point of view, and explain that not only still dividing cells but also cells that are unable to divide, both can be targeted by aging (Kirkwood TBL. & Austad SN. 2000).

1.1.1. Free radical theory

The free radicals theory postulates that the aging process is the initiation of free radical reactions (Harman D. 2003) and in hyperglycemic patients may rise due to increased free radicals production. The theory suggests that most of free radicals are initiated and produced by mitochondria and a life span is determined by the rate of free radical damage to the mitochondria (Harman D. 1983).

1.1.2. Glycation theory

The theory is based on non-enzymatic reaction - glycation. The theory suggests that glucose acts a mediator of aging. The cross-links between glucose and proteins lead to stable intra- and inter-molecular changes which can influence cells, tissues and organs (Soškić V. et al., 2008). Thus the glycation may have tremendous cumulative effect during a person's life leading to shorter life span in diabetics.

1.1.3. Caloric restriction

The theory proposes that life span can be prolonged by lover calorie intake but the compounds are the full qualitative (Vitetta L. & Anton B. 2007). Decreases in calorie intake reduce free radicals production – lower oxidative stress and decreased inflammatory processes (Ungvari Z. et al., 2008).

Patients with hyperglycemia may present more than one reason of increased aging process.

1.2. Late complications of hyperglycemia

As hyperglycemia starts (prediabetes, diabetes mellitus) late metabolic complications, caused by glucose toxicity (Robertson RP. & Harmon JS. 2006), oxidative stress (Cumaoğlu

A. et al., 2010), dyslipidemia (Gordon L. et al., 2010), increased polyol pathway (Obrosova I.G. 2005) and glycation of protein (Xie X. et a., 2010), increase.

1.3. Protein glycation

Protein glycation and oxidative stress in a context of aging is widely discussed (Robertson RP. 2004; Muller F.L. et al., 2007; Soškić V., et al. 2008). Protein glycation depends on duration of hyperglycemia and increase in aging and co-morbidities (Peppa M. & Vlassara H. 2005).

Non-enzymatic glycation of proteins leads trough Amadori products such as glycated albumine (fructosamine), glycated hemoglobine (HbA_{1c}) to Advanced Glycation End Products (AGEs) eg. N^{ε}-carboxymethyllysine (CML) (figure 1), bio-active molecules which accumulate with age. AGEs are produced in human as a part of normal metabolism, but are elevated in diabetic patients, and depends on hyperglycemia duration and level (higher and longer hyperglycemia leads to higher AGEs concentration).

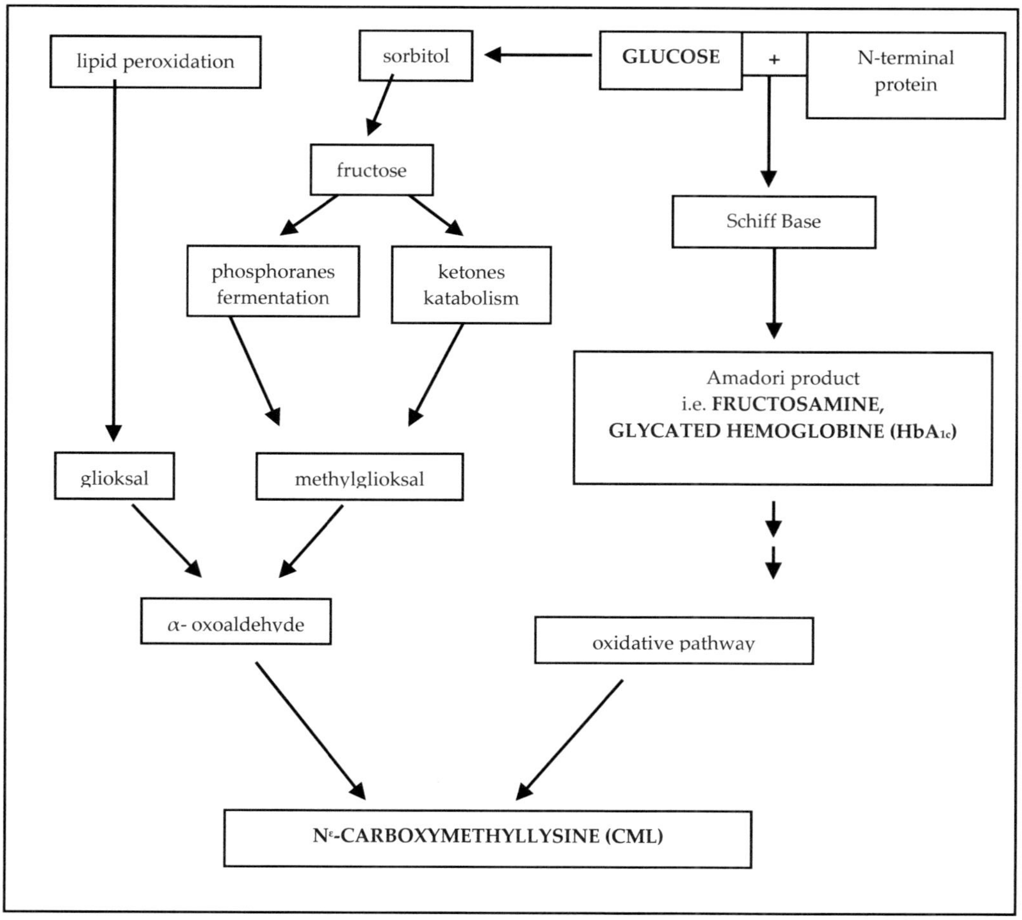

Figure 1. Pathways for the Advanced End Products Formation i.e. N^{ε}-carboxymethyllysine.

1.3.1. Fructosamine

Fructosamine is an Amadori product that is formed as a result of lysine side chain of protein modification by glucose and its serum level is reported to increase in diabetes. The product serves as short term marker (2-3 weeks) of glycemic control (Armbruster DA.1987; True MW. 2009). Fructosamine can undergo oxidative cleavage leading to the formation of Avanced Glycation End products (AGEs), which are implicated in long-term complications of diabetes mellitus.

1.3.2. Glycated hemoglobin, HbA_{1c}

Glycated hemoglobin, HbA_{1c}, is an Amadori product that is now recognized as a marker of glycemic control. Glycated hemoglobine, HbA_{1c} measures blood glucose control over a period of eight to twelve weeks (Rohlfing CL. et al., 2002). The results from different trials (The ACCORD trial (ACCORD Group 2008), the Veterans Affairs Diabetes Trial (VADT Investigators 2009), the Action in Diabetes and Vascular Disease—PreterAx and DiamicroN Modified Release Controlled Evaluation (ADVANCE) trial (ADVANCE Collaborative Group 2009)), have created a debate about the optimal choice of glycated hemoglobine target. The International Diabetes Federation recommends a level of less than 6.5% (IDF 2006) whereas the American Diabetes Association recommends an HbA_{1c} level of less than 7.0% as the standard of glycemic treatment goal (ADA 2010). the American Diabetes Association recommends a HbA_{1c} level of less than 8.0% as the glycemic treatment goal for the elderly diabetic persons. Nowadays the HbA_{1c} is also recommended for diagnosis of diabetes (ADA 2010).

1.3.3. Advanced glycation end products - N^{ε}-carboxymethyllysine, CML

N^{ε}-carboxymethyllysine, {(2S)-2-amino-6-(carboxymethylamino)hexanoic acid}, (CML), (figure 2) one of dominant Advanced Glycation End products (AGEs), is formed in vivo by oxidative cleavage of the Amadori product threulosyl-lysine (combined non-enzymatic glycation and glycoxidation) and of metal-catalyzed oxidation of LDL or peroxidation of polyunsaturated fatty acids in the presence of fructose-lysine (Fu M.X. et al., 1996) (As in figure 1). Thus CML may serve as bio-marker of oxidative stress and protein damage in aging, diabetes mellitus and atherosclerosis (Southern L. et al., 2007; Semba R. D. et al., 2009). Excessive formation of CML has been proposed to be an important mechanism for accelerated atherogenesis in patients with hyperglycemia.

There are many evidences indicating that protein glycation and oxidative stress may accompany and explain metabolic late diabetic complications. Investigation of glycated proteins (fructosamine, HbA_{1c}) and AGEs (i.e. CML), in early stages of glucose metabolism problems, may explain metabolic complications in hyperglycemic elderly persons.

The aim of the study was to analyze fructosamine in plasma, HbA_{1c} in blood and CML serum concentrations among elderly patients with increased risk for type 2 diabetes mellitus (prediabetes) and normal glucose tolerance.

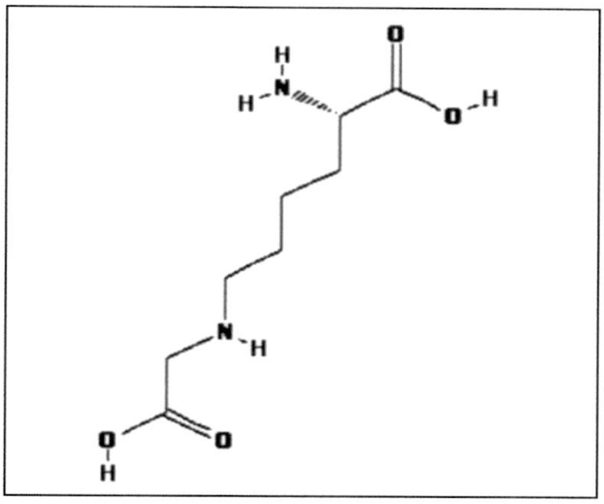

Figure 2. Chemical structure of N^{ε}-carboxymethyllysine, (2S)-2-amino-6-(carboxymethylamino)hexanoic acid, (CML) – one of the Advanced Glycation End product.

2. Material and methods

The study was performed in the Department of Clinical Biochemistry and Laboratory Medicine, Chair of Chemistry and Clinical Biochemistry of Poznan University of Medical Sciences under the permission from local ethics group in accordance with the Declaration of Helsinki of 1975 for Human Research and the study protocol was approved by the Bioethics Committee of Poznan University of Medical Sciences in Poznan, Poland.

Subjects and Settings: This study population consisted of 313 elderly Caucasians (65 and older) from Poznan metropolitan area, and after following exclusion criteria (below), 58 of them with no acute diseases or severe chronic disorder were enrolled to the study. They were performed complete physical examination including the measurement of waist circumference (WC) in centimeters, percentage of body fat (FAT) by bioimpedance using BodyStat equipment and the calculation of body mass index (BMI=kg/m^2). Arterial blood pressure: systolic (SBP) and diastolic (DBP) were measured twice by sphyngomanometer MEDEL PALM PRO No: 91431 (Novamedica Ltd, Birmingham, United Kingdom) in sitting position, after at least 5 minutes rest. The arterial blood pressure was expressed than as mean value.

The exclusion criteria were the presence of following conditions: a coronary artery disease, a history of diabetes, the neoplastic diseases, the inflammatory diseases, a previous therapy, use of anti- and oxidant drugs, alcohol use, smoking and electrocardiography findings specific for myocardial ischaemia/infarct.

Additional biochemical exclusion criteria were microalbuminuria and macroalbuminuria as albumin/creatinin ratio > 30 mg of albumin/1 g of creatinin in fresh morning urine sample and decreased estimated Glomerular Filtration Rate (eGFR) less than 60 ml/min/m^2 based on Modified Diet in Renal Diseases (MDRD) formula:

$$\text{eGFR (ml/min/1.75m}^2\text{)} =$$
$$= \{186 \times [\text{creatynin}]^{-1,154} \times [\text{age}]^{-0,203} \times 0,742\ [\text{for women}] \times 1,210\ [\text{for Afroamerican}]\}$$

Blood sampling and biochemical analysis: The studied subjects were collected ulnar venous blood twice: at 0 minute (fasting) and at 120 minute of the 75,0-g OGTT. Fasting plasma samples without hemolysis were used for glucose and lipid determinations. Fasting serum samples designated for fructosamine and N^{ε}-carboxymethyllysine measurements were frozen and stored at –25° C until assayed, separately. Blood collected at 120 minute of OGTT was used for plasma glucose determination.

Glucose and lipids assay. Oral glucose tolerance test (OGTT) was performed according to WHO recommendations (WHO 1999) between 7.00-9.00 am. Glucose concentration was determined at 0 min (fasting) and 120 min (postprandial) following a standard dose of 75 g glucose load. Glucose and lipid parameters including total cholesterol (T-C), high density lipoproteins cholesterol (HDL-C), triacyloglycerydes (TG) concentrations were evaluated by enzymatic methods using bioMerieux reagent kit (Marcy-l'Etoile, France) and the UV-160A Shimadzu spectrophotometer (Shimadzu Co., Kyoto, Japan). Low density lipoproteins cholesterol (LDL-C) was calculated using the Friedewald formula:

$$\text{LDL-C [mmol/l]}=\{[(\text{T-C})-(\text{HDL-C})]-(\text{TG}/2{,}2)\}$$

The reference sera: RANDOX Assayed Human Multi Sera Level 1 (as normal) and RANDOX Assayed Human Multi Sera Level 2 (as pathological) (Randox, Crumlin, United Kingdom) were used for monitoring the accuracy of the determinations.

Results of OGTT allowed to classify subjects for normal glucose tolerance (NGT) (n=30, mean age 69,5 years) and prediabetic (PRE) (n=20, mean age 70,0 years) categories, while newly diagnosed type 2 diabetes mellitus (T2DM) patients were excluded from the study. The interpretation of oral glucose tolerance test is presented in Table 2 (ADA 2012).

Categories of glycemia during OGTT		Plasma glucose concentration	
		Fasting (at 0 min.)	at 120 min.
Normal glucose tolerance (NGT)		< 5,6 mmol/l < 100 mg/dl	< 7,8 mmol/l < 140 mg/dl
High risk of diabetes (Prediabetes, PRE)	Impaired Fasting Glycemia (IFG)	5,6 – 6,9 mmol/l 100 – 125 mg/dl	< 7,8 mmol/l < 140 mg/dl
	Impaired Glucose Tolerance (IGT)	< 7,0 mmol/l < 126 mg/dl	7,8 – 11,0 mmol/l 140 –199 mg/dl
Diabetes mellitus (DM)		< 7,0 mmol/l < 126 mg/dl	≥ 11,1 mmol/l ≥ 200 mg/dl

Table 2. The interpretation of oral glucose tolerance test (OGTT)

Fructosamine assay. Glycated albumine (fructosamine) was determined using calorymetric metod based on the ability of ketoamines to reduce nitrotetrazolium-blue (NBT) to formazan in an alkaline solution. The rate of formation of formazan is directly proportional to the concentration of fructosamine. The measurement was done by Cobas 400 (Roche Diagnostics, Mannheim, Germany).

The sensitivity of this assay was 0,14 μmol/l with intra-assay coefficient of variation (CV) and inter-assay CV precision at 2,8% and 0,65% respectively.

HbA1c assay. Glycated hemoglobin, (HbA_{1c}) was determined using ion exchange high performance liquid chromatography (HPLC), D-10 (BioRad, Heidelberg, Germany). Using a specific standardized measurement set established through the National Glycohemoglobin Standardization Program (NGSP). The sensitivity of this assay was 0,05% with intra-assay coefficient of variation (CV) and inter-assay coefficient of variation (CV) precision at 2,35% and 2,66% respectively.

N^{ε}-carboxymethyllysine {(2S)-2-amino-6-(carboxymethylamino)hexanoic acid} assay. Fasting plasma samples were drown and the concentration of N^{ε}-carboxymethyllysine (CML) was measured with a novel competition-based ELISA assay using a CML-specific monoclonal antibody ELISA kit (MicroCoat, Bernried am Starnberger See, Germany). Absorbance was read using a microtitre ELISA plate reader (Sunrise™, Tecan Group Ltd, Männedorf, Switzerland) at 405 nm. CML concentrations were obtained from standard curve (linear/linear plot method) and expressed in ng/ml. All samples were run in triplicate. The sensitivity of this competitive ELISA assay was 5 ng/ml with intra-assay coefficient of variation (CV) and inter-assay CV precision at 5% and 6,8% respectively.

Statistical Analysis Statistica (version 6.0) for Windows was used for statistical analysis. The normality of value distribution was checked by Shapiro-Wilk test. Then, the results with a Gaussian distribution were analyzed with Student's t test, and those with a non-Gaussian distribution with a nonparametric Mann-Whitney U test to assess the differences between studied groups. The Spearman rank correlation test was used to evaluate the strength of association between two variables. A $p<0.05$ was considered statistically significant.

Sensitivity, specificity and the highest diagnostic value for the fructosamine, HbA_{1c}, CML level we obtain based on ROC curves analysis using MedCalc® v. 9.3.7.0 for Windows. ROC curves analyses were used to determine the optimal values of fructosamine, glycated hemoglobine (HbA_{1c}) and N^{ε}-carboxymethyllysine (CML) distinguishing between normal and disturbed glucose tolerance groups.

All results are shown as mean ± standard deviation (SD) and median (in brackets).

3. Results

In our study group, after ruling out those with any disease, patients were divided into: normoglycemic (n=30), prediabetes (n=20) and as newly diagnosed diabetes mellitus type 2 (n=8) (based on oral glucose tolerance test, see methods). The newly diagnosed diabetes type 2 were excluded than. All investigated patients were normoalbuminuria staged and eGFR > 60ml/min/m^2.

3.1. Comparison of normoglycemic (NGT) and prediabetic (PRE) subjects

Table 3 shows the baseline characteristics and clinical parameters of the elderly normal glucose tolerance subjects (NGT) and elderly prediabetes patients (PRE) according to Oral

Glucose Tolerance Test (OGTT). The groups by definition were different as far as glucose concentration was concerned (both fasting and postprandial) (p=0,0000002 and p=0,000009 respectively).

The investigated groups did not differ in clinical parameters such as arterial blood pressure and anthropometric factors (BMI, body fat, waist circumference) as well as plasma lipids.

	NGT (n=30) Mean ± SD (Median)	PRE (n=20) Mean ± SD (Median)	p
Age [years]	70,6 ± 8,4 (69,5)	70,2 ± 5,27 (70,0)	NS
BMI [kg/m^2]	27,9 ± 4,4 (26,6)	30,8 ± 5,5 (30,0)	NS
Waist [cm]	91,0 ± 7,1 (92,0)	95,5 ± 12,8 (93,0)	NS
FAT [%]	36,1 ± 17,6 (45,0)	38,3 ± 11,8 (41,5)	NS
SBP [mmHg]	136,4 ± 13,8 (135,0)	142,9 ± 11,0 (140,0)	NS
DBP[mmHg]	83,2 ± 8,8 (85,0)	78,2 ± 8,5 (80,0)	NS
G0' [mmol/l]	5,0 ± 0,5 (5,0)	5,8 ± 0,5 (5,8)	by def.: p=0,000002
G120' [mmol/l]	5,2 ± 1,2 (5,2)	7,2 ± 1,3 (7,2)	by def.: p=0,000009
Fructosamine [µmol/l]	253,5 ± 26,6 (255,0)	258,3 ± 27,8 (253,5)	NS
HbA_{1c} [%]	5,85 ± 0,40 (5,85)	6,22 ± 0,47 (6,30)	p<0,005
CML [ng/ml]	2248,7 ± 375,9 (2292,4)	2079,9 ± 418,9 (1987,0)	NS
TC [mmol/l]	4,98 ± 0,72 (5,01)	5,05 ± 0,89 (5,00)	NS
TG [mmol/l]	1,16 ± 0,50 (0,94)	1,54 ± 0,98 (1,24)	NS
HDL-C [mmol/l]	1,65 ± 0,36 (1,66)	1,46 ± 0,30 (1,44)	NS
LDL-C[mmol/l]	2,82 ± 0,71 (2,88)	2,90 ± 0,72 (2,82)	NS

p – the probability of obtaining a test statistic, SD – standard deviation, NS – not significant, by def. - by definition, NGT – normoglycemic group, PRE – prediabetic group, BMI – Body Mass Index, FAT – body fat, SBP – systolic blood pressure, DBP – diastolic blood pressure, G0' – fasting glucose, G120' - postprandial glucose, measured at 120 min after 75 grams glucose load, HbA_{1c} – glycated hemoglobin, CML – N^{ε}carboxymethyllysine, TC – total cholesterol, TG – triglycerides, HDL-C – high density lipoproteins cholesterol, LDL-C – low density lipoproteins cholesterol,

Table 3. Baseline characteristics and clinical parameters of the normal glucose tolerance subjects (NGT) and prediabetes patients (PRE) according to Oral Glucose Tolerance Test (OGTT).

The glycated albumin - fructosamine did not differ between investigated groups (Figure 3) whereas glycated hemoglobin HbA_{1c} were higher in the prediabetes individuals (p<0,005) (Figure 4).

The CML did not differentiate normoglycemic and prediabetes elderly persons (Figure 5).

Different correlations between glycated proteins (fructosamine and HbA_{1c}) and metabolic parameters were found in analyzed subgroups (table 4 and 5 respectively) at p<0,01. There were no correlations in any investigated groups for the CML (table 6).

ROC curve analysis yielded a fructosamine concentration of the highest diagnostic value in distinguishing PRE and NGT (<=237 µmol/l, 29.0% sensitivity and 88,2% specificity,

AUC=0,511) based on OGTT (Figure 6). ROC curve analysis yielded a HbA_{1c} percentage of the highest diagnostic value in distinguishing PRE and NGT (>6,1 %, 54,8% sensitivity and 88,2% specificity, AUC=0,679) based on OGTT (Figure 7). ROC curve analysis yielded a CML concentration of the highest diagnostic value in distinguishing PRE and NGT (<=2403,2 ng/ml, 76.7% sensitivity and 41,2% specificity, AUC=0,548) based on OGTT (Figure 8).

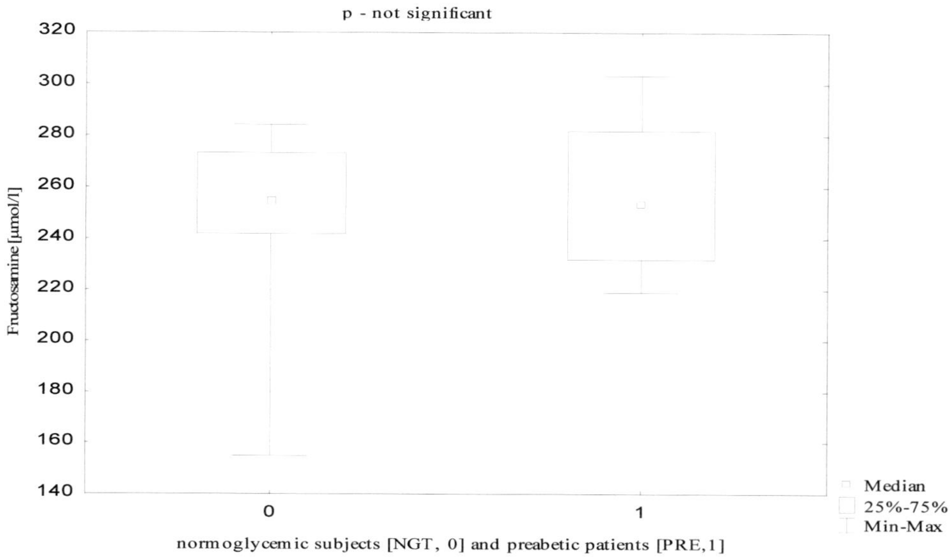

Figure 3. Comparison of fructosamine between normoglycemic subjects (NGT, 0) and prediabetic patients (PRE, 1).

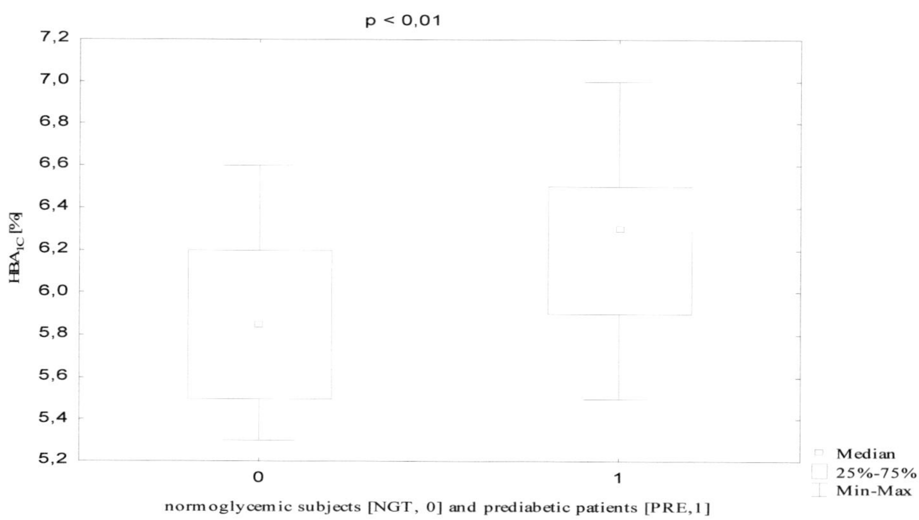

Figure 4. Comparison of glycated hemoglobin (HbA_{1c}) between normoglycemic subjects (NGT, 0) and prediabetic patients (PRE, 1).

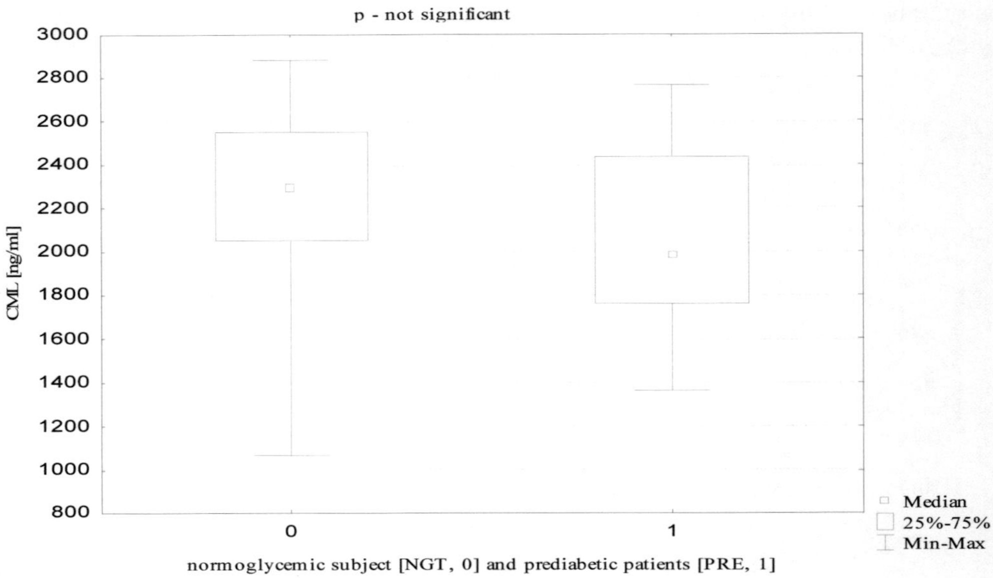

Figure 5. Comparison of CML between normoglycemic subjects (NGT, 0) and prediabetic patients (PRE, 1).

p<0,01	All persons (n=50)	NGT (n=30)	PRE (n=20)
Fructosamine & BMI	NS	NS	NS
Fructosamne & waist	NS	NS	NS
Fructosamine & FAT	R=0,39	NS	NS
Fructosamine & SBP	NS	NS	NS
Fructosamine & DBP	NS	NS	NS
Fructosamine & G0'	NS	NS	NS
Fructosamine & G120'	NS	R=0,48	NS
Fructosamine & TC	NS	NS	NS
Fructosamine & TG	NS	NS	NS
Fructosamine & HDL-C	NS	NS	NS
Fructosamine & LDL-C	NS	NS	NS

p – the probability of obtaining a test statistic, NS – not significant, NGT – normoglycemic group, PRE – prediabetic group, BMI – Body Mass Index, FAT – body fat, SBP – systolic blood pressure, DBP – diastolic blood pressure, G0' – fasting glucose, G120' (postprandial glucose) measured at 120 min after 75 grams glucose load, TC – total cholesterol, TG – triglycerides, HDL-C – high density lipoproteins cholesterol, LDL-C – low density lipoproteins cholesterol,

Table 4. Correlation for fructosamine in all investigated persons, NGT and PRE groups.

$p<0,01$	All (n=50)	NGT (n=30)	PRE (n=20)
HbA_{1c} BMI	NS	NS	R=-0,78
HbA_{1c} and waist	R=0,39	NS	NS
HbA_{1c} and FAT	NS	NS	NS
HbA_{1c} and SBP	NS	NS	NS
HbA_{1c} and DBP	NS	NS	NS
HbA_{1c} and G0'	R=0,45	NS	NS
HbA_{1c} and G120'	R=0,58	0,51	NS
HbA_{1c} and TC	NS	NS	NS
HbA_{1c} and TG	NS	NS	NS
HbA_{1c} and HDL-C	R=-0,47	NS	NS
HbA_{1c} and LDL-C	NS	NS	NS

p – the probability of obtaining a test statistic, NS – not significant, NGT – normoglycemic group, PRE – prediabetic group, BMI – Body Mass Index, FAT – body fat, SBP – systolic blood pressure, DBP – diastolic blood pressure, G0' – fasting glucose, G120' (postprandial glucose) measured at 120 min after 75 grams glucose load, HbA_{1c} – glycated hemoglobin, TC – total cholesterol, TG – triglycerides, HDL-C – high density lipoproteins cholesterol, LDL-C – low density lipoproteins cholesterol,

Table 5. Correlation for HbA_{1c} in all investigated persons, NGT and PRE groups.

$p<0,01$	All (n=50)	NGT (n=30)	PRE (n=20)
CML and BMI	NS	NS	NS
CML and waist	NS	NS	NS
CML and FAT	NS	NS	NS
CML and SBP	NS	NS	NS
CML and DBP	NS	NS	NS
CML and G0'	NS	NS	NS
CML and G120'	NS	NS	NS
CML and TC	NS	NS	NS
CML and TG	NS	NS	NS
CML and HDL-C	NS	NS	NS
CML and LDL-C	NS	NS	NS

p – the probability of obtaining a test statistic, NS – not significant, NGT – normoglycemic group, PRE – prediabetic group, BMI – Body Mass Index, FAT – body fat, SBP – systolic blood pressure, DBP – diastolic blood pressure, G0' – fasting glucose, G120' (postprandial glucose) measured at 120 min after 75 grams glucose load, CML – N^{ε}-carboxymethyllysine, TC – total cholesterol, TG – triglycerides, HDL-C – high density lipoproteins cholesterol, LDL-C – low density lipoproteins cholesterol,

Table 6. Correlation for CML in all investigated persons, NGT and PRE groups.

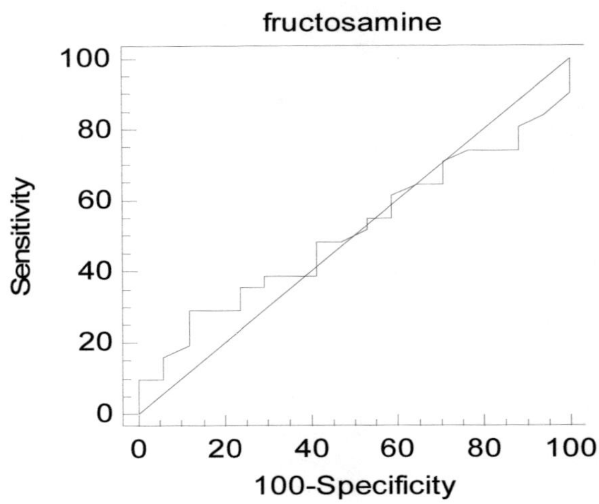

Figure 6. Receiver operating characteristic (ROC) curve for fructosamine diagnostic value (sensitivity and specificity) in distinguishing between normal glucose tolerance subjects (NGT) and prediabetic patients (PRE) classified according to OGGT results.

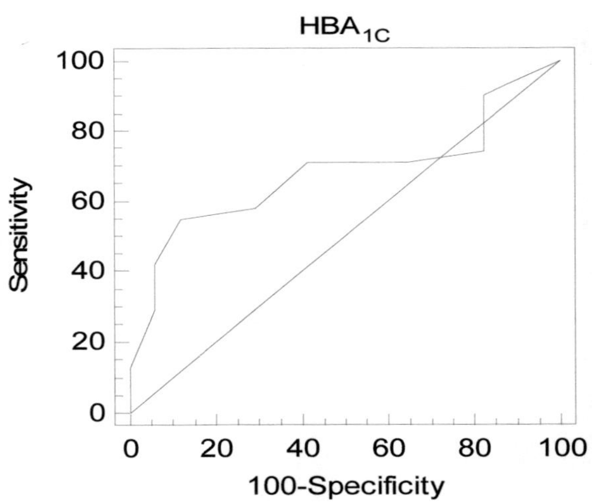

Figure 7. Receiver operating characteristic (ROC) curve for HbA_{1c} diagnostic value (sensitivity and specificity) in distinguishing between normal glucose tolerance subjects (NGT) and prediabetic patients (PRE) classified according to OGGT results.

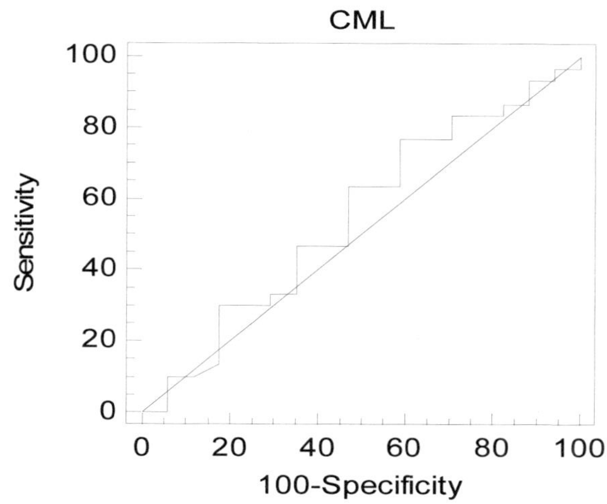

Figure 8. Receiver operating characteristic (ROC) curve for CML diagnostic value (sensitivity and specificity) in distinguishing between normal glucose tolerance subjects (NGT) and prediabetic patients (PRE) classified according to OGGT results.

3.2. Comparison of two prediabetic (PRE) subgroups: Impaired Fasting Glucose (IFG) and Impaired Glucose Tolerance (IGT) subjects

Table 7 shows the baseline characteristics and clinical parameters of the Impaired Fasting Glucose subjects (IFG) and Impaired Glucose Tolerance subjects (IGT) subgroups of prediabetic elderly patients according to Oral Glucose Tolerance Test (OGTT). The subgroups by definition were different as far as glucose concentration was concerned (both fasting and postprandial) (p=0,01 and p=0,001 respectively). Otherwise the prediabetic subgroups did not differ in clinical parameters as well as biochemical factors. However the glycated hemoglobin (HbA_{1c}) had tendency to be higher in the Impaired Glucose Tolerance individuals and the glycated albumin - fructosamine and Advanced Glycation End Product - N^{ε}-carboxymethyllysine had tendency to be higher in Impaired Fasting Glucose subjects.

4. Disscusion

One of the fundamental elements for establishing prevention, treatment and prognosis of diabetes mellitus is an assessment of the clinical stage of glucose metabolism problems.

Dysglycemia population is recognized with increased cardiovascular morbidity and mortality [Khaw KT. Et al., 2004; Sung J. et al. 2009). The cumulative effect of many metabolic risk factors (clinical and biochemical) in one individual which influenced cardiovascular risk are widely discussed (Selvin E. et al., 2005; Gerstein HC. et al., 2005). In our study we investigated elderly otherwise healthy persons. We found that in those with the increased risk for the type 2 diabetes mellitus (prediabetes) there were more (but not significant) indicators for the metabolic syndrome (obesity, abdominal obesity, systolic hypertension).

	IFG (n=8) Mean ± SD (Median)	IGT (n=12) Mean ± SD (Median)	p
Age [years]	69,8 ± 3,8 (69,0)	70,2 ± 6,56 (70,0)	NS
BMI [kg/m^2]	30,4 ± 6,8 (29,0)	31,7 ± 4,6 (30,5)	NS
Waist [cm]	96,0 ± 13,8 (91,5)	96,5 ± 12,9 (94,0)	NS
FAT [%]	35,3 ± 12,6 (38,8)	39,8 ± 12,2 (44,4)	NS
SBP [mmHg]	141,7 ± 12,1 (142,5)	142,0 ± 10,8 (140,0)	NS
DBP[mmHg]	76,7 ± 8,8 (72,5)	79,0 ± 9,1 (80,0)	NS
G0' [mmol/l]	6,3 ± 0,5 (6,4)	6,3 ± 0,5 (6,8)	by def.: p=0,01
G120' [mmol/l]	6,6 ± 1,0 (7,0)	8,8 ± 1,0 (9,1)	by def.: p=0,001
Fructosamine [μmol/l]	261,8 ± 27,5 (267,0)	257,0 ± 30,5 (253,5)	NS
HbA_{1c} [%]	6,04 ± 0,60 (5,90)	6,35 ± 0,37 (6,40)	NS
CML [ng/ml]	2123,9 ± 375,5 (2122,7)	2053,4 ± 443,1 (1987,0)	NS
TC [mmol/l]	4,85 ± 0,86 (4,74)	5,41 ± 0,89 (5,25)	NS
TG [mmol/l]	1,22 ± 0,47 (1,18)	1,73 ± 1,2 (1,14)	NS
HDL-C [mmol/l]	1,53 ± 0,42 (1,50)	1,51 ± 0,32 (1,50)	NS
LDL-C[mmol/l]	2,76 ± 0,83 (2,92)	3,09 ± 0,61 (2,87)	NS

p – the probability of obtaining a test statistic, SD – standard deviation, NS – not significant, by def. - by definition, NGT – normoglycemic group, PRE – prediabetic group, BMI – Body Mass Index, FAT – body fat, SBP – systolic blood pressure, DBP – diastolic blood pressure, G0' – fasting glucose, G120' - postprandial glucose, measured at 120 min after 75 grams glucose load, HbA_{1c} – glycated hemoglobin, CML – N^{ε}-carboxymethyllysine, TC – total cholesterol, TG – triglycerides, HDL-C – high density lipoproteins cholesterol, LDL-C – low density lipoproteins cholesterol,

Table 7. Baseline characteristics and clinical parameters of the prediabetes (PRE) subgroups the Impaired Fasting Glucose subjects (IFG) and the Impaired Glucose Tolerance subjects (IGT) according to Oral Glucose Tolerance Test (OGTT).

We had hoped while performing those analysis to find a set of laboratory measures that would provide a better indicator of a prediabetic elderly persons for glycemic control than any one measure alone.

The amount of glycated proteins (fructosamine and HbA_{1c}) depend on time-averaged glucose concentration. Thus fructosamine and HbA_{1c} reflect the extent of exposure to glucose in the 2-4 and 8-12 weeks before testing, respectively. Since 2010, American Diabetes Association has added a new recommendation for diagnosis of diabetes mellitus, concerning not only based on hyperglycemia (random, fasting or due to OGTT) but also glycated hemoglobin HbA_{1c} (ADA 2010).

The primary aim of the study was to evaluate the blood levels of glycated proteins and CML in two clinical situations, normal glucose tolerance and prediabetic state in elderly patients. Our study showed that the glycated hemoglobin corresponded better in distinguishing the NGT from PRE in the investigated elderly persons than fructosamine or advanced glycation end product – N^{ε}-carboxymeethyllysine.

Hyperglycemia and oxidative stress accelerate not only glycation of proteins such as hemoglobin but also leads to Advanced Glycated End Products (AGEs) such as N^{ε}-carboxymethyllysine (CML). During natural aging AGEs accumulate and the concentration of formers depends on time and progressive reduction in the capacity to neutralise oxidative stress and may leads to many complications such as atherosclerosis and dementia (Hipkiss AR., 2006; Semba RD. et al., 2010). In 2003 Hamelin M. and collegues established that CML are increased in the rat serum with aging (Hamelin M. et al., 2003). So is CML independent risk factor for aging or rather diseases? Our study focused on CML in elderly group at the earliest stages of hyperglycemia. Our investigated groups had no known clinical and laboratory complications, in all subgroups CML concentration is very high in comparison with others investigators. Ahmed K.A. et al. excluded the effect of age on CML concentration in type 2 diabetic patients with ischemic heart disease (Ahmed K.A. et al., 2007). They argued that increased CML concentration was an independent from other risk factors for the coronary artery disease (CAD) in type 2 diabetes mellitus and ha significant predictive power to CAD especially in type 2 diabetes mellitus (Ahmed K.A. et al., 2008). In our investigated groups CML concentration were higher in comparison with CML concentration in Ahmed work. Our investigated study patients were either with normal glucose metabolism or prediabetes stage, both elderly patients with no clinical complications such as CAD or kidney failure. CML concentration depends on proteins glycation but also is directly proportional to creatinine concentration and inversely proportional to glomerular filtration rate. Hirata K. work showed that CML is increased in type 2 diabetes mellitus patients with kidney failure in comparison with type 2 diabetes mellitus patients with normo-, micro- or even macroalbumnuria (Hirata K. & Kubo K. 2004). While Wagner Z. et collegues demonstrated normal levels of CML and AGEs (fluorescence) in patients with type 2 diabetes mellitus who had normal renal function (Wagner Z. et al., 2001). Since we excluded patients with CAD or kidney disturbances, those factors did not influences CML concentration, in plasma in our investigated groups. Thus, the determined CML concentration in plasma did not follow increased accumulation in the body. Baumann M. and colleagues found that CML might be accumulated in tissues, what could lead to different metabolic complications (Baumann M., 2009).

Interesting work showed Dworacka M. et colleagues. Their results revealed significantly higher CML in non-diabetic patients with coronary heart disease than in healthy control subjects and were comparable to serum CML in patients with type 2 diabetes mellitus without late complications and coronary heart disease (Dworacka M. et al., 2002). In our study we realized higher (but not significant) CML concentration in subgroup defined as normoglycemic. This patients had lower total cholesterol, LDL-C and triglicerydes and higher HDL-C in comparison with prediabetics. Thus it is possible that complications of diabetes mellitus are themselves related to pathobiochemical alterations other than protein glycation i.e. oxidative stress and lipids peroxidation.

There is no doubt that elevated CML are closely associated with late complication of hyperglycemia in patients with type 2 diabetes mellitus or atherosclerotic angiopathies.

Further studies should be performed in patients with the very early stages of dysglycemia to find when the pathology starts.

Different tendencies for HbA_{1c} and fructosamine and CML were observed while IFG or IGT were separated (as in table 7). Based on HbA_{1c} IGT group seems to be more advanced on the way to diabetes. However IFG individuals tended to present higher fructosamine and CML which may reflect not only glycation. There is no literature data concerning different metabolic aspect of IFG or IGT in elderly, but in middle aged population Faerch K. et al. showed different insulin action and incretin hormone concentration suggesting different management according to the prediabitic subgroup diagnosis (Faerch K. et al., 2008).

Despite some answers our study has brought, that there are some challenges for the future investigations that should be coped. What biomarker could predict the increased risk related to dysglycemia in elderly patients? Does the kind of prediabetes state matter, in a context of metabolic complications, especially in elderly patients?

5. Conclusions

There is no doubt that elevated fructosamine, HbA_{1c} and CML are closely associated with late complication of hyperglycemia in patients with type 2 diabetes mellitus or atherosclerotic angiopathy. The best marker in dysglycemic but not yet diabetic elderly patients seems to be only glycated hemoglobin. When N^{ε}-carboxymethyllysine and fructosamine as a single marker seem to be not good enough prognostic indicators of dysglycemia. In apparently healthy elderly people otherwise with no diagnosed comorbidities but with hyperglycemia, clinical assessment and laboratory investigations of hyperglycemia complications may help in prevention all global complications. In our opinion CML and/or fructosamine may result from different metabolic pathways (i.e. glycation and oxidative stress).

Author details

Sylwia Dzięgielewska-Gęsiak and Ewa Wysocka
Department of Clinical Biochemistry and Laboratory Medicine, Chair of General Chemistry and Clinical Biochemistry, Poznan University of Medical Sciences, Poznan, Poland

Acknowledgement

This work was supported by Poznan University of Medical Sciences research project No 501-01-2228369-00260 and No 501-01-2228369-008636. No conflict of interest was declared with relation to this work.

6. References

ACCORD Diabetes Study Group (2008); *Effects of intensive glucose lowering in type 2 diabetes*. N Engl J Med 2008; 358: 2545-559.

ADA (2010); *Standards of medical care in diabetes—2010.* Diabetes Care 2010; 33: S11- S61.

ADA (2012); The Expert Committee on the Diagnosis and Classification of Diabetes; Standards of Medical Care in Diabetes – 2012. Diabetes Care 2012; 35: Supplement1, S11-S63.

ADVANCE Collaborative Group (2009); *Cognitive function and risks of cardiovascular disease and hypoglycaemia in patients with type 2 diabetes: the Action in Diabetes and Vascular Disease: Preterax and Diamicron Modified Release Controlled Evaluation (ADVANCE) trial.* Diabetologia. 2009 Nov; 52 (11): 2328-2336.

Ahmed K.A., Muniandy S., Ismail I.S. (2007); *Role of N^{ε}-carboxymethyllysine in the dvelopmentof ischemic heart disease in type 2 diabetes mellitus.* J. Clin. Biochem Nutr. 41, 97-105.

Ahmed K.A., Muniandy S., Ismail I.S. (2008); *Implications of N^{ε}-carboxymethyllysine in altered metabolism of low density lipoproteins in patients with type 2 diabetes and coronary artery disease.* J. Med. Sci., 2008, 8, 152-161.

Armbruster DA. (1987); *Fructosamine: structure, analysis, and clinical usefulness.* Clin Chem. 1987 Dec; 33 (12): 2153-2163.

Barnett T. (1998) Epidemiology, complications and costs of diabetes mellitus scale. In.: The insulin treatment of diabetes: a practical guide, London, Halthcare: 6–9, 1998.

Baumann M., Richart T., Sollinger D., Pelisek J., Roos M., Kouznetsova T., Eckstein HH., Heemann U., Staessen JA (2009); *Association between carotid diameter and the advanced glycation end product N-epsilon-carboxymethyllysine (CML).* Cardiovasc. Diabetol. (2009) 6; 8: 45, doi:10.1186/1475-2840-8-45.

Cumaoğlu A., Rackova L, Stefek M., Kartal M., Maechler P, Karasu C. (2010); *Effects of olive leaf poly phenols against H2O2 toxicity in insulin secreting β-cells.* ABP 2010, 58, 1/2011, 45-50.

Dworacka M., Winiarska H., Szymańska M., Szczawińska K., Wierusz-Wysocka B. (2002); *Serum N-epsilon-(carboxymethyl)lysine is elevated in nondiabetic coronary heart disease patients.* J. Basic. Clin. Physiol. Pharmacol. 2002, 13(3):201-213.

Faerch K., Vaag A, Holst JJ, Glumer C, Pedersen O, Borch-Johnsen K. (2008); Impaired fasting glycaemia vs impaired glucose tolerance: similar impairment of pancreatic alpha and beta cell function but differential roles of incretin hormones and insulin action. Diabetologia 2008, 51, 853-861.

Fu M.X., Requena R., Jenkins A., Lyons T., Baynes J.W., Thorpe S.R. (1996); The advanced glycation end product, N^{ε}(Carboxymethyl)lysine, is a product of both lipid peroxidation and glycoxidation reactions. *J. Biol. Chem. 1996, 271: 9982–9986.*

Gerstein HC, Pogue J, Mann JF, Lonn E, Dagenais GR, McQueen M, Yusuf S. (2005); *The relationship between dysglycaemia and cardiovascular and renal risk in diabetic and non-diabetic participants in the HOPE study: a prospective epidemiological analysis.* Diabetologia. 2005; 48: 1749–1755.

Gordon L., Ragoobirsingh D., Morrison E., McGrowder D., Choo-Kang E., Martorell E., (2010); *Dyslipidaemia in hypertensive obese type 2 diabetic patients in Jamaica.* Arch. Med. Sci. 2010, 6, 5: 701-708.

Hamelin M., Borot-Laloi C., Friguet B., Bakala H. (2003); *Increased level of glycoxidation product N$^{\varepsilon}$-carboxymethyl-lysine in rat serum and urine proteins with aging: link with glycoxidative Damage accumulation in kidney.* Arch. Biochem. Biophys. (2003) 411, 215-222.

Harman D. (1983); *Free radical theory of aging: consequences of mitochondrial aging*. Age 6: 86–94.

Harman D. (2003); The free radical theory of aging. Antioxid Redox Signal., 2003, 5(5), 557-561.

Harris M. (1996); Impaired glucose tolerance – Prevalence and conversion to NIDDM, Diabet Med., 1996, 13 (Suppl 2), 9-11.

Hipkiss AR. (2006); Accumulation of altered proteins and aging: causes and effects. Exp. Gerontol. (2006), 41 (5): 464-473.

Hirata K., Kubo K. (2004); *Relationship between blod levels of N$^{\varepsilon}$-carboxymethyllysine and pentosidine and the severity of microangiopathy in type 2 diabetes.* Endocr. J.51(6):537-44.

IDF (2006); Global guideline for type 2 diabetes: recommendations for standard, comprehensive, and minimal care. *Diabet Med 2006; 23: 579-593.*

Khaw KT, Wareham N, Bingham S, Luben R, Welch A, Day N. (2004); *Association of Hemoglobin A1c with cardiovascular disease and mortality in adults: the European Prospective Investigation Into Cancer in Norfolk.* Ann Intern Med. 2004; 141: 413–420.

Kirkwood TBL., Austad SN. (2000) Why do we age? Nature, 2000, 408, 233-238.

Matthews D.R. (1999); The natural history of diabetes-related complications: the UKPDS experience. United Kingdom Prospective Diabetes Study. Diabetes Obes Metab., Suppl 2, 7-13.

Muller F.L., Lustgarten M.S., Jang Y., Richardson A, Van Remmen H. (2007); *Trends in oxidative aging theories.* Free. Radic. Biol. Med. (2007) 15, 43(4), 477-503,

Nuttal F.Q. (1999); *Effect of age on the percentage of hemoglobin A1c and the percentage of total glycohemoglobin in non-diabetic persons.* J. Lab. Clin. Med. 1999, 134, 451-453.

Obrosova I.G. (2005); *Increased sorbitol pathway activity generates oxidative stress in tissue sites for diabetic complications*. Antioxid. Redox Signal. 2005, 7: 1543–1552.

Okereke OI., Kang JH., Cook NR., Gaziano JM., Manson AE., Buring JE., Grodstein F. (2008); Type 2 diabetes mellitus and cognitive decline in two large cohorts of community-dwelling older adults. J Am Geriatr Soc 2008, Jun; 56 (6): 1028-1036.

Peppa M. Vlassara H. (2005); *Advanced glycation end products and diabetic complications: A general overview.* Hormones, 2005, 4 (1), 28-37.

Robertson RP. (2004); *Chronic oxidative stress as a central mechanism for glucose toxicity in pancreatic islet beta cells in diabetes.* J Biol Chem. 2004; 279: 42351-42354.

Robertson RP, Harmon JS. (2006); *Diabetes, glucose toxicity, and oxidative stress: A case of double jeopardy for the pancreatic islet beta cell.* Free Rad. Biol. Med. 2006. 41: 177–184.

Rohlfing CL., Wiedmeyer HM., Little RR., England JD., Tennill A., Goldstein DE. (2002); *Defining the relationship between plasma glucose and HbA1c: analysis of glucose profiles and HbA1c in Diabetes Control and Complications Trial.* Diabetes Care 2002: 25: 275-278.

Selvin E, Coresh J, Golden SH, Brancati FL, Folsom AR, Steffes MW. (2005); *Glycemic control and coronary heart disease risk in persons with and without diabetes: the Atherosclerosis Risk in Communities Study.* Arch Intern Med. 2005; 165: 1910–1916

Semba RD., Ferrucci L., Sun K., Beck J., Dalal M., Varadhan R., Walston J., Guralnik J.M., Fried L.P. (2009); *Advanced glycation end products and their circulating receptors predict cardiovascular disease mortality in older communitydwelling women* Aging Clin. Exp. Res. 2009, 21 (2): 182–190.

Semba RD, Nicklett EJ, Ferrucci L. (2010); *Does accumulation of advanced glycation end products contribute to the aging phenotype?* J. Gerontol. A Biol. Sci. Med. Sci., 2010, 65 (9): 963-975.

Šoškić V., Groebe K., Schrattenholz A. (2008); *Nonenzymatic posttranslational protein modifications in ageing.* Exp Gerontol., 2008 Apr;43 (4): 247-57

Southern L., Williams J., Esiri M.M. (2007); Immunohistochemical study of N-epsilon-carboxymethyl lysine (CML) in human brain: relation to vascular dementia, *BMC Neurology 2007, 7: 35 doi:10.1186/1471-2377-7-35.*

Sung J, Song Y-M, Ebrahim S, Lawlor D. (2009); *Fasting blood glucose and the risk of stroke And myocardial infarction.* Circulation. 2009; 119: 812–819.

True MW. (2009); *Circulating biomarkers of glycemia in diabetes management and implications for personalized medicine.* J Diabetes Sci Technol. 2009 Jul 1; 3(4): 743-747.

Turner R.C., Millns H., Neil H.A.W., Stratton I.M., Manley S.E., Matthews D.R., Holman R.R. for the United Kingdom Prospective Diabetes Study Group (1998); *Risk factors for coronary artery disease in non-insulin dependent diabetes mellitus: United Kingdom prospective diabetes study (UKPDS: 23)* BMJ (1998) 316; 823-828.

Ungvari Z., Parrado-Fernandez C., Csiszar A., de Cabo R. (2008); *Mechanisms underlying caloric restriction and lifespan regulation: implications for vascular aging.* Circ Res., 2008, 14, 102(5), 519-528.

VADT Investigators. (2009) Duckworth W., Abraira C., Moritz T., Reda D., Emanuele N., Reaven P.D., Zieve F.J., Marks J., Davis S.N., Hayward R., Warren S.R., Goldman S., McCarren M., Vitek M.E., Henderson W.G., Huang G.D. (2009); *Glucose control and vascular complications in veterans with type 2 diabetes.* N Engl J Med. 2009 Jan 8; 360 (2): 129-139.

Vitetta L., Anton B. (2007); *Lifestyle and nutrition, caloric restriction, mitochondrial health and hormones: scientific interventions for anti-aging.* Clin Interv Aging., 2007, 2(4), 537-543.

Wagner Z., Wittman I., Mazak I., Schinzel R. Heidland A., Kientsch-Engel R., Nagy J. (2001); *N^{ε}-carboxymethyllysine levels in patients with type 2 diabetes: role of renal function.* Am. J. Kidney Dis. 2001, 38: 785-791.

Wild S., Roglic G., Green A., Sicree R., King H. (2004); Global Prevalence Of Diabetes; Diab. Care, 2004, 27, 1047–1053.

Winger JM, Hornick T. (1996); Age-associated changes in the endocrine system. Nurs Clin North Am. 1996 Dec;31(4):827-44.

World Health Organization. (1999) Definition, Diagnosis and Classification of Diabetes Mellitus and its Complications.

Raport of a WHO Consultation. Part 1: Diagnosis and Classification of Diabetes Mellitus. Geneva: WHO Department of Non-communicable Disease Surveillance, 1999: 1-59, http://www.who.int

Xie X., Chowdhury S.R., Sangle G., Shen G.X. (2010) *Impact of diabetes-associated lipoproteins on oxygen consumption and mitochondrial enzymes in porcine aortic endothelial cells,* ABP 2010, 57, 4, 393-398.

Chapter 7

The Relationship Between Chronic Alcohol Use and Type 2 Diabetes Mellitus: New Insights into Mechanisms of Appetite-Regulating Peptides

Soo-Jeong Kim and Dai-Jin Kim

Additional information is available at the end of the chapter

http://dx.doi.org/10.5772/51795

1. Introduction

Appetite regulating peptides, particularly ghrelin and leptin in alcohol dependence are significantly related with abnormal glucose tolerance or insulin resistance which contribute to Type 2 diabetes mellitus (T2DM) [1-5]. Available evidence consistently indicates that altered levels of ghrelin and leptin are linked to overall diabetogentc effects of chronic alcohol comsumption, and have important mediating roles in the deteriorated pathophysiology of T2DM in alcoholic patients [6]. Moreover, these peptides in the regulation of food seeking behavior have a similar mechanism of controlling of alcohol craving behavior [7, 8]. Threrefore, alterations of the peptides modulating numerous metabolic processes could present an intriguing biological mechanism on the relationship between chronic alcohol consumption and risk of T2DM. However, the manner in which the peptides contribute to the development or maintenance of T2DM with alcohol dependence is not clear. This review describes ghrelin and leptin implicated in the elevated risk of developing T2DM with chronic use of alcohol that attributes to the impact of glucose and insulin metabolism. Additionally, to identify whether these two peptides are relevant to the increase in the clustering of metabolic disturbance and progression of T2DM, the background information on the peptides, their role in glucose homeostasis and insulin function in addition to their mechanism of action are discussed. This review on the relationship between chronic use of alcohol and T2DM may further clarify the role of the peptides and provides an insight into the effects of chronic alcohol use in the pathophysiology of T2DM.

2. Pathophysiology of T2DM

T2DM, known as "non-insulin-dependent DM," is a complex, multifactorial metabolic disorder. Characteristic features of T2DM include chronic hyperglycemia and declining pancreatic β-cell effectiveness, leading to the absence of a first-phase insulin response to nutrient ingestion. Further, slower glucose absorption and higher fasting glucose levels occur from factors such as a reduced insulin-mediated glucose uptake in muscle, impaired hepatic insulin sensitivity, defective insulin action and/or secretion in liver and a disruption of secretary function of adipocytes [9-11]. Glucose levels rise and hyperglycemia develops from deteriorated insulin secretion [12]. Mechanistically, the manifestation of T2DM features a relative decrease in insulin secretion suggesting that this may be in accordance with a decreased β-cell mass failing to compensate for peripheral insulin resistance [13-16]. In the last two decades, declining pancreatic β-cell effectiveness has been a criterion for the development of hyperglycemia and T2DM; its progressive character also determines the course of the disease [17]. Impaired glucose-stimulated insulin secretion, defective β-cell gene expression and disrupted mitochondrial ultrastructure is thought to be due to lipid accumulation and 'lipoapoptosis' is observed in pancreatic β-cells from type 2 diabetic animals [18]. This is also supported by reports that chronic, high glucose administration generates the combination of hyperglycemia and chronic dislipidemia, termed 'glucolipotoxicity,' driving a vicious cycle by which metabolic abnormalities impair insulin secretion, which further aggravates metabolic disturbances in β-cell lines and isolated rat islets [19].

There is mounting evidence that chronically elevated circulating levels of glucose and fatty acids, critical characteristics of T2DM, contribute to relentless β-cell function decline, by endorsing glucolipotoxicity, which induces endoplasmic reticulum (ER) stress [20, 21], oxidative stress [22, 23], mitochondrial dysfunction [23, 24] and islet inflammation [25, 26]. Several studies have provided evidence that prolonged exposure to increased concentrations of fatty acids is associated with reduction of glucose induced insulin secretion [27], impairment of insulin gene expression [28, 29] and induction of β-cells death [30, 31]. Importantly, lipoapoptosis only occurs in the presence of concomitant elevation in insulin secretion [32, 33]. Thus, hyperglycemia and hyperlipidemia have been postulated to conduct to the worsening of insulin secretary capacity and β-cell mass observed in T2DM [16]. It is to note, that during feeding, insulin secretion occurs in two phases. An elevation of insulin synthesis in pancreatic β-cells following an initial rapid release of insulin (i.e. first phase) to nutrient ingestion occurs primarily in response to elevated circulating glucose concentrations. The insulin level stimulates glucose uptake into striated muscle tissues through glucose transport type 4 (GLUT-4) for utilization as a source of energy and into adipose tissues for glycerol synthesis; it also affects liver cells thereby activating glycogen formation. Consequently, glucose utilization by these different tissues contributes to a decrease in concentrations of glucose in blood. Long term release of insulin occurs in response to continuously high glucose concentrations as part of the second phase of insulin response. On the other hand, during this period of hypoglycemia there is an altered interaction between pancreatic islets and glucagon-producing α cells, causing increased plasma glucagon, and residual β-cell function largely preserves the first-line defence against hypoglycemia in T2DM [34].

3. Interplay between alcohol consumption and T2DM

Chronic, heavy alcohol consumption, an independent risk factor for T2DM [35-37], disrupts glucose homeostasis and is associated with development of insulin resistance [38-40].

3.1. Epidemiological evidence

The association between alcohol consumption and DM was demonstrated early in 1971 by Phillips et al. [41]. This study suggested that alcohol with doses of 266 to 513 ml produced glucose intolerance and insulin resistance in three of six healthy subjects. Later, this relationship was also demonstrated in a cross-sectional health screening survey of 636 individuals with negative urine glucose, suggesting that alcohol dependence was one of the malignant factors in individuals with impaired glucose tolerance diagnosed by performing a 75-g oral glucose tolerance test (OGTT) [42]. Moreover, alcohol consumption influenced fasting plasma glucose levels along with obesity after analysis of 434 pairs of adult female nondiabetic twins [43]. These results implied that alcohol might impair fasting and postprandial glycemic controls and thus may be a risk factor for T2DM, sharing common genetic factors. Indeed, alcohol consumption within the past week appears to be an independent risk factor of the development of T2DM after a 10 year, prospective population-based study [44]. This significant association was observed only in men and remained significant after adjusting for other hazards of T2DM.

However, there also have been studies with negative or opposite findings explaining the relationship between alcohol consumption and the development of T2DM. Alcohol consumptions of 5-14.9g/d and more than 15g/d were associated with a decreased relative risk of DM in women [45]. In a later study worked on younger women, light to moderate drinking (<14.9g/d) was also associated with a lower risk of T2DM compared to lifelong abstinence, whereas heavy drinking showed a significantly increased diabetic risk [46]. Similarly, moderate amount of alcohol consumption (30.0-49.9 g/d) was associated with reduced risk of the development of DM in 41,810 male health professionals [47]. Lowering the incidence of T2DM by light to moderate drinking, T2DM was also observed in older adults [48]. On the other hand, no effect of alcohol consumption on the development of T2DM was reported in large population-based survey [49]. The aforementioned results suggest the presence of possible influencing factors, such as gender [44, 50] and amount of alcohol consumption [46, 50].

Regarding drinking patterns, Conigrave et al. [51] found that more frequent drinking is more protective against T2DM. A later study [50] also showed that binge drinking for 1-3 days increased the risk of T2DM compared to non-drinking, while drinking the same amount over a week did not increase the risk. Meanwhile, there has been controversy on the type of alcoholic beverage and the risk of T2DM. Some studies noted protective effects of wine on T2DM than other alcoholic beverages [52]. However, other studies presented no significant difference with various alcoholic liquors [48, 51]. In addition, obesity may also influence the relationship between alcohol consumption and T2DM. A systematic review of studies in Japanese showed that alcohol consumption is a risk factor for DM, whereas moderate drinking is associated with a reduced diabetic risk in higher body mass index (BMI) men in some studies [53]. Although the mediating effects of obesity are supported by a positive association between alcohol intake, adiponectin levels and insulin sensitivity [54, 55], more studies will be needed to confirm this issue.

To date, 3 meta-analyses were performed in an attempt to draw a possible conclusion. Carlson et al. [56] analyzed data from 13 cohorts and suggested a U-shaped relationship between the amount of alcohol consumption and risk of T2DM. Moderate drinking, corresponding to about 5-30g/d was associated with a reduced risk of DM (relative risk: RR=0.72, 95% CI=0.67-0.77) in both men and women. This U-shaped relationship in both sexes was also demonstrated in a meta-analysis by Koppes et al. [57] in which lowest risk was in alcohol drinkers of 6-48g/d. Drinkers of ≥48g/d showed equal RR to that of nondrinkers. In their study, adjustment for confounding factors including diagnostic measures of T2DM (self-reported versus tested) and BMI (low- versus high-BMI) was performed. Results of a self-reported diagnosis were associated with lower RR than using a diagnostic test, whereas BMI did not affect the RR of T2DM. A third meta-analysis of Bauliunas et al. [58] additionally identified a deleterious effect of heavy drinking (≥60 g/d for men and ≥50g/d for women) in addition to the protective effect of moderate drinking in both sexes.

3.2. Alcohol consumption and risk of T2DM

Along with the epidemiological data on the relationship between alcohol consumption and T2DM, studies exploring underlying mechanisms between them have been performed. Most directly, alcohol can induce acute and chronic pancreatitis and result in DM as in T1DM [59]. However, there is a growing body of evidence suggesting that the diabetogenic effect of alcohol does not seem to be mediated by decreased insulin secretion [41]. The priming effect of ethanol-enhanced insulin secretion in pancreatic β-cells might be caused by an early defence mechanism used to compensate for alcohol-inhibited basal insulin secretion. In contrast, a limited number of studies have reported deleterious effects of alcohol on β-cells in which alcohol inhibited insulin secretion [60].

Excessive heavy alcohol use increases ROS production and may be a mechanism of pancreatic β-cells dysfunction in T2DM. The reason is that ROS production is one of the earliest events in glucose intolerance through mitochondrial dysfunction and β-cells are very sensitive to oxidative stress [61]. Previous studies of alcohol dependence have shown that alcohol elevated the level of β-cell apoptosis and increased insulin resistance in the liver and skeletal muscle, which is among the earliest detectable alterations in humans with T2DM [62]. In addition, the mechanisms by which this occurs are often multifactorial and quite complex, involving many cell signaling pathways. A common result of DM is hyperglycemia, which in turn contributes to the progression and maintenance of an overall oxidative environment [63]. In obesity, oxidative stress is now recognized to be an important feature in dysregulation of adipokines and inflammation [64].

Among potential mediators of alcohol-induced insulin resistance including acetate, lactate, acetaldehyde, free fatty acids and triglycerides, hepatic insulin sensitizing substance (HISS) and glutathione need to be considered. Alcohol suppresses the release or action of HISS and meal-induced insulin sensitization in rats [65]. Moreover, in animal models, acute alcohol administration also reduces glutathione [66] which is important for HISS release [67]. As with acute alcohol consumption, hepatic glutathione and HISS seem to be involved. In contrast to the acute alcohol effect, chronic ethanol consumption increased hepatic glutathione levels and HISS release in cases of moderate dose, whereas decreased glutathione and HISS were reported at high doses [68].

On the other hand, results on the effect of chronic ethanol consumption on insulin sensitivity showed that insulin sensitivity was improved [66, 69-72] or unchanged [73-75] after chronic alcohol consumption. The mechanism by which chronic alcohol consumption enhances insulin sensitivity also remains elusive. Alcohol consumption is proposed to increase plasma adiponectin levels, which subsequently lowers plasma TNF-α, which interferes with insulin signaling [76]. Taken together, alcohol might induce alterations in insulin resistance mediated by lipids, inflammation oxidative stress and altered metabolism. Moreover, the effect of alcohol on insulin sensitivity may be influenced by periods of and amount of alcohol consumption. Impaired suppression of hepatic glucose production by insulin is likely due to impaired insulin signaling in liver after chronic alcohol exposure. For instance, chronic ethanol consumption decreases tyrosine phosphorylation of insulin receptor substrate-1 as well as activities of PI 3-kinase and Akt (protein kinase B) in the liver [77].

3.3. Ghrelin and leptin correlated with risk of T2DM in alcoholic patients

It has been investigated that ghrelin may be associated with β-cell hypofunction and the first-phase insulin secretion defects in T2DM and exert to regulate glucose homeostasis with glucagon and insulin [78]. Additionally, abnormal glucose tolerance and insulin resistance, which are main characteristics of T2DM, through performing 75g OGTT seemed to be affected by leptin as well as, the levels of leptin were higher in diabetic patients independently of body fat mass when it compared with healthy control patients [4]. Thus, ghrelin and leptin have been regarded to have influence on T2DM. Valuable efficacy of plasma ghrelin and leptin levels by the development of T2DM in patients with alcohol dependence were changed [6]. The data showed that ghrelin levels did not differ among the groups, even though there was a tendency towards decreased ghrelin levels; whereas the leptin level increased significantly with development of T2DM (Fig. 1).

The demographic characteristics of each group were shown in Table 1. The three groups exhibited similar values of age, height, weight, BMI and lipid profiles such as HDL-cholesterol, LDL-cholesterol, and triglyceride. Fasting glucose concentration and hemoglobin A1c, HOMA-IR in the DM group had significantly higher levels than NGT and Pre-DM groups.

Clinical characteristics	NGT	Pre-DM	DM
Alcohol history			
Alcohol use disorder identification test	21.7 ± 1.09	21.17 ± 1.61	24.3 ± 1.23
Alcohol dependency scale	42.29 ± 1.38	38.86 ± 1.74	43.83 ± 1.79
Onset age of problematic drinking (years)	36.58 ± 1.89	37.56 ± 1.68	40.05 ± 2.88
General characteristics			
Age (years)	47.35 ± 1.37	48.87 ± 1.57	52.77 ± 1.84
Weight (kg)	66.83 ± 1.46	65.39 ± 1.25	63.96 ± 1.92
Height (cm)	169.57 ± 0.81	167.76 ± 0.8	167.38 ± 0.85
BMI (kg/m^2)	23.19 ± 0.42	23.2 ± 0.36	22.77 ± 0.57
HDL-Cholesterol (mg/dl)	56.91 ± 2.27	51.08 ± 2.36	55.19 ± 4.44
LDL-Cholesterol (mg/dl)	113.09 ± 3.87	104.63 ± 4.95	101.96 ± 4.72
Triglyceride (mg/dl)	115.02 ± 10.31	135.33 ± 13.06	139.88 ± 15.54
GOT (IU/l)	69.5 ± 11.53	71.7 ± 9.19	52.54 ± 6.96
GPT (IU/l)	40.93 ± 5.25	50.07 ± 8.66	34 ± 6.19
γ-GTP (IU/l)	178.87 ± 45.33	205.07 ± 32.64	254.96 ± 67.99
Clinical characteristics related to glucose tolerance			
Fasting Glucose (mg/dl)	86.09 ± 1.05	91.48 ± 1.45	124.19 ± 7.01**
Fasting Insulin (μU/ml)	4.8 ± 0.84	4.73 ± 0.69	6.22 ± 1.4
HemoglobinA1c (%Hb A1c)	5.5 ± 0.05	5.64 ± 0.08	7.13 ± 0.36**
HOMA-IR	1.02 ± 0.17	1.05 ± 0.15	1.87 ± 0.36*
HOMA-β	83.56 ± 18.56	66.13 ± 11.55	54.91 ± 14.87

Table 1. Characteristics of subjects classified by oral glucose tolerance test among patients with alcohol dependence BMI, body mass index; HDL-cholesterol, high density lipoprotein-cholesterol; LDL-cholesterol, low density lipoprotein-cholesterol; GOT, glutamate oxaloacetate transaminase; GPT, glutamate pyruvate transaminase; γ-GTP, γ-glutamyl transferase; HOMA-IR, homeostasis model assessment-insulin resistance; HOMA-β, homeostasis model assessment-β-cell function (*, p<0.05 and **, p<0.01 compared with NGT).

Moreover, this study demonstrated that leptin was significantly correlated with BMI, fasting insulin concentration and HOMA-IR reflecting insulin resistance (Table 2). The BMI was similar in the groups and the subjects were regarded as a non-obese group. The leptin produced by adipocytes increased in proportion to fat mass [79, 80]. The plasma leptin levels are highly correlated with BMI in both obese and normal weight subjects [81]. In spite of the correlation between BMI and leptin, covarying for BMI in our statistical analyses did not alter our findings.

Leptin also has been shown to be correlated with insulin concentration and insulin sensitivity [82-84]. The direct relationship between leptin and insulin seemed to be mutual. Insulin also had a role in the regulation of leptin concentrations [85]. Among all patients with chronic alcoholism, significant quadratic association of leptin level with insulin concentration and HOMA-IR were observed using simple regression analysis (Fig. 2, Table 3).

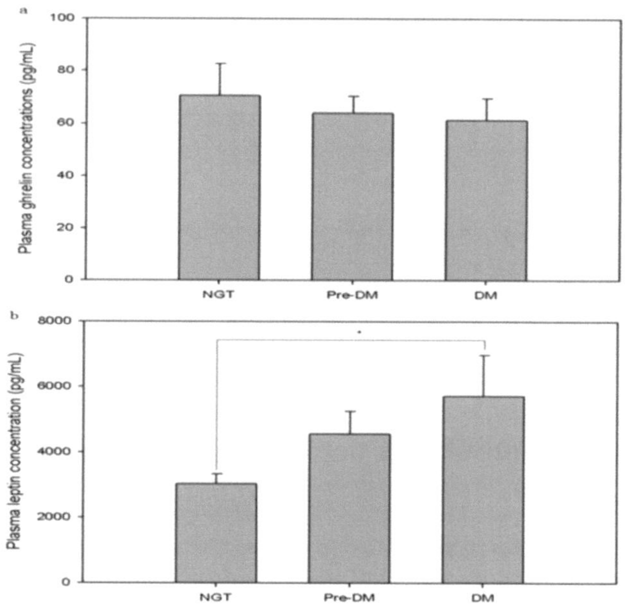

Figure 1. Comparison of plasma (a) ghrelin and (b) leptin levels among three groups classified by oral glucose tolerance test (OGTT) among alcoholic patients (*, $p<0.05$ compared with NGT).

	BMI	Insulin	Leptin	Ghrelin	HOMA-IR
BMI					
Insulin	0.17				
Leptin	0.334**	0.379**			
Ghrelin	-0.066	-0.168	-0.171*		
HOMA-IR	0.195*	0.960**	0.388**	-0.173	

Table 2. Correlation of BMI, fasting insulin, leptin and ghrelin levels and HOMA-IR (*, $p<0.05$ and **, $p<0.01$).

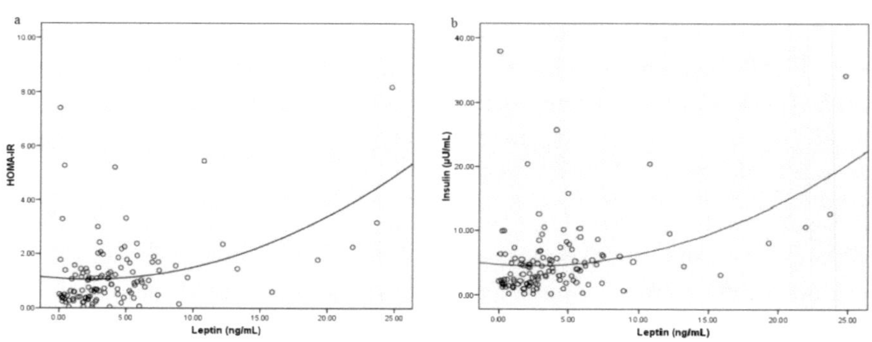

Figure 2. Quadratic regression plots of plasma leptin levels with both insulin resistance index (a) and fasting insulin level (b) in chronic alcoholic subjects. The quadratic regression equation was $y = 0.007x^2 - 0.037x + 1.075$ for fasting leptin level and HOMA-IR (A) and $y = 0.031x^2 - 0.141x + 4.509$ for fasting leptin and insulin level (B).

Independent-Dependent	Linear	Quadratic
Leptin-HOMA-IR	0.390**	0.437**
Lepin-Insulin	0.363**	0.409**

Table 3. Comparison of various kinds of regression models to find better model to fit the relationship of leptin with HOMA-IR and insulin level (**, $p<0.01$).

In conclusion, leptin can play a role in the pathogenesis of T2DM in patients with alcohol dependence. Chronic alcohol consumption might produce leptin resistance, which produces a significant correlation between leptin and the fasting insulin concentration, β-cell function and insulin resistance. However, more study will be needed to determine the mechanism of the relationship between alcohol intake and leptin resistance.

4. Role of the appetite regulating peptides in alcohol dependence and prevalence of T2DM

The neuropeptide, ghrelin secreted from cells of the gastric oxyntic glands in stomach, and leptin excreted from white adipose cells, have received attention due their roles in the neurobiology of alcohol dependence [2, 6]. Many studies have suggested that ghrelin and leptin predominantly produce variations of glucose and insulin concentrations, which may initiate metabolic disorders [86, 87]. In addition, recent research regarding neuroendocrinological alterations of ghrelin and leptin in patients with alcohol dependence has showed that chronic use of alcohol represents a potentially crucial risk factor for T2DM prevalence as ghrelin reduces insulin secretion stimulated by the increased level of blood glucose in the β cells of pancreas, while in contrast, leptin increases insulin secretion and action [88-90]. In regards to the diabetogenic effects of chronic use of alcohol, development of pancreatic β-cell dysfunction, insulin resistance, obesity, impairment of liver function in glucose metabolism have been noted [35]. Indeed, alcoholic patients with T2DM have repeatedly been found to have deregulation of the ghrelin and leptin systems, as indicated by impaired insulin secretion, increased hepatic glucose production and decreased peripheral glucose utilization [38-40]. Moreover, these peptides are regarded to have an influence on T2DM-mediated alcohol cravings and relapses in alcoholism during alcohol abstinace [91-94]. Therefore, it is conceivable that alterations of appetite peptides provoked by chronic alcohol use might contribute to the development of T2DM, including defective glucose tolerance and impaired insulin resistance.

The decreases in ghrelin are paralleled by increases in leptin and rises in insulin [87, 95]. Leptin, which is elevated in the plasma of obese subjects, controls fat cell secretary productions on ghrelin secretion due to leptin-related decreases in ghrelin levels. [96-98]. It has been suggested that leptin is significantly associated with BMI and alcohol consumption, influencing fasting insulin concentration and HOMA-IR, and the passible mechamism of alcohol leptin interaction may be attributable to a direct noxious effect of alcohol on the pancreatic islet cells, or may reflect a truncal fat pattern related to heavy use of alcohol [44]. Thus, the adverse effect of heavy use of alcohol on serum insulin concentrations, a risk for DM, seems to be partially mediated through its effect on BMI. Interestingly, it has been proposed that elevated peripheral insulin resistance may produce increased leptin concentrations regardless of body fat profiles, suggesting that leptin released from fat tissue in alcohol dependence patients may be abundant irrespective of body fat content [6]. Therefore, altered leptin concentrations in alcoholic patients contribute to the incidence of T2DM mainly due to chronic alcohol consumption rather than body fat mass.

In the clinical studies, increases of mean body weights and leptin concentrations resulted from therapeutic treatment of insulin for 1 year in T2DM patients. [99], suggesting that insulin prompted leptin secretion, which was believed to exert influence on the increased body weight. Further, decrease of insulin-stimulated glucose utilization in skeletal muscle was exibited by long periods of leptin exposure. This is to the fact that insulin-stimulated p38 mitogen-activated protein kinase (MAPK) activation was inhibited and GLUT4 activation was decreased by leptin [100]. Leptin also can interfere with insulin signaling and induce gluconeogenesis in hepatocytes directly [83]. Insulin-stimulated glucose uptake into isolated adipocytes was inhibited by chronic alcohol feeding via vitiation of the fusion of GLUT4 vesicles at the plasma membrane of rats. Chronically fed with alcohol sustains insulin signaling through PI 3-kinase in adipocytes [101] but results in the disruption of insulin mediated Cbl/TC10 signaling pathway which leads to attenuated insulin-stimulated glucose transport [102]. Thus, a combination of decreased GLUT4 expression and impaired insulin-stimulated GLUT4 trafficking to the plasma membrane contributes to reduced glucose uptake in response to insulin in adipocytes. Hence, the possibility that ghrelin and leptin can be related with deteriorated pathophysiology of T2DM, aligned with defective insulin signaling pathway, including change in kinase activity, glucose transporter translocation and intracellular enzyme activity, in alcoholic patients exists.

5. Ghrelin in glucose and insulin homeostasis

Ghrelin was originally isolated from the stomach, but ghrelin has also been identified in other peripheral tissues, such as the gastrointestinal tract, pancreas, ovary and adrenal cortex [3, 103-105]. Regulation of ghrelin secretion, as well as its biological effects, appears to be opposite those of leptin and antagonize leptin's effects in appetite regulation [95, 106-108]. A suppressive role of ghrelin in insulin secretion from pancreatic islets is supported by the observation that ghrelin inhibits glucose-stimulated insulin secretion and disrupts glucose tolerance in normal subjects [109]. There is evidence that ghrelin may have proliferative or protective roles on β-cells [110] and stimulates insulin secretion, which primarily occurs in response to increased circulating glucose levels, whereas insulin reduces plasma ghrelin in normal controls and T2DM patients [111]. Moreover, ghrelin may be associated with β-cell hypofunction and first-phase insulin secretion defects in T2DM as well as regulates glucose homeostasis with glucagon and insulin [78]. Furthermore, it has been noted that deficiency of the genes encoding ghrelin and its receptor (GHS-R1a) enhances insulin levels, increases glucose-stimulated insulin secretion, improves peripheral insulin sensitivity and prevents high-fat diets from inducing obesity [112]. Similarly, ghrelin receptor antagonists which inhibit ghrelin signaling have been shown to improve the diabetic condition by promoting glucose-dependent insulin secretion [113]. Ghrelin can also inhibit the activity of glucose-sensing neurons in the dorsal vagal complex of rats, indicating that ghrelin manipulates the sensitivity of glucose-sensing neurons [114, 115].

The pathophysiological role of ghrelin in glucose homeostasis was strengthened by the fact that ghrelin may decline endogenous glucose production through suppression of insulin secretory capacity [116], while reinforcing insulin action on glucose disposal [112]. A recent study demonstrated that acylated ghrelin has a positive correlation with insulin resistance, as indicated by the increased insulin and glucose concentrations, whereas correlation between des-acylated ghrelin and HOMA-IR was shown to be negative [117]. On the other hand, it has been reported that fasting ghrelin levels at any other point might be impossible to use for predicting the development of impaired glucose regulation [118]. The reduction of ghrelin levels were shown to be associated independently with T2DM, agreeing with the results of studies demonstrating that ghrelin has an inverse correlation with insulin resistance evaluated by HOMA-IR [119]. Moreover, increases in ghrelin during chronic alcohol use suggested that a role of ghrelin may contribute significantly to the overall alcohol response. It has likewise been reported that ghrelin is not only a regulator of glucose and insulin metabolism in the central nervous system (CNS), but also a modulator of those in the periphery. In the periphery, ghrelin has been shown to stimulate hepatic glucose production [120] and inhibit insulin release from pancreatic islets [121, 122]. Peripheral ghrelin produced in the gastrointestinal tract [103, 123] reaches ghrelin-receptors in the anterior pituitary and potentially in the mediobasal and mediolateral hypothalamus through the general circulation to stimulate GH release and to regulate energy homeostasis [124]. Therefore, it can be postulated that decreases in ghrelin concentrations as well as facilitation of the development of perturbations in glucose metabolism resulting from deregulation of the CNS and the periphery might lead to perseverance of T2DM. Besides, low blood ghrelin concentrations appears to influence growth hormone/insulin like growth facor-1-axis which may, in turn, affect increased insulin resistance and ultimately manifest T2DM [125].

6. Leptin in glucose and insulin homeostasis

Leptin, an adipocyte-derived anorexic peptide plays a primary role in regulation of energy homeostasis including food intake and energy expenditure involved in obesity, regulating overall metabolism and particularly glucose metabolism. Leptin is transported across the blood brain barrier (BBB) by binding to its receptor in the arcuate nucleus of the hypothalamus to regulate glucose metabolism via central leptin signaling, which modulates sympathetic and neuroendocrine activities [126, 127], as well as though peripheral signaling in insulin-sensitive tissues such as liver and muscle [128, 129]. A previous study demonstrated that serum leptin was positively correlated with fasting blood glucose in obese patients with DM, suggesting that resistance to insulin and leptin may have participated in increasing food intake in T2DM. Additionally, leptin has to be considered as a possible regulator of the gastrohypothalamic axis involved in short-term feeding regulation [130] and may have a central role in islet cell growth and insulin secretion [131]. In addition, several other appetite-related hormones such as anorexigenic neuropeptides, alpha-melanocyte-stimulating hormone (alpha-MSH), proopiomelanocortin (POMC), cocaine and amphetamine regulated transcript (CART) and corticotropin-releasing hormone (CRH) are stimulated by leptin. Conversely, orexigenic neuropeptides NPY, melanin-concentrating hormone (MCH), orexins and agouti-related peptide (AgRP) are inhibited by leptin which suppresses food intake and enhances energy expenditure through these central interactions, which is associated with T2DM [132-135].

In the brain, obesity and T2DM typified by both insulin and leptin resistance, on account of either reduced BBB transport or impaired neuronal capacity to sense peripheral signals, causes increased concentrations of anorexigenic neuropeptides and reduced concentrations of orexigenic ones [136]. It has been postulated that leptin resistance might be due to defective leptin transport across the BBB [137]. Leptin enters the brain by a satiable transport system and that capacity of leptin transport is lower in obese individuals, thereby providing a mechanism for leptin resistance [138]. The development leptin resistance most likely involves a period of excess caloric intake, resulting in a disturbance of the leptin system, leading to sustained defects. The hypothalamus exposed to high leptin levels becomes less sensitive to leptin, resulting in a sustained increase in leptin levels [139]. Leptin resistance may also have functional implications in peripheral tissues expressing leptin receptors, such as pancreatic β cells, where insulin is synthesized and secreted; leptin may also affect hepatocytes, muscle and adipose tissue, where insulin exerts its function [140]. In all these tissues, an effect of leptin has been demonstrated on insulin secretion and on insulin-induced activities such as glucose utilization [83, 141]. Also, increased leptin levels, probably reflecting leptin resistance, was shown to be strongly related to insulin resistance [142]. Moreover, peripheral leptin inhibits insulin secretion in pancreatic β-cells [83], whereas insulin stimulates leptin production in adipocytes [85]. Therefore, reciprocal interaction of leptin and insulin called 'adipo-insular axis' is central under physiological conditions.

However, in few studies, glucose and insulin levels were able to increase circulating leptin levels, indicating that the capacity of leptin to suppress insulin secretion in pancreatic β-cell might be a possible involvement of T2DM [143, 144]. Interestingly, reduced leptin sensitivity of the pancreatic β-cell occurs concurrently with hyperinsulinemia resulting from not only decreased insulin sensitivity, but also increased insulin secretion, and consequently hyperleptimia as part of a vicious cycle that promotes both and insulin resistance [145]). Leptin has been shown to increase whole-body glucose utilization, decrease glycogen stores and inhibit insulin-stimulated glucose uptake [146], implying that increased leptin levels contribute to increased glycemia and altered glucose homeostasis [147]. Therefore, the capacity of leptin to suppress insulin secretion in pancreatic β-cell suggests a possible involvement in T2DM. Moreover, obese *(ob)* gene depleted mice exhibited susceptibility to the development of obesity and diabetic disorders, indicating that leptin-(an *ob* gene product) induced insulin resistance may be considered a major influence in developing T2DM [148]. Thus, animal models that are used to elucidate mechanisms underlying obesity and T2DM often display an altered diabetogenic imbalance, involving leptin. This suggests that dysfunction of leptin's ability in T2DM may not only represent a consequence of the disease, but also plays an important role in its cause.

7. Inverse interactions between leptin and ghrelin

Leptin is important for the negative feedback regulation of ghrelin in states of moderate body weight increase, whereas recombinant leptin administration is ineffective on altering ghrelin levels in healthy subjects [149]. There is currently evidence that ghrelin and leptin exert antagonistic effects via their specific receptors in the CNS and in peripheral tissues. Ghrelin increases appetite and food intake via centrally mediating actions but, peripherally it modulates pancreatic β-cells function as well as glucose and lipid metabolism [150]. The satiety inducing effects of leptin include the suppression of ghrelin secretion to induce anorexic effects [97]. Adipogenic as well as orexigenic effects of ghrelin are also most likely mediated by a specific central network of neurons that is also mediated by leptin [124, 151-153].

In the brain, ghrelin may transfort the BBB and bind to its receptors in the hypothalamus after secretion into the bloodstream from the stomach [105, 154, 155]. Ghrelin reaches the brain via the vagal nerve and nucleus tractus solitarus [154, 156] and is released locally in the hypothalamus, where it may directly affect various hypothalamic nuclei [154, 157]. In addition, central ghrelin may affect the energy centre in the hypothalamus and both ghrelin and leptin stimulate and suppress, respectively hypothalamic neurons containing various neuropeptides, resulting in anorexic or orexic effects on energy balance. Ghrelin thus stimulates the activity of neurons expressing NPY, AgRP and orexin [158-160] and inhibits POMC neurons and CRH-producing neurons [157]. The interaction between ghrelin and leptin in the hypothalamus indicates that these peptides have different effects in the hypothalamic neurons producing various orexigenic and anorexigenic peptides, presenting more or less opposing effects on energy balance.

In hepatocytes, ghrelin reduces and leptin augments insulin signal transduction, resulting in increased and decreased glucose production, respectively [120]. In pancreatic β-cells, insulin release was stimulated by ghrelin but inhibited by leptin administration [3]. Insulin was postulated to act indirectly via ghrelin and leptin to suppress appetite [5]. However, attenuated suppressive action of insulin on ghrelin and particular association between insulin resistance and leptin resistance were shown in T2DM [5, 142]. Thus, leptin seems to the major determinant of ghrelin effects on progression of metabolic syndromes.

8. Conclusion

The studies discussed here demonstrate that the role of appetite regulating peptides, ghrelin and leptin, in alcohol patients with T2DM may be of high importance for clinical research and practice. The extensive functional interactions between these peptides, which may contribute significantly to the overall defecting glucose tolerance with regard to alcoholism, may have a new insight into mechanism of T2DM. Therefore, understanding of mechanisms underlying the pivotal relations between ghrelin, leptin and glucose homeostasis during chronic use of alcohol represents an additional therapeutic intervention for T2DM.

Author details

Soo-Jeong Kim and Dai-Jin Kim
The Catholic University of Korea College of Medicine, Republic of Korea

Acknowledgement

This study was supported by a grant of the Korea Health 21R&D Project, Ministry for Health, Welfare and Family Affairs, Republic of Korea (A111378).

9. References

[1] Nicolas JM, Fernandez-Sola J, Fatjo F, Casamitjana R, Bataller R, Sacanella E, et al. Increased circulating leptin levels in chronic alcoholism. Journ. 2001;25(1):83-8.
[2] Kraus T, Schanze A, Groschl M, Bayerlein K, Hillemacher T, Reulbach U, et al. Ghrelin levels are increased in alcoholism. Journ. 2005;29(12):2154-7.
[3] Date Y, Nakazato M, Hashiguchi S, Dezaki K, Mondal MS, Hosoda H, et al. Ghrelin is present in pancreatic alpha-cells of humans and rats and stimulates insulin secretion. Journ. 2002;51(1):124-9.
[4] Fischer S, Hanefeld M, Haffner SM, Fusch C, Schwanebeck U, Kohler C, et al. Insulin-resistant patients with type 2 diabetes mellitus have higher serum leptin levels independently of body fat mass. Journ. 2002;39(3):105-10.
[5] Erdmann J, Lippl F, Wagenpfeil S, Schusdziarra V. Differential association of basal and postprandial plasma ghrelin with leptin, insulin, and type 2 diabetes. Journ. 2005;54(5):1371-8.
[6] Ju A, Cheon YH, Lee KS, Lee SS, Lee WY, Won WY, et al. The change of plasma ghrelin and leptin levels by the development of type 2 diabetes mellitus in patients with alcohol dependence. Journ. 2011;35(5):905-11.
[7] Thiele TE, Navarro M, Sparta DR, Fee JR, Knapp DJ, Cubero I. Alcoholism and obesity: overlapping neuropeptide pathways? Journ. 2003;37(6):321-37.
[8] Kalra SP, Kalra PS. Overlapping and interactive pathways regulating appetite and craving. Journ. 2004;23(3):5-21.
[9] Kahn CR. Banting Lecture. Insulin action, diabetogenes, and the cause of type II diabetes. Journ. 1994;43(8):1066-84.
[10] Lin Y, Sun Z. Current views on type 2 diabetes. Journ.;204(1):1-11.
[11] Lin Y, Sun Z. Current views on type 2 diabetes. Journ. 2010;204(1):1-11.
[12] Reaven GM. Role of insulin resistance in human disease (syndrome X): an expanded definition. Journ. 1993;44:121-31.
[13] Rhodes ET, Ferrari LR, Wolfsdorf JI. Perioperative management of pediatric surgical patients with diabetes mellitus. Journ. 2005;101(4):986-99, table of contents.

[14] Kumari M, Brunner E, Fuhrer R. Minireview: mechanisms by which the metabolic syndrome and diabetes impair memory. Journ. 2000;55(5):B228-32.
[15] Falkmer S. Role of sulfhydryl inhibitors in the pathogenesis of diabets mellitus. Journ. 1962;Suppl 154:106-7.
[16] Butler AE, Janson J, Bonner-Weir S, Ritzel R, Rizza RA, Butler PC. Beta-cell deficit and increased beta-cell apoptosis in humans with type 2 diabetes. Journ. 2003;52(1):102-10.
[17] Harmon JS, Gleason CE, Tanaka Y, Poitout V, Robertson RP. Antecedent hyperglycemia, not hyperlipidemia, is associated with increased islet triacylglycerol content and decreased insulin gene mRNA level in Zucker diabetic fatty rats. Journ. 2001;50(11):2481-6.
[18] Unger RH, Orci L. Lipoapoptosis: its mechanism and its diseases. Journ. 2002;1585(2-3):202-12.
[19] Roche E, Farfari S, Witters LA, Assimacopoulos-Jeannet F, Thumelin S, Brun T, et al. Long-term exposure of beta-INS cells to high glucose concentrations increases anaplerosis, lipogenesis, and lipogenic gene expression. Journ. 1998;47(7):1086-94.
[20] Eizirik DL, Cardozo AK, Cnop M. The role for endoplasmic reticulum stress in diabetes mellitus. Journ. 2008;29(1):42-61.
[21] Marchetti P, Bugliani M, Lupi R, Marselli L, Masini M, Boggi U, et al. The endoplasmic reticulum in pancreatic beta cells of type 2 diabetes patients. Journ. 2007;50(12):2486-94.
[22] Wajchenberg BL. beta-cell failure in diabetes and preservation by clinical treatment. Journ. 2007;28(2):187-218.
[23] Prentki M, Nolan CJ. Islet beta cell failure in type 2 diabetes. Journ. 2006;116(7):1802-12.
[24] Li N, Brun T, Cnop M, Cunha DA, Eizirik DL, Maechler P. Transient oxidative stress damages mitochondrial machinery inducing persistent beta-cell dysfunction. Journ. 2009;284(35):23602-12.
[25] Maedler K, Sergeev P, Ris F, Oberholzer J, Joller-Jemelka HI, Spinas GA, et al. Glucose-induced beta cell production of IL-1beta contributes to glucotoxicity in human pancreatic islets. Journ. 2002;110(6):851-60.
[26] Cnop M, Welsh N, Jonas JC, Jorns A, Lenzen S, Eizirik DL. Mechanisms of pancreatic beta-cell death in type 1 and type 2 diabetes: many differences, few similarities. Journ. 2005;54 Suppl 2:S97-107.
[27] Zhou YP, Grill VE. Long-term exposure of rat pancreatic islets to fatty acids inhibits glucose-induced insulin secretion and biosynthesis through a glucose fatty acid cycle. Journ. 1994;93(2):870-6.
[28] Ritz-Laser B, Meda P, Constant I, Klages N, Charollais A, Morales A, et al. Glucose-induced preproinsulin gene expression is inhibited by the free fatty acid palmitate. Journ. 1999;140(9):4005-14.
[29] Kelpe CL, Moore PC, Parazzoli SD, Wicksteed B, Rhodes CJ, Poitout V. Palmitate inhibition of insulin gene expression is mediated at the transcriptional level via ceramide synthesis. Journ. 2003;278(32):30015-21.
[30] Poitout V. Glucolipotoxicity of the pancreatic beta-cell: myth or reality? Journ. 2008;36(Pt 5):901-4.

[31] Cnop M, Hannaert JC, Hoorens A, Eizirik DL, Pipeleers DG. Inverse relationship between cytotoxicity of free fatty acids in pancreatic islet cells and cellular triglyceride accumulation. Journ. 2001;50(8):1771-7.

[32] Jacqueminet S, Briaud I, Rouault C, Reach G, Poitout V. Inhibition of insulin gene expression by long-term exposure of pancreatic beta cells to palmitate is dependent on the presence of a stimulatory glucose concentration. Journ. 2000;49(4):532-6.

[33] Briaud I, Harmon JS, Kelpe CL, Segu VB, Poitout V. Lipotoxicity of the pancreatic beta-cell is associated with glucose-dependent esterification of fatty acids into neutral lipids. Journ. 2001;50(2):315-21.

[34] Salehi M, Aulinger BA, D'Alessio DA. Targeting beta-cell mass in type 2 diabetes: promise and limitations of new drugs based on incretins. Journ. 2008;29(3):367-79.

[35] Kao WH, Puddey IB, Boland LL, Watson RL, Brancati FL. Alcohol consumption and the risk of type 2 diabetes mellitus: atherosclerosis risk in communities study. Journ. 2001;154(8):748-57.

[36] Wannamethee SG, Shaper AG, Perry IJ, Alberti KG. Alcohol consumption and the incidence of type II diabetes. Journ. 2002;56(7):542-8.

[37] Wei M, Gibbons LW, Mitchell TL, Kampert JB, Blair SN. Alcohol intake and incidence of type 2 diabetes in men. Journ. 2000;23(1):18-22.

[38] Onishi Y, Honda M, Ogihara T, Sakoda H, Anai M, Fujishiro M, et al. Ethanol feeding induces insulin resistance with enhanced PI 3-kinase activation. Journ. 2003;303(3):788-94.

[39] Wan Q, Liu Y, Guan Q, Gao L, Lee KO, Zhao J. Ethanol feeding impairs insulin-stimulated glucose uptake in isolated rat skeletal muscle: role of Gs alpha and cAMP. Journ. 2005;29(8):1450-6.

[40] Sotaniemi EA, Keinanen K, Lahtela JT, Arranto AJ, Kairaluoma M. Carbohydrate intolerance associated with reduced hepatic glucose phosphorylating and releasing enzyme activities and peripheral insulin resistance in alcoholics with liver cirrhosis. Journ. 1985;1(3):277-90.

[41] Phillips GB, Safrit HF. Alcoholic diabetes. Induction of glucose intolerance with alcohol. Journ. 1971;217(11):1513-9.

[42] Umeki S, Hisamoto N, Hara Y. Study on background factors associated with impaired glucose tolerance and/or diabetes mellitus. Journ. 1989;120(6):729-34.

[43] Selby JV, Newman B, King MC, Friedman GD. Environmental and behavioral determinants of fasting plasma glucose in women. A matched co-twin analysis. Journ. 1987;125(6):979-88.

[44] Holbrook TL, Barrett-Connor E, Wingard DL. A prospective population-based study of alcohol use and non-insulin-dependent diabetes mellitus. Journ. 1990;132(5):902-9.

[45] Stampfer MJ, Colditz GA, Willett WC, Manson JE, Arky RA, Hennekens CH, et al. A prospective study of moderate alcohol drinking and risk of diabetes in women. Journ. 1988;128(3):549-58.

[46] Wannamethee SG, Camargo CA, Jr., Manson JE, Willett WC, Rimm EB. Alcohol drinking patterns and risk of type 2 diabetes mellitus among younger women. Journ. 2003;163(11):1329-36.

[47] Rimm EB, Chan J, Stampfer MJ, Colditz GA, Willett WC. Prospective study of cigarette smoking, alcohol use, and the risk of diabetes in men. Journ. 1995;310(6979):555-9.

[48] Djousse L, Biggs ML, Mukamal KJ, Siscovick DS. Alcohol consumption and type 2 diabetes among older adults: the Cardiovascular Health Study. Journ. 2007;15(7):1758-65.

[49] Hodge AM, Dowse GK, Collins VR, Zimmet PZ. Abnormal glucose tolerance and alcohol consumption in three populations at high risk of non-insulin-dependent diabetes mellitus. Journ. 1993;137(2):178-89.

[50] Hodge AM, English DR, O'Dea K, Giles GG. Alcohol intake, consumption pattern and beverage type, and the risk of Type 2 diabetes. Journ. 2006;23(6):690-7.

[51] Conigrave KM, Hu BF, Camargo CA, Jr., Stampfer MJ, Willett WC, Rimm EB. A prospective study of drinking patterns in relation to risk of type 2 diabetes among men. Journ. 2001;50(10):2390-5.

[52] Goldberg DM, Soleas GJ, Levesque M. Moderate alcohol consumption: the gentle face of Janus. Journ. 1999;32(7):505-18.

[53] Seike N, Noda M, Kadowaki T. Alcohol consumption and risk of type 2 diabetes mellitus in Japanese: a systematic review. Journ. 2008;17(4):545-51.

[54] Thamer C, Haap M, Fritsche A, Haering H, Stumvoll M. Relationship between moderate alcohol consumption and adiponectin and insulin sensitivity in a large heterogeneous population. Journ. 2004;27(5):1240.

[55] Englund Ogge L, Brohall G, Behre CJ, Schmidt C, Fagerberg B. Alcohol consumption in relation to metabolic regulation, inflammation, and adiponectin in 64-year-old Caucasian women: a population-based study with a focus on impaired glucose regulation. Journ. 2006;29(4):908-13.

[56] Carlsson S, Hammar N, Grill V. Alcohol consumption and type 2 diabetes Meta-analysis of epidemiological studies indicates a U-shaped relationship. Journ. 2005;48(6):1051-4.

[57] Koppes LL, Dekker JM, Hendriks HF, Bouter LM, Heine RJ. Moderate alcohol consumption lowers the risk of type 2 diabetes: a meta-analysis of prospective observational studies. Journ. 2005;28(3):719-25.

[58] Baliunas DO, Taylor BJ, Irving H, Roerecke M, Patra J, Mohapatra S, et al. Alcohol as a risk factor for type 2 diabetes: A systematic review and meta-analysis. Journ. 2009;32(11):2123-32.

[59] Sjoberg RJ, Kidd GS. Pancreatic diabetes mellitus. Journ. 1989;12(10):715-24.

[60] Rosengren A, Wilhelmsen L, Wedel H. Separate and combined effects of smoking and alcohol abuse in middle-aged men. Journ. 1988;223(2):111-8.

[61] Hurt RD, Patten CA. Treatment of tobacco dependence in alcoholics. Journ. 2003;16:335-59.

[62] Mauvais-Jarvis F, Kahn CR. Understanding the pathogenesis and treatment of insulin resistance and type 2 diabetes mellitus: what can we learn from transgenic and knockout mice? Journ. 2000;26(6):433-48.

[63] Sesti G. Pathophysiology of insulin resistance. Journ. 2006;20(4):665-79.

[64] Gustafson B. Adipose tissue, inflammation and atherosclerosis. Journ.;17(4):332-41.

[65] Lautt WW, Legare DJ, Reid MA, Sadri P, Ting JW, Prieditis H. Alcohol suppresses meal-induced insulin sensitization. Journ. 2005;3(1):51-9.

[66] Kiechl S, Willeit J, Poewe W, Egger G, Oberhollenzer F, Muggeo M, et al. Insulin sensitivity and regular alcohol consumption: large, prospective, cross sectional population study (Bruneck study). Journ. 1996;313(7064):1040-4.

[67] Guarino MP, Afonso RA, Raimundo N, Raposo JF, Macedo MP. Hepatic glutathione and nitric oxide are critical for hepatic insulin-sensitizing substance action. Journ. 2003;284(4):G588-94.

[68] Shaw S, Rubin KP, Lieber CS. Depressed hepatic glutathione and increased diene conjugates in alcoholic liver disease. Evidence of lipid peroxidation. Journ. 1983;28(7):585-9.

[69] Mayer EJ, Newman B, Quesenberry CP, Jr., Friedman GD, Selby JV. Alcohol consumption and insulin concentrations. Role of insulin in associations of alcohol intake with high-density lipoprotein cholesterol and triglycerides. Journ. 1993;88(5 Pt 1):2190-7.

[70] Flanagan DE, Moore VM, Godsland IF, Cockington RA, Robinson JS, Phillips DI. Alcohol consumption and insulin resistance in young adults. Journ. 2000;30(4):297-301.

[71] Goude D, Fagerberg B, Hulthe J. Alcohol consumption, the metabolic syndrome and insulin resistance in 58-year-old clinically healthy men (AIR study). Journ. 2002;102(3):345-52.

[72] Davies MJ, Baer DJ, Judd JT, Brown ED, Campbell WS, Taylor PR. Effects of moderate alcohol intake on fasting insulin and glucose concentrations and insulin sensitivity in postmenopausal women: a randomized controlled trial. Journ. 2002;287(19):2559-62.

[73] Bell DS. Alcohol and the NIDDM patient. Journ. 1996;19(5):509-13.

[74] Cordain L, Melby CL, Hamamoto AE, O'Neill DS, Cornier MA, Barakat HA, et al. Influence of moderate chronic wine consumption on insulin sensitivity and other correlates of syndrome X in moderately obese women. Journ. 2000;49(11):1473-8.

[75] Flanagan DE, Pratt E, Murphy J, Vaile JC, Petley GW, Godsland IF, et al. Alcohol consumption alters insulin secretion and cardiac autonomic activity. Journ. 2002;32(3):187-92.

[76] Hotamisligil GS, Murray DL, Choy LN, Spiegelman BM. Tumor necrosis factor alpha inhibits signaling from the insulin receptor. Journ. 1994;91(11):4854-8.

[77] Yeon JE, Califano S, Xu J, Wands JR, De La Monte SM. Potential role of PTEN phosphatase in ethanol-impaired survival signaling in the liver. Journ. 2003;38(3):703-14.

[78] Fromenty B, Vadrot N, Massart J, Turlin B, Barri-Ova N, Letteron P, et al. Chronic ethanol consumption lessens the gain of body weight, liver triglycerides, and diabetes in obese ob/ob mice. Journ. 2009;331(1):23-34.

[79] Considine RV, Sinha MK, Heiman ML, Kriauciunas A, Stephens TW, Nyce MR, et al. Serum immunoreactive-leptin concentrations in normal-weight and obese humans. Journ. 1996;334(5):292-5.

[80] Frederich RC, Hamann A, Anderson S, Lollmann B, Lowell BB, Flier JS. Leptin levels reflect body lipid content in mice: evidence for diet-induced resistance to leptin action. Journ. 1995;1(12):1311-4.
[81] Havel PJ, Kasim-Karakas S, Mueller W, Johnson PR, Gingerich RL, Stern JS. Relationship of plasma leptin to plasma insulin and adiposity in normal weight and overweight women: effects of dietary fat content and sustained weight loss. Journ. 1996;81(12):4406-13.
[82] Segal KR, Landt M, Klein S. Relationship between insulin sensitivity and plasma leptin concentration in lean and obese men. Journ. 1996;45(7):988-91.
[83] Cohen B, Novick D, Rubinstein M. Modulation of insulin activities by leptin. Journ. 1996;274(5290):1185-8.
[84] Seufert J, Kieffer TJ, Leech CA, Holz GG, Moritz W, Ricordi C, et al. Leptin suppression of insulin secretion and gene expression in human pancreatic islets: implications for the development of adipogenic diabetes mellitus. Journ. 1999;84(2):670-6.
[85] Widjaja A, Stratton IM, Horn R, Holman RR, Turner R, Brabant G. UKPDS 20: plasma leptin, obesity, and plasma insulin in type 2 diabetic subjects. Journ. 1997;82(2):654-7.
[86] Flanagan DE, Evans ML, Monsod TP, Rife F, Heptulla RA, Tamborlane WV, et al. The influence of insulin on circulating ghrelin. Journ. 2003;284(2):E313-6.
[87] Saad MF, Bernaba B, Hwu CM, Jinagouda S, Fahmi S, Kogosov E, et al. Insulin regulates plasma ghrelin concentration. Journ. 2002;87(8):3997-4000.
[88] Berkelman RL, Ralston M, Herndon J, Gwinn M, Bertolucci D, Dufour M. Patterns of alcohol consumption and alcohol-related morbidity and mortality. Journ. 1986;35(2):1SS-5SS.
[89] Magis DC, Jandrain BJ, Scheen AJ. [Alcohol, insulin sensitivity and diabetes]. Journ. 2003;58(7-8):501-7.
[90] van de Wiel A. Diabetes mellitus and alcohol. Journ. 2004;20(4):263-7.
[91] Kraus T, Reulbach U, Bayerlein K, Mugele B, Hillemacher T, Sperling W, et al. Leptin is associated with craving in females with alcoholism. Journ. 2004;9(3-4):213-9.
[92] Addolorato G, Capristo E, Leggio L, Ferrulli A, Abenavoli L, Malandrino N, et al. Relationship between ghrelin levels, alcohol craving, and nutritional status in current alcoholic patients. Journ. 2006;30(11):1933-7.
[93] Kiefer F, Jahn H, Kellner M, Naber D, Wiedemann K. Leptin as a possible modulator of craving for alcohol. Journ. 2001;58(5):509-10.
[94] Kim DJ, Yoon SJ, Choi B, Kim TS, Woo YS, Kim W, et al. Increased fasting plasma ghrelin levels during alcohol abstinence. Journ. 2005;40(1):76-9.
[95] Weigle DS, Cummings DE, Newby PD, Breen PA, Frayo RS, Matthys CC, et al. Roles of leptin and ghrelin in the loss of body weight caused by a low fat, high carbohydrate diet. Journ. 2003;88(4):1577-86.
[96] Barazzoni R, Zanetti M, Stebel M, Biolo G, Cattin L, Guarnieri G. Hyperleptinemia prevents increased plasma ghrelin concentration during short-term moderate caloric restriction in rats. Journ. 2003;124(5):1188-92.
[97] Bagnasco M, Kalra PS, Kalra SP. Ghrelin and leptin pulse discharge in fed and fasted rats. Journ. 2002;143(2):726-9.

[98] Lippl F, Erdmann J, Atmatzidis S, Schusdziarra V. Direct effect of leptin on gastric ghrelin secretion. Journ. 2005;37(2):123-5.

[99] Aas AM, Hanssen KF, Berg JP, Thorsby PM, Birkeland KI. Insulin-stimulated increase in serum leptin levels precedes and correlates with weight gain during insulin therapy in type 2 diabetes. Journ. 2009;94(8):2900-6.

[100] Sweeney G, Keen J, Somwar R, Konrad D, Garg R, Klip A. High leptin levels acutely inhibit insulin-stimulated glucose uptake without affecting glucose transporter 4 translocation in l6 rat skeletal muscle cells. Journ. 2001;142(11):4806-12.

[101] Poirier LA, Rachdaoui N, Nagy LE. GLUT4 vesicle trafficking in rat adipocytes after ethanol feeding: regulation by heterotrimeric G-proteins. Journ. 2001;354(Pt 2):323-30.

[102] Sebastian BM, Nagy LE. Decreased insulin-dependent glucose transport by chronic ethanol feeding is associated with dysregulation of the Cbl/TC10 pathway in rat adipocytes. Journ. 2005;289(6):E1077-84.

[103] Kojima M, Hosoda H, Date Y, Nakazato M, Matsuo H, Kangawa K. Ghrelin is a growth-hormone-releasing acylated peptide from stomach. Journ. 1999;402(6762):656-60.

[104] Date Y, Kojima M, Hosoda H, Sawaguchi A, Mondal MS, Suganuma T, et al. Ghrelin, a novel growth hormone-releasing acylated peptide, is synthesized in a distinct endocrine cell type in the gastrointestinal tracts of rats and humans. Journ. 2000;141(11):4255-61.

[105] Tortorella C, Macchi C, Spinazzi R, Malendowicz LK, Trejter M, Nussdorfer GG. Ghrelin, an endogenous ligand for the growth hormone-secretagogue receptor, is expressed in the human adrenal cortex. Journ. 2003;12(2):213-7.

[106] Horvath TL, Diano S, Sotonyi P, Heiman M, Tschop M. Minireview: ghrelin and the regulation of energy balance--a hypothalamic perspective. Journ. 2001;142(10):4163-9.

[107] Klok MD, Jakobsdottir S, Drent ML. The role of leptin and ghrelin in the regulation of food intake and body weight in humans: a review. Journ. 2007;8(1):21-34.

[108] Tolle V, Kadem M, Bluet-Pajot MT, Frere D, Foulon C, Bossu C, et al. Balance in ghrelin and leptin plasma levels in anorexia nervosa patients and constitutionally thin women. Journ. 2003;88(1):109-16.

[109] Tong J, Prigeon RL, Davis HW, Bidlingmaier M, Kahn SE, Cummings DE, et al. Ghrelin suppresses glucose-stimulated insulin secretion and deteriorates glucose tolerance in healthy humans. Journ. 2010;59(9):2145-51.

[110] Irako T, Akamizu T, Hosoda H, Iwakura H, Ariyasu H, Tojo K, et al. Ghrelin prevents development of diabetes at adult age in streptozotocin-treated newborn rats. Journ. 2006;49(6):1264-73.

[111] Anderwald C, Brabant G, Bernroider E, Horn R, Brehm A, Waldhausl W, et al. Insulin-dependent modulation of plasma ghrelin and leptin concentrations is less pronounced in type 2 diabetic patients. Journ. 2003;52(7):1792-8.

[112] Yada T, Dezaki K, Sone H, Koizumi M, Damdindorj B, Nakata M, et al. Ghrelin regulates insulin release and glycemia: physiological role and therapeutic potential. Journ. 2008;4(1):18-23.

[113] Zorrilla EP, Iwasaki S, Moss JA, Chang J, Otsuji J, Inoue K, et al. Vaccination against weight gain. Journ. 2006;103(35):13226-31.

[114] Penicaud L, Leloup C, Fioramonti X, Lorsignol A, Benani A. Brain glucose sensing: a subtle mechanism. Journ. 2006;9(4):458-62.

[115] Wang WG, Chen X, Jiang H, Jiang ZY. Effects of ghrelin on glucose-sensing and gastric distension sensitive neurons in rat dorsal vagal complex. Journ. 2008;146(1-3):169-75.

[116] Sun Y, Asnicar M, Smith RG. Central and peripheral roles of ghrelin on glucose homeostasis. Journ. 2007;86(3):215-28.

[117] Barazzoni R, Zanetti M, Ferreira C, Vinci P, Pirulli A, Mucci M, et al. Relationships between desacylated and acylated ghrelin and insulin sensitivity in the metabolic syndrome. Journ. 2007;92(10):3935-40.

[118] Vartiainen J, Rajala U, Jokelainen J, Keinanen-Kiukaanniemi S, Kesaniemi YA, Ukkola O. Serum ghrelin and the prediction of the development of impaired glucose regulation and Type 2 diabetes in middle-aged subjects. Journ. 2010;33(7):496-500.

[119] Schofl C, Horn R, Schill T, Schlosser HW, Muller MJ, Brabant G. Circulating ghrelin levels in patients with polycystic ovary syndrome. Journ. 2002;87(10):4607-10.

[120] Murata M, Okimura Y, Iida K, Matsumoto M, Sowa H, Kaji H, et al. Ghrelin modulates the downstream molecules of insulin signaling in hepatoma cells. Journ. 2002;277(7):5667-74.

[121] Dezaki K, Sone H, Yada T. Ghrelin is a physiological regulator of insulin release in pancreatic islets and glucose homeostasis. Journ. 2008;118(2):239-49.

[122] Broglio F, Arvat E, Benso A, Gottero C, Muccioli G, Papotti M, et al. Ghrelin, a natural GH secretagogue produced by the stomach, induces hyperglycemia and reduces insulin secretion in humans. Journ. 2001;86(10):5083-6.

[123] Kojima M, Hosoda H, Matsuo H, Kangawa K. Ghrelin: discovery of the natural endogenous ligand for the growth hormone secretagogue receptor. Journ. 2001;12(3):118-22.

[124] Tschop M, Smiley DL, Heiman ML. Ghrelin induces adiposity in rodents. Journ. 2000;407(6806):908-13.

[125] Gauna C, Delhanty PJ, Hofland LJ, Janssen JA, Broglio F, Ross RJ, et al. Ghrelin stimulates, whereas des-octanoyl ghrelin inhibits, glucose output by primary hepatocytes. Journ. 2005;90(2):1055-60.

[126] Zsombok A, Smith BN. Plasticity of central autonomic neural circuits in diabetes. Journ. 2009;1792(5):423-31.

[127] German JP, Thaler JP, Wisse BE, Oh IS, Sarruf DA, Matsen ME, et al. Leptin activates a novel CNS mechanism for insulin-independent normalization of severe diabetic hyperglycemia. Journ. 2010;152(2):394-404.

[128] Honmura A, Yanase M, Saito H, Iguchi A. Effect of intrahypothalamic injection of neostigmine on the secretion of epinephrine and norepinephrine and on plasma glucose level. Journ. 1992;130(5):2997-3002.

[129] Iguchi A, Burleson PD, Szabo AJ. Decrease in plasma glucose concentration after microinjection of insulin into VMN. Journ. 1981;240(2):E95-100.

[130] Trayhurn P, Hoggard N, Mercer JG, Rayner DV. Leptin: fundamental aspects. Journ. 1999;23 Suppl 1:22-8.

[131] Ruhl CE, Everhart JE. Leptin concentrations in the United States: relations with demographic and anthropometric measures. Journ. 2001;74(3):295-301.

[132] de Lecea L, Kilduff TS, Peyron C, Gao X, Foye PE, Danielson PE, et al. The hypocretins: hypothalamus-specific peptides with neuroexcitatory activity. Journ. 1998;95(1):322-7.

[133] Sakurai T, Amemiya A, Ishii M, Matsuzaki I, Chemelli RM, Tanaka H, et al. Orexins and orexin receptors: a family of hypothalamic neuropeptides and G protein-coupled receptors that regulate feeding behavior. Journ. 1998;92(5):1 page following 696.

[134] Bittencourt JC, Presse F, Arias C, Peto C, Vaughan J, Nahon JL, et al. The melanin-concentrating hormone system of the rat brain: an immuno- and hybridization histochemical characterization. Journ. 1992;319(2):218-45.

[135] Date Y, Nakazato M, Matsukura S. [A role for orexins and melanin-concentrating hormone in the central regulation of feeding behavior]. Journ. 2001;59(3):427-30.

[136] Kastin AJ, Pan W. Dynamic regulation of leptin entry into brain by the blood-brain barrier. Journ. 2000;92(1-3):37-43.

[137] Schwartz MW, Peskind E, Raskind M, Boyko EJ, Porte D, Jr. Cerebrospinal fluid leptin levels: relationship to plasma levels and to adiposity in humans. Journ. 1996;2(5):589-93.

[138] Caro JF, Kolaczynski JW, Nyce MR, Ohannesian JP, Opentanova I, Goldman WH, et al. Decreased cerebrospinal-fluid/serum leptin ratio in obesity: a possible mechanism for leptin resistance. Journ. 1996;348(9021):159-61.

[139] Kolaczynski JW, Ohannesian JP, Considine RV, Marco CC, Caro JF. Response of leptin to short-term and prolonged overfeeding in humans. Journ. 1996;81(11):4162-5.

[140] Kieffer TJ, Heller RS, Habener JF. Leptin receptors expressed on pancreatic beta-cells. Journ. 1996;224(2):522-7.

[141] Emilsson V, Liu YL, Cawthorne MA, Morton NM, Davenport M. Expression of the functional leptin receptor mRNA in pancreatic islets and direct inhibitory action of leptin on insulin secretion. Journ. 1997;46(2):313-6.

[142] Wauters M, Considine RV, Yudkin JS, Peiffer F, De Leeuw I, Van Gaal LF. Leptin levels in type 2 diabetes: associations with measures of insulin resistance and insulin secretion. Journ. 2003;35(2):92-6.

[143] Wellhoener P, Fruehwald-Schultes B, Kern W, Dantz D, Kerner W, Born J, et al. Glucose metabolism rather than insulin is a main determinant of leptin secretion in humans. Journ. 2000;85(3):1267-71.

[144] Sonnenberg GE, Krakower GR, Hoffmann RG, Maas DL, Hennes MM, Kissebah AH. Plasma leptin concentrations during extended fasting and graded glucose infusions: relationships with changes in glucose, insulin, and FFA. Journ. 2001;86(10):4895-900.

[145] Seufert J. Leptin effects on pancreatic beta-cell gene expression and function. Journ. 2004;53 Suppl 1:S152-8.

[146] Kamohara S, Burcelin R, Halaas JL, Friedman JM, Charron MJ. Acute stimulation of glucose metabolism in mice by leptin treatment. Journ. 1997;389(6649):374-7.

[147] Pravdova E, Macho L, Fickova M. Alcohol intake modifies leptin, adiponectin and resistin serum levels and their mRNA expressions in adipose tissue of rats. Journ. 2009;43(3):117-25.

[148] Srinivasan K, Ramarao P. Animal models in type 2 diabetes research: an overview. Journ. 2007;125(3):451-72.

[149] Chan JL, Moschos SJ, Bullen J, Heist K, Li X, Kim YB, et al. Recombinant methionyl human leptin administration activates signal transducer and activator of transcription 3 signaling in peripheral blood mononuclear cells in vivo and regulates soluble tumor necrosis factor-alpha receptor levels in humans with relative leptin deficiency. Journ. 2005;90(3):1625-31.

[150] Higgins SC, Gueorguiev M, Korbonits M. Ghrelin, the peripheral hunger hormone. Journ. 2007;39(2):116-36.

[151] Kalra SP, Dube MG, Pu S, Xu B, Horvath TL, Kalra PS. Interacting appetite-regulating pathways in the hypothalamic regulation of body weight. Journ. 1999;20(1):68-100.

[152] Bowers CY. Unnatural growth hormone-releasing peptide begets natural ghrelin. Journ. 2001;86(4):1464-9.

[153] Shintani M, Ogawa Y, Ebihara K, Aizawa-Abe M, Miyanaga F, Takaya K, et al. Ghrelin, an endogenous growth hormone secretagogue, is a novel orexigenic peptide that antagonizes leptin action through the activation of hypothalamic neuropeptide Y/Y1 receptor pathway. Journ. 2001;50(2):227-32.

[154] Korbonits M, Goldstone AP, Gueorguiev M, Grossman AB. Ghrelin--a hormone with multiple functions. Journ. 2004;25(1):27-68.

[155] Banks WA, Tschop M, Robinson SM, Heiman ML. Extent and direction of ghrelin transport across the blood-brain barrier is determined by its unique primary structure. Journ. 2002;302(2):822-7.

[156] Ueno H, Yamaguchi H, Kangawa K, Nakazato M. Ghrelin: a gastric peptide that regulates food intake and energy homeostasis. Journ. 2005;126(1-2):11-9.

[157] Cowley MA, Smith RG, Diano S, Tschop M, Pronchuk N, Grove KL, et al. The distribution and mechanism of action of ghrelin in the CNS demonstrates a novel hypothalamic circuit regulating energy homeostasis. Journ. 2003;37(4):649-61.

[158] Nakazato M, Murakami N, Date Y, Kojima M, Matsuo H, Kangawa K, et al. A role for ghrelin in the central regulation of feeding. Journ. 2001;409(6817):194-8.

[159] Kamegai J, Tamura H, Shimizu T, Ishii S, Sugihara H, Wakabayashi I. Chronic central infusion of ghrelin increases hypothalamic neuropeptide Y and Agouti-related protein mRNA levels and body weight in rats. Journ. 2001;50(11):2438-43.

[160] Toshinai K, Date Y, Murakami N, Shimada M, Mondal MS, Shimbara T, et al. Ghrelin-induced food intake is mediated via the orexin pathway. Journ. 2003;144(4):1506-12.

Section 3

Dietary Constituents and Insulin Resistance

Chapter 8

Importance of Dietary Fatty Acid Profile and Experimental Conditions in the Obese Insulin-Resistant Rodent Model of Metabolic Syndrome

Annadie Krygsman

Additional information is available at the end of the chapter

http://dx.doi.org/10.5772/53805

1. Introduction

Obesity is currently regarded as one of the most alarming pandemic diseases worldwide as it is closely related to, and in many cases causative of, Type 2 Diabetes (T2D), coronary heart disease (CHD), cancer and other pathophysiological disturbances. A cluster of these disorders are linked together under the term Metabolic Syndrome (MetS). These factors include impaired glucose tolerance and/or insulin resistance, dyslipidemia (high plasma levels of triglycerides and low density lipoproteins), central obesity and hypertension [1]. In the USA a recent Health and Nutrition Examination Survey (NHANES) reported that 68.3% of study subjects were considered as overweight (BMI ≥ 25) and 33.9% obese (BMI ≥ 30) [2]. The rising incidence of childhood obesity and T2D, high blood pressure, hyperinsulinemia and dyslipidemia are particularly worrisome as these children often mature to be obese adults [3]. This risk of developing obesity and T2D has largely been blamed on the increased consumption of energy dense foods and fat intake, particularly saturated fat, but it is interesting to know that the mean fat intake of the human population has not increased much in the past 50 years [4]. It is true that the vast advancement in technological developments has led to a reduction in physical activity worldwide, but as obesity now involves infants and the populations of developing countries [5], this obesity pandemic cannot be attributed to this alone. In addition, laboratory and other domesticated animals have also been subject to the increased prevalence of obesity, despite having largely unchanged living conditions for many years [5].

Obesity and MetS have nevertheless been blamed on excess intake of fat leading to excess energy intake exceeding energy expenditure, which causes the deposition of this energy in the format of greater numbers of excessively enlarged fat cells. When this fat deposition occurs in the central trunk (visceral fat accumulation) it is highly causative and suggestive of the risk of developing MetS, due to associated high levels of blood cholesterol and triglycerides [6]. It is especially dietary saturated fat acid (SFA) consumption that has been thought to lead to the elevation of these blood factors which are highly indicative of CHD risk. Most recently, through meta-analyses of large international studies, the consumption of SFA has been de-vilified and the causal link between these parameters and CHD disproven [7-9]. The question thus arises which changes in the dietary composition in the past half-century is causing this obesogenic outcome? Although the total fat content of the diet has not changed significantly, a growing number of reports are making it quite clear that the dietary fatty acid quality may be responsible for the differential influence on obesity and pathophysiological outcome.

The main alteration within the fatty acid profile of the modern diet has been the increased use of vegetable oil, both as a cheaper and more accessible alternative to animal fats, but also as a substitute to animal fats to reduce the intake of SFAs. Vegetable oils, although higher in monounsaturated fatty acids, are very high in omega-6 fatty acids (100-fold larger) compared with animal fat [10]. These oils are also much lower in omega-3 fatty acids, leading to an increase in the ratio of dietary omega-6:omega-3 fatty acids. In the past few years a growing number of studies and meta-analyses have focused on the influence of dietary omega-6:omega-3 ratio, and the role of omega-3 fatty acids in the development of T2D and CHD [11-13] and a clear link between a high ratio of omega-6:omega-3 fatty acids and the development of these pathologies illustrated (Fig. 1). These effects are, to a large extent, believed to be due to the pro-inflammatory functions of the omega-6 arachidonic acid (AA) cascade which has deleterious effects in a variety of tissues due to chronic low-grade systemic inflammation. This inflammatory environment is now considered a key component of MetS, as the enlarged adipocytes are known to secrete many relevant pre-inflammatory adipokines [14]. These pro-inflammatory adipokines are to a great extent responsible for insulin resistance, hallmarked by decreased fatty acid oxidation and an increase in triglyceride and free fatty acid (FFA) synthesis. These FFAs are then deposited within the adipocytes, leading to and worsening obesity and the perpetual further effect on metabolic dysregulation of fat and glucose homeostasis. Conversely, the omega-3 fatty acids eicosapentanoic acid (EPA) and docohexanoic acid (DHA) have anti-inflammatory properties, and serve as protection against MetS and CHD [15]. In adipocytes, these omega-3 fatty acids prevent insulin resistance mediated by the AA-induced increase in pro-inflammatory eicosanoids, via modulation of adiponectin levels and function [16-18]. This positive effect can only occur when an excess of omega-6 fatty acids is not present, as high levels of omega-6 fatty acids prevent the synthesis of omega-3 fatty acids in tissues [19], and it is thus arguable whether supplementation or dietary increase of omega-3 fatty acids would effectively attenuate the deleterious effects of omega-6 mediated inflammatory mechanisms without a decrease in the intake of omega-6 fatty acids [20-22].

Close scrutiny of the modern Western diet in epidemiological studies have brought to attention the role of the fatty acid profile of certain native and regional diets in the prevention of the development of MetS and all of its associated symptoms [8, 9, 23, 24]. In populations consuming diets rich in omega-3 fatty acids, the prevalence of impaired glucose tolerance and CHD is much lower than those populations consuming the Western diet.

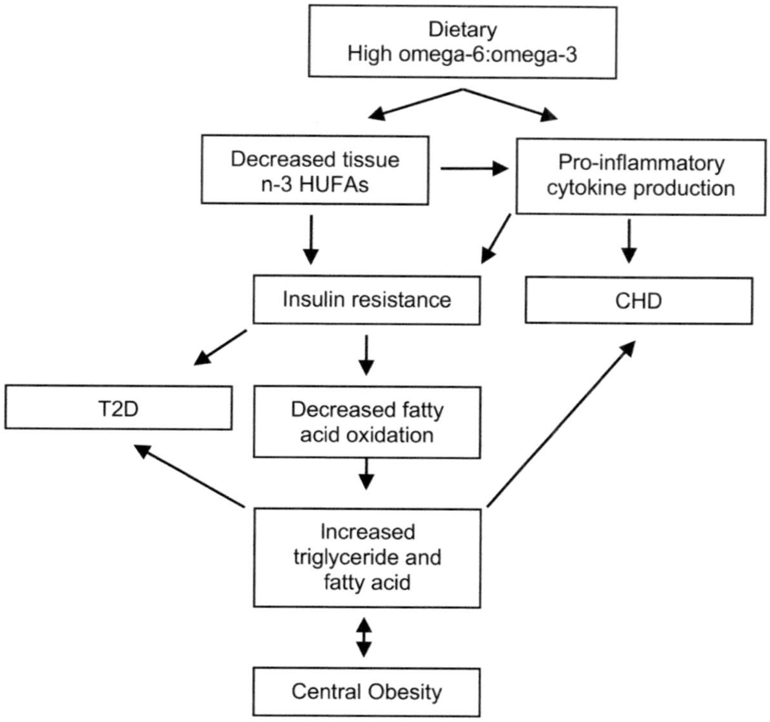

Figure 1. The role of dietary omega-6:omega-3 ratio on the development of obesity, T2D and CHD.

Japanese island-dwellers and Alaskan natives, who adopt the Western diets through migration, forsake the consumption of their native high omega-3 foods in lieu of high omega-6 Western foods leading to as much as an 80% increase in T2D. Icelandic natives have a very low incidence of T2D, despite their high prevalence of overweight and obesity [25], found to be due to an inverse association with the omega-3 content of reindeer milk, and thus positively associated with its omega-6:omega-3 fatty acid ratio. Furthermore, Icelandic animal fodder contains fish meal which greatly reduces the omega-6:omega-3 content of the milk, and this provides a protective factor against MetS and T2D. This is contrast to other Norwegian countries, as well the rest of the Western world, where animal fodder contains high amounts of omega-6 fatty acids.

Animal feeds were also subject to the change from a low to high omega-6 content with the incorporation of vegetable oils, and this has led to and increase in obesity in domestic and laboratory animals [5]. Laboratory animals, whose housing and husbandry practices have no changed much in the last 50 years, now have a much increased mid-life bodyweight.

This is proposed to be due to the substitution of dietary fat source from lard to soy bean oil (or soy meal) and hence the omega-6:omega-3 ratio has increased from 2:1 to 12.5:1 [26]. This is very concerning as these feeds serve as control and maintenance diets and are utilized in most rodent research colonies worldwide. Maternal programming is a well-described field, especially in the development of T2D, and animals exposed to pro-diabetic diets during pregnancy give rise to offspring with a higher propensity of developing metabolic perturbations [27]. The 'control' diet used in the majority of studies thus in fact may represent a high omega-6 treatment diet, which casts a degree of doubt on the accuracy of results obtained from such experiments. More careful scrutiny and transparency of rodent dietary composition is needed in order to make valid comparisons with other dietary interventions in the study of MetS components.

Animal models of MetS are not only influenced by dietary fatty acid composition, and other husbandry-associated factors such as day/night cycle and time-of-day experimental procedures can also influence the outcome of such studies. Rodents, by nature, are nocturnally active animals, but sampling and experimental procedures commonly take place in the day time which is the inactive rest phase of these animals. The circadian clock, which is regulated by daylight exposure, plays a critical role in many physiological processes associated with insulin, fatty acid and glucose metabolism. In the rat, insulin levels are low during its inactive diurnal phase, and high during the nocturnal phase with high glucose utilization [28]. Sampling of blood and performance of glucose tolerance tests usually take place in the morning, as it represents the most convenient time for the scientist, following a 6-12 h overnight fast during the animal's active phase. This causes a rapid fall in blood glucose levels, whereas fasting during the day in the animal's rest phase causes a much less significant drop in blood glucose levels. In addition, stress induction due to this food deprivation, causes a rise in corticosteroid levels which mobilizes fatty acids from triglyceride stores [29] giving an inaccurate reflection of the blood levels of these compounds. This of course is not desirable in an experimental setting and undue bias is incorporated. A solution is to reverse the light-dark cycle, so that all animal procedures are carried out during the animal's active phase. This creates the most effective scenario, but is critically dependent on the absence of dark-phase light contamination, as even dim light during the dark phase causes the inhibition of the circadian rhythms in blood glucose, lactic acid, insulin and corticosteroid levels [29] which would compromise or alter the outcome of scientific investigations.

Creating and using accurate and comparable models for research into MetS and associated CHD is essential in providing relevant and applicable data that may be extended to human disease state research. Basic principles such as dietary composition and fatty acids profile, together with appropriate husbandry practices are thus of major importance in the design an execution of research studies using animal models. This chapter will endeavor to highlight some of the crucial aspects surrounding dietary fat composition and use of the rodent model of diet-induced obesity and metabolic syndrome.

2. Role of omega-6 and omega-3 fatty acids in insulin resistance and CHD

Fatty acids are important sources of fuel as they yield large quantities of ATP when metabolized and the heart and skeletal muscle prefer fatty acids to glucose as fuel [30]. Fatty acids consist of a long aliphatic chain with a carboxylic acid group at one end and may be saturated or unsaturated (those that contain no double bonds are saturated, and those that have double bonds are unsaturated). The biological reactivity of these compounds are dependent on both the length of the fatty acid chains as well as the number and positional location of double bonds prevalent (n-3, n-6, n-7 and n-9). An 18-carbon fatty acid containing two or more double bonds is referred to as being polyunsaturated fatty acids (PUFA), whereas fatty acids consisting of 20 or 22 carbons are termed highly unsaturated fatty acids (HUFA). It is especially the n-3 and n-6 HUFA that are considered to be major role-players affecting diet-dependent disease. These fatty acids are responsible for maintaining correct cell membrane protein function and fluidity and cellular functioning. The more highly unsaturated fatty acids, such as the n-6 arachidonic acid, are converted to eicosanoid derivatives which have a hormone-like action and are involved inflammatory pathologies such as obesity, insulin resistance and atherosclerosis [31-33]. In contrast, the n-3 fatty acid-derived eicosanoids have anti-inflammatory and anti-thrombotic activities [34, 35]. It is this action of the n-6 derived eicosanoids that is of particular importance as they are major role-players in diet-associated pathologies through their pro-inflammatory actions (Fig. 2).

A number of studies, including the Seven Countries Study, have shown the Mediterranean Diet to be preventative of insulin resistance and CHD and protective against certain cancers [19, 36, 37]. This diet is characterized by a high intake of unsaturated fatty acids in the form of virgin olive oil containing a very low ratio of omega-6:omega-3 fatty acids (2:1). In these

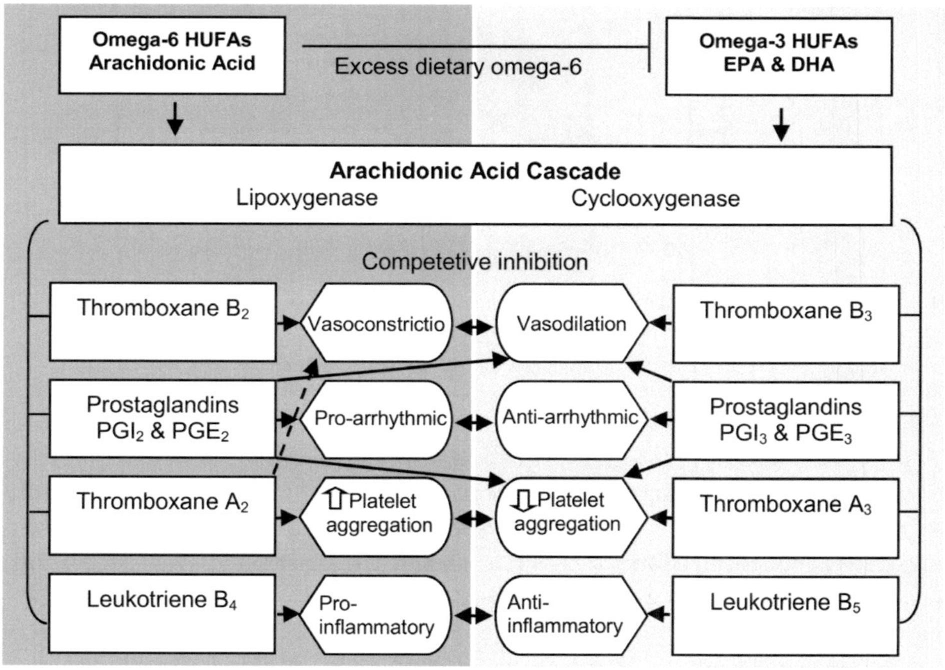

Figure 2. The effects of omega-6 vs. omega-3 conversion pathways on inflammation in coronary heart disease (adapted from [45])

studies, Western diets of non-Mediterranean countries (USA, Western Europe and Scandinavia), and containing omega-6:omega-3 fatty acid ratios in excess of 15:1, was associated with significant higher incidences of insulin resistance and CHD. More importantly, the lack of detrimental effect of SFA and cholesterol intake, in the presence of optimal omega-3 intake, was simultaneously indicated [38, 39], as was the failure to document a relationship between dietary cholesterol and CHD (reviewed by [9]). Reducing SFA intake or replacing SFA with MUFA was found to not improve cardiovascular risk [40, 41]. Moreover, blood cholesterol levels alone do not predict absolute CHD mortality rates observed for different groups worldwide (Fig. 3) and these death rates differ at each cholesterol level. In fact, the elevations in blood cholesterol are fatal only to the magnitude that omega-6 exceeds omega-3 in tissue HUFA [19]. It is thus not surprising that it has recently been proposed that omega-6 HUFA blood levels are more indicative of heart disease risk than total cholesterol level, where high omega-6 HUFA levels inhibits omega-3 synthesis [42, 43]. The authors of the 25-year follow-up of the Seven Countries Study considered factors affecting inflammatory oxidative processes and thrombosis to be of great importance [44].

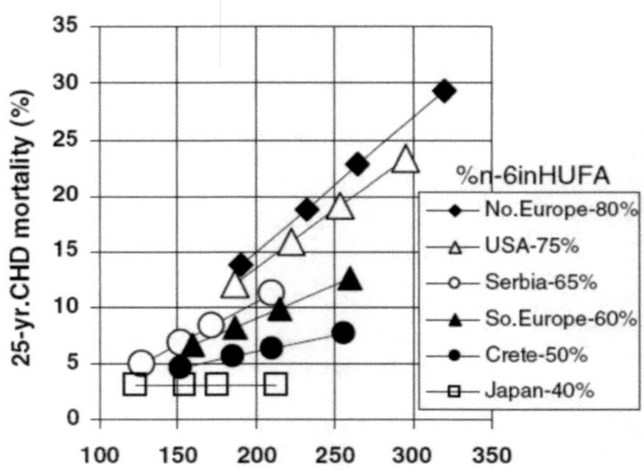

Figure 3. Dietary fatty acid imbalances which elevate blood cholesterol are fatal only to the magnitude that omega-6 exceeds omega-3 in tissue HUFA (From [19]).

Omega-6 fatty acids are further known to amplify post-prandial oxidative stress leading to these elevations in inflammatory vascular lesions and atherosclerosis. High percentages of HUFA in plasma and adipose tissue of obese children have been reported, associated with higher concentrations of inflammatory markers [46]. In contrast, omega-3 HUFAs prevent and reverse high fat diet-induced insulin resistance, in part via modulation of adipose tissue inflammatory product secretion patterns [11, 20, 47]. The omega-3 HUFAs act via different pathways to establish this protective effect by, amongst others, inhibiting the pro-inflammatory NFKB pathway due to its inhibition of SFA-activation of Toll like receptors (TLR) 2 and -4, with DHA being the most potent inhibitor of this pathway. The omega-3 HUFA EPA competes for cyclooxygenase and lipooxygenase enzymes in the AA cascade, and in this manner reduces the production of pro-inflammatory AA-derived eicosanoids.

Furthermore, EPA and DHA inhibits the release of AA by inhibiting phopholipase-A2, and thus also reduces activation of the pro-inflammatory AA-cascade [48]. Inflammation, mediated via AA-derived eicosanoids, also plays a critical role in the pathophysiology of atherosclerosis with coronary plaques being highly inflamed with a core rich in lipids [49]. Recently published studies reported that the blood plasma ratio of omega-6:omega-3 plays an important role in endothelial function and vascular tone, and that a high ratio is significantly associated with a high prevalence of coronary artery lesions [50]. The plasma EPA/AA ratio and high-sensitivity CRP levels were further found to be independent predictors of the presence of complex coronary lesion. In addition, the fact that omega-3 fatty acid supplementation improves endothelium-dependent vasodilation further supports the recommendation that modulation of dietary omega-6 and omega-3 fatty acids is a safe and necessary approach to improving vascular health and reducing the risk of CHD [51, 52].

3. Evolution of the omega-6:omega-3 fatty acid dietary ratio

Studies in Paleolithic nutrition and modern-day hunter-gatherer populations estimate that humans evolved on a diet that was much lower in saturated fatty acids than is today's diet, and contained small but roughly equal amounts of omega 6 and omega 3 fats [10]. The Paleolithic diet, also known as the Cave Man or Hunter-Gatherer diet, prevailed for about 2.5 million years and ended 10 000 years ago with the development of agriculture [53, 54]. These stone age humans centered their diet on foods that could be hunted and fished, such as meat, offal and seafood, and could be gathered, such as eggs, insects, fruit, nuts, seeds, vegetables, mushrooms, herbs and spices. The proportion of nutrients, although dependent on latitude and other influences, consisted of roughly 20-35% each protein and carbohydrates and 30-60% fat. Of the total food intake 45-65% came from animal products and 35-55% from plant products, but it is debatable whether any grains or tubers were consumed [54]. Omega-3 fatty acids were found in all of these foods, and a balance existed between omega-3 and omega-6 for this entire period. Hunters tended to target herbivores, and the total carcass fat of such animals averaged about 7% compared with domesticated beef cows 40%, and with 35% PUFA compared with the current 7% in grain-fed beef [55]. Carbohydrates nearly all came from fruit and vegetables, and a small proportion from honey [56], thus consisting overall of low glycemic load carbohydrates.

The modern human inherited characteristics by genetic adaptation accrued over millions of years of the Paleolithic Period, and the vast majority of our biochemistry and physiology are adapted to life conditions that existed prior to the advent of agriculture about 10 000 years ago. At this time humans began to cultivate plants and later to domesticate animals constituting the Agricultural Revolution leading to the Neolithic Period. The gradual spread of agriculture throughout the Old and New Worlds generally led to an increase in population, and demand for foodstuffs which soon led to difficulties in exploitation of game and wild plant food. The main dietary innovation that accompanied agriculture involved the introduction of cereal grains. Crop cultivation became necessary to supply in the increased demand for foodstuffs, leading to cereal grains becoming staple food – a departure from native nutrition unparalleled and unseen in other free-living primates of that period [57]. Before that time, early humans did recognize that grains could be consumed in times of shortage, but the labor involved in milling the grains discouraged frequent use. The almost 60% intake of fruits and vegetables soon declined to an estimated 20% of daily caloric intake, with cereal grains consumed in place thereof. Grains are high in omega-6 fatty acids and low in omega-3, and this led to the increased dietary ratio of omega-6:omega-3 (Fig 4).

Since this major change in the human diet, natural selection has had too little time to make the optimal genetic adaptations to the new dietary composition, leading to physiological and metabolic maladaptation [58]. These incomplete genetic changes are not seen in modern hunter-gatherer populations it is thus reasonable to conclude that humans are maladapted to diets of domesticated and processed plant foods, contributing too many of the current diseases of civilization. What has compounded these maladaptive consequences of the agricultural age, is the fact that the demand for meat in the past 50 years has led to the implementation of large cattle and poultry feedlots in order to provide in the increased demand for meat. Prior to that time, animals were pasture-reared and consumed a diet of green leaves high in the omega-3 fatty acid α-linolenic acid (ALA) resulting in a meat ratio of omega-6:omega-3 of 2:1, vs. 4:1 in grain-fed meat in beef and poultry as well as eggs. Cattle moved from pasture to feedlots for fattening prior to slaughter lose this valuable ALA store, as well as EPA and DHA with the supply diminishing each day the animal spends in the feedlot (Fig. 5 [59]).

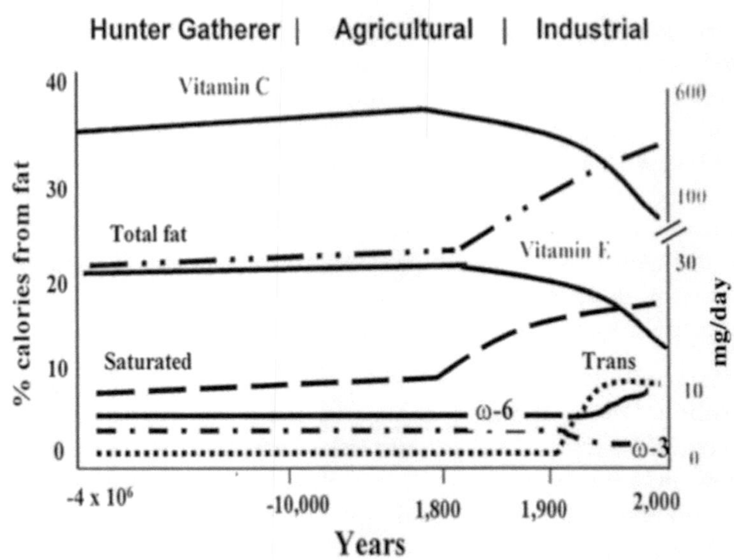

Figure 4. Change in dietary omega-6:omega-3 ratio from the Paleolithic Period to the current dietary composition [10].

In addition to the new emphasis on grain feeds for domestic livestock, the first part of the 20th century marked the onset of the industrial vegetable oil industry [60]. Technological advancements after World War I made large-scale production of vegetable oil more efficient and economic. With the advent of hydrogenation of oils to increase solidification, the ALA content was greatly reduced leaving a high concentration LA, and hence a high omega-6:omega-3 ratio, with similar changes in the production of other oils such as cottonseed oil, safflower oil and sunflower seed oil. Soy bean meal/oil forms the main constituent of livestock and poultry feed, shortening and margarine and it thus forms a large proportion of the average daily fat intake in most countries. These changes in the consumption of essential fatty acids throughout the 20th century was recently (2011) reported for the first time as a detailed quantitative analysis (Fig. 6 [61]). They found that the estimated consumption of soy bean oil increased in excess of 1000-fold from 1909 to 1999. This consequently led to a 3-fold increase in the intake of LA which was the primary determinant for the declining percentages of omega-3 HUFAs in tissue throughout the 20th century.

Animals have not been spared the fate of this deleterious dietary transformation, as presented in a very recent study which investigated the mid-life body weight of animal species living with or around humans in industrialized societies [5]. The authors found that the body weight of primates and rodents living in controlled laboratory environments, as well as feral rodents and domestic dogs and cats, has increased over the past few decades similarly to humans. Although in this study it was speculated that certain viral pathogens and epigenetic factors possibly could have contributed to this obesogenic effect, it is also highly likely that it could be due to the deleterious transformation to a high omega-6 intake in chow. As in the human diet, the fat content of chow has remained constant during the time period o.n which this study was focused.

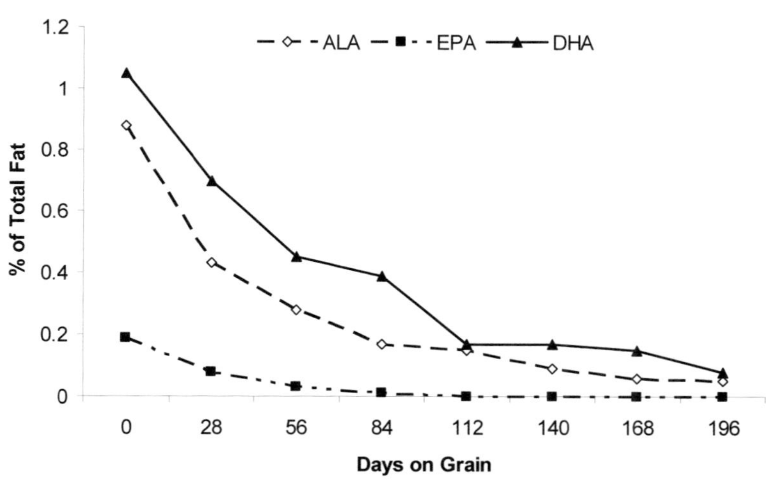

Figure 5. Rapid decline in fat-derived omega-3 stores of beef cattle receiving grain after being moved from pasture to feedlot (from [59])

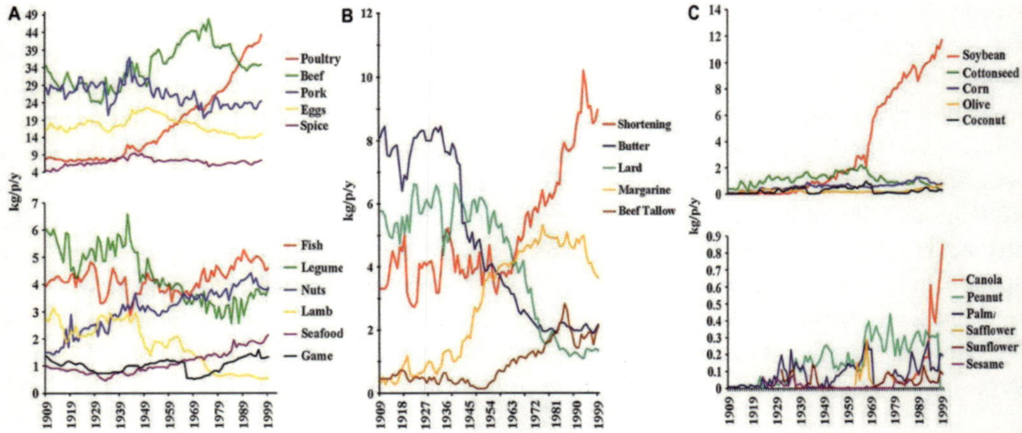

Figure 6. Changes in the estimated per capita consumption (kg/person/year) in the USA between 1909 and 1999 of A: of major food commodities; B: Major fat commodities; C: Vegetable and seed oils (from [61])

Indeed the fatty acid composition of standard rodent chow has changed similarly to that of humans, with comparable effects on the omega-6:omega-3 ratio [62-64]. Fifty years ago, laboratory chow fat content consisted of the lard of animals grazing on grass which had an omega-6:omega-3 of less than 6:1, but since then the omega6:omega-3 ratio in the control rodent diet has changed from 6:1 in 1998, to 9:1 in 2002, 12.5:1 in 2006 [26]. Standard high fat research diets now contain omega-6:omega-3 ratios in excess of 11:1 [51]. All maintenance diets contain soy bean oil as their main fat source with omega-6:omega-3 ratio of 8:1 which is much higher than lard produced from grass-reared beef at 2:1 used before the change to soy bean oil (Table 1). Hydrogenated soy bean oil produces severe insulin resistance [65], and is thus not suitable as a source of fat for rodent maintenance diets.

Fat/Oil	Omega-6:omega-3
Sunflower seed	Omega-6 only
Safflower	253:1
Corn	83:1
Lard	10:1
Soy Bean	8:1
Beef Tallow (Grain-fed)	8:1
Milk Fat (Grain-fed)	5:1
Beef Tallow (Grass-finished)	2:1
Canola	2:1
Milk Fat (Grass-finished)	1:1
Flax Seed	0.2:1

Table 1. Omega-6:omega-3 ratios of commonly-consumed fat sources in the USA [66, 67]

Although the evidence is now mounting and the clear link between excessive omega-6 intake and modern Western diseases of lifestyle established, formal dietary recommendations (Institute of Medicine, National Academies of Science), have not incorporated these alarming findings. Dietary Reference Intakes (Food and Nutrition Board) in 2006 recommended an adequate intake of omega-6:omega-3 of 10:1, a ratio now proven to be deleterious to especially cardiovascular health [67]. These recommended dietary intake guidelines are thus in urgent need of revision to include the levels and profiles based on the evidence now available in literature.

4. Rodent models for the study of insulin resistance and CHD

Model organisms have extensive value as sentinels informing us about environmental factors which may potentially have an impact on humans [68]. The severity of the obesity epidemic has created an urgent need to study the causes and progression of the pathologies associated therewith such as MetS. Animal models that sufficiently mimic all the aspects of this syndrome, including obesity, insulin resistance, dyslipidemia and hypertension are required for such studies.

A large variety of animal species have been used as models to study MetS, with varying degrees of success. The ideal model should be small and economical, but large enough to perform the required experimental procedures. Non-human primates are in many respects the ideal models as they are phylogenetically close to humans, consume a comparable omnivorous diet, and develop MetS and CHD as they age [69], but in addition to important ethical issues, they have an extended lifespan, are expensive to house and carry viral zoonoses dangerous to humans. Other animals, such as the domestic pig, the dog and the rabbit all provide potential as models for MetS and CHD research, but cost, cultural status and species-specific vulnerabilities to dietary modulation [70], place doubt on their efficacy for this research field. The rat, in particular, resembles the human both in physiology and metabolism, and follows an omnivorous diet similar to humans with whom the rat has spread worldwide [71]. Since the development of the first defined rat strain at the Wistar Institute in the 1920s, the rat has been used regularly and to great effectivity for the study of diet-induced obesity, insulin resistance and the disease states associated therewith, such as CHD [70, 72].

Standard laboratory rat species, such as the Wistar or Sprague-Dawley strains, are successfully utilized for diet-induced MetS models [73]. The diets aim at reproducing high fat diets (HFD) similar to what is ingested in the Westernized society, i.e. a high percentage total fat (of calories) with a high SFA content with or without high carbohydrate content. Varying combinations and amounts of carbohydrates and fats are used in different studies [72, 74, 75], with the carbohydrates fructose or sucrose standardly used, but the fat source varying. Long-term feeding of these diets induce obesity, increased abdominal fat deposition, hyperinsulinemia, hypertension and impaired glucose tolerance in most rat and mouse strains [76]. Fat fractions in these diets range between 20% and 60% of energy as fat as either animal-derived lard or beef tallow, or plant oils such as soy bean oil, coconut oil, olive oil, safflower oil [73]. The problem is that in many cases, these constituents or profile of the fatty acid element in the diet are not available, not taken into account or not reported in published literature. In fact, standard chow prepared by commercial companies contains fats obtained from a variety of sources, both animal and vegetable, which, considering the variation in omega-6:omega-3 fatty acid ratio between such foodstuffs can have far-reaching implications for the outcomes of studies employing these diets. This complicates the study of the effects of dietary fats on obesity and insulin resistance and associated disease states, and makes comparison between studies almost impossible. A rodent high fat diet high in SFA content, in the presence of a low omega-6:omega-3 ratio would not give the same results as a diet similar in total fat and SFA content, but with a high omega-6:omega-3 ratio. Even with low to moderate fat percentages (20-30%) in the presence of the recommended SFA content (10%), high omega-6:omega-3 ratios can lead to glucose intolerance in rodents indicated by decreased insulin response to intravenous glucose tolerance tests [77].

Rodent models share many traits with human diabetic cardiomyopathy, such as left ventricular hypertrophy, increased ventricular stiffness, ventricular dilatation, decreased fatty acid uptake, cardiac inflammation and fibrosis, decreased cardiac function and endothelial dysfunction [72]. In the Wistar rat the onset of cardiomyopathy occurs within 7 weeks of receiving the diet, and leads to cardiac steatosis, impaired contractile function and mitochondrial degeneration with increased myocardial fatty acid uptake [78]. Simple high fat feeding with caloric excess is thus sufficient to induce metabolic defects that area associated with diabetic cardiomyopathy, but isocaloric high fat diets based on saturated fats alone do not induce insulin resistance and in fact improve cardiac function [79, 80]. This could point to both the deleterious role of hyperinsulinemia and impaired glucose homeostasis on the development of cardiac defects due to the consumption of the Western Diet, or could indicate the failure to take into account the PUFA profile of said diets used in these studies.

It is worthy to note the normal rat is resistant to the development of atherosclerosis, and simple Western high fat diets do not induce atherosclerosis in these animals. Induction of atherosclerosis is less easily achieved, and generally requires addition of cholesterol to the animal's diet. Atherosclerosis can be induced by increasing the oxidized form of LDL in the blood by either increasing the total LDL while maintaining the proportion of oxidized LDL, or by increasing the proportion of oxidized LDL. Linoleic acid may be a factor in the susceptibility of LDL to oxidation as LDL is rich in LA, but the dietary content of LA differs in its ability to cause LDL oxidation depending on its effect on the blood lipid profile which in turn varies according to species. Saturated fat feeding only exacerbates an increase in LDL when excessive cholesterol is consumed, and in the absence of cholesterol SFA does not cause a rise in LDL both in rats and humans and atherosclerosis does not result [81] (reviewed in [82]).

Although rodent models play a very important role in, and indeed have advanced the understanding of the underlying pathological mechanisms of human MetS and CHD, these models do have limitation and none exist that exactly phenocopies the human MetS disease condition. By adding dietary inconsistencies these models cannot be used to their full potential and clear and transparent dietary formulations, which include the fatty acid profile, are crucial for providing comparable studies and thus results. Maintenance and Control diets should consist of the correct recommended balance of omega-6:omega-3 fatty acids to provide a 'healthy' model and control group as reference with which to compare dietary interventions.

5. The circadian clock in animal models of insulin resistance and fatty acid metabolism

Nutrient homeostasis in many species of vertebrates is intricately controlled by coordinated interactions of daily rhythms of activity and rest, feeding behavior and energy expenditure and storage across the daily 24h light-and-dark cycles [83]. This circadian clock, under the control of molecular mechanisms cycling in the suprachiasmatic nuclei (SCN) of the hypothalamus, plays a critical role in a diverse group of physiological processes in different cell types associated with insulin, glucose and fatty acid metabolism. The main factor responsible for synchronization of the circadian rhythm is sun light, which determines the precise length of the day and night in the 24 h period. This serves to orient the human or animal in relation to the point of day, and light is thus one of the most powerful synchronizers of the circadian rhythm. In the absence of pronounced SCN signals the circadian rhythm in peripheral tissues becomes uncoupled, resulting in aberrant cellular metabolism and disease risk [29, 83]. The changes in lifestyle during the past 50 years has, in addition to an increased intake of inappropriate, energy-dense and poor fat- and nutrient-quality foods, also led to increased time spent awake and hence disrupted pattern of eating, sleeping and physical activity. This causes an asynchrony with the circadian rhythm with profound effects on glucose and fatty acid metabolism, which is well-described in the human and linked to metabolic derangements associated with and leading to increased adiposity and BMI [84].

The main synchronizers of the peripheral circadian clocks are food restriction, glucocorticoids and melatonin [85]. Of the peripheral tissues, the adipose tissue circadian clock plays a fundamental role in glucose and lipid metabolism [86, 87]. Any disturbances of the adipocyte circadian clock van alter adipocyte responsiveness to different stimuli, i.e. levels of glucose, insulin and fatty acids, and can alter the level of lipogenesis and lipolysis. The adipokine, adiponectin, which plays an important role in insulin sensitivity, inflammation and fatty acid oxidation, presents a circadian rhythm similar to insulin, with peak levels in the early active phase and low levels in the inactive phase (Table 2). The early hours of the active phase are characterized by higher glucose levels and thus higher insulin demand in anticipation of the onset of stimulus [88-90]. At the end of the active phase and the start of the rest phase, insulin levels and sensitivity are low and oral or intravenous glucose (or consumption of a meal) leads to a significantly higher plasma glucose response. Accordingly, rodents respond differently by day and night to insulin and 2-deoxy-D-glucose with a rapid fall in blood glucose levels occurring at the end of the active phase after a 6h overnight fast in contrast to delayed and diminished hypoglycemia following a day time (inactive phase) fast [89]. Furthermore, the circulating FFA levels follow the same circadian pattern as glucose and are low in the active phase and high in the inactive phase in both humans and rats, with an increased turnover present in humans with T2D [90, 91]. The role of adiponectin in FFA, insulin and glucose metabolism in context of the circadian rhythm is shown in Figure 7. Under normal condition, i.e. healthy diet and daily sleep-wake cycle, adiponectin levels are high in the early active phase which stimulates AMPK, resulting in increased fatty acid oxidation and energy yield, with resultant low triglyceride levels. Adiponectin also upregulates PI3K which further downstream contributes to the improvement and optimization of insulin action, thus counteracting any pro-obesogenic and insulin-resistance inducing effects.

	Active phase	**Inactive phase**
Glucose	Low	High
Insulin	High	Low
FFAs	Low	High
- Omega-6	Low	High
- Omega-3	High	Low
- Eicosanoids	High	Low
Adiponectin	High	Low
O-GlcNAc	High	Low

Table 2. Circadian pattern of compounds involved in the regulation metabolic processes linked with metabolic homeostasis related to the development of insulin resistance and CHD. [88, 92-94].

Both obesity and dysregulated circadian rhythms can profoundly modulate adiponectin from various perspectives, all which may have bearing on the application of the rodent model of insulin resistance. Peak levels of corticosteroids occur at the start of the active/dark phase, and then fall during the light/inactive phase, reaching the lowest level just before the dark/light transition. Any stressor experienced at this time, be it anxiety, starvation, fear or pain would cause an increase in corticosteroid levels and hence release of FFAs from fat stores.

The circadian rhythm of specific PUFAs is largely lacking in literature, and to our knowledge, only one study has been published in which the daily variation of omega-6 and omega-3 fatty acid levels was reported [94]. In this study only preliminary evidence is presented, but the fact that a differential circadian rhythm for these fatty acids was identified is of great possible importance and deserves further exploration. This also supports earlier findings that a circadian rhythm for eicosanoid production exists, with low levels during the inactive phase and high levels present during the active phase [92]. In light of the fact the plasma FFA profile represents the dietary FFA profile [77], it is likely that the levels omega-6 HUFAs will be increased when a diet high in omega-6 fatty acids is followed. As arachidonic acid, via NFkB and eicosanoid conversions products, causes a suppression of adiponectin, this would exaggerate and amplify the pro-diabetic, insulin resistance and hyperglycemic propensity of the hormonal profile of the inactive phase. This further suppression of adiponectin, already low at the active/inactive phase transition,

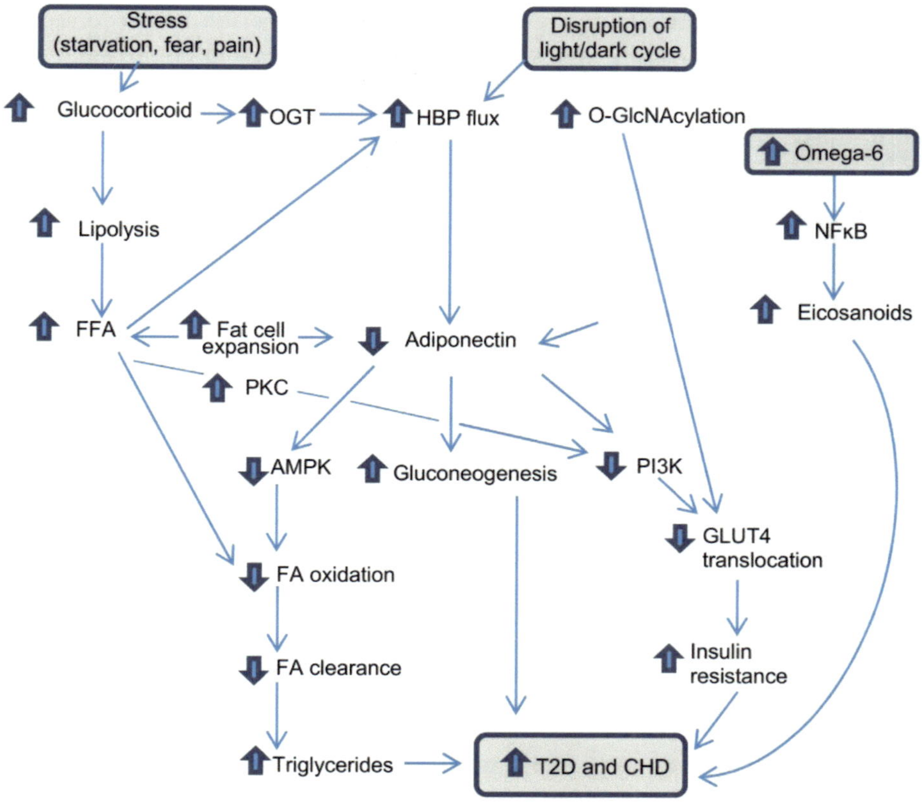

Figure 7. A simplified representation of the interrelation of obesity, circadian rhythm disruption and dietary fatty acid intake on development of metabolic perturbations related to T2D and CHD.

would lead to down regulation of AMPK and hence increased triglyceride levels due to decreased fatty acid oxidation and clearance. Furthermore, this would ultimately lead to hyperglycemia due to the increased fatty acid-induced flux through the hexosamine biosynthetic pathway (HBP) which further decreases adiponectin levels, and thus increases its stimulating effect on liver gluconeogenesis.

It is known that a glucose-fatty acid cycle operates in the heart and diaphragm muscle by decreasing the rate of oxidation of the alternative substrate in the presence of increased availability of the other substrate [95, 96]. In the presence of high circulating levels of FFAs, a decrease in the rate of carbohydrate oxidation is seen, and vice versa when high circulating levels of glucose prevail. It is in this context that the HBP serves as a nutrient-sensing mechanism and both excess FFA and glucose can lead to augmented flux through this pathway, which ultimately plays a role in causing insulin resistance in the adipocyte, liver, muscle and pancreatic β-cell via reduced recruitment and translocation of GLUT4 to the plasma membrane [97, 98]. In the presence of excess FFA, glycolysis is inhibited distal to fructose-6-phosphate by increased levels of acetyl-CoA, leading to inhibition of pyruvatedehydrogenase, which in turn increases fructose-6-phosphate availability and thus increased flux via catalyzation of glutamine:fructose 6-phosphate amido transferase (GFAT). This ultimately leads to accumulation of uridine-5′-disphospho-N-acetylglucosamine (UDP-GlcNAc) levels in tissues and this is directly correlated with the degree of insulin resistance. UDP-GlcNAc is the end product of the HBP, and serves as a substrate for O-linked glycosylation (O-GlcNAc) of proteins. It is thus regarded as the mediator of the HBP flux and thus insulin resistance by posttranslational protein modification of the insulin receptor proteins (IRS-1 and IRS-2) as well as GLUT4 (reviewed in [99]). There have, however, been conflicting reports in literature in which the lipid supplement Intralipid (a fat emulsion used intravenously as source of calories for patients requiring extended periods of parenteral nutrition regarded as 'safe' by the FDA) was found to induce insulin resistance without increasing HBP products [100], but as Intralipid consists mainly of soy bean oil with a ratio of omega-6:omega-3 of 7:1 [101] it is likely that insulin resistance was mediated mainly through the pro-inflammatory effects of the arachidonic acid cycle (Fig. 7) and to a lesser extent via flux through the HBP. Circulating FFAs also invoke insulin resistance via upregulation of PKC/PTEN which has an inhibitory effect on IRS-1 and IRS-2, which then further downstream prevents translocation of GLUT4 to the plasma membrane due to downregulation of PI3K [102]. This places increased emphasis on the critical need of clear definition of the profile of fats used in research studies, as it is probable that high levels of omega-6 fatty acids have a differential influence on these metabolic pathways in addition to being intricately involved in the circadian time structure of organisms.

In the heart, the cardiomyocyte circadian clock, in a time-of-day-dependent manner, regulates metabolism and ischemic tolerance similar to the regulatory roles of that of protein O-GlcNAcylation [93]. These variations mediate the clock-dependent regulation of O-GlcNAc transferase and O-GlcNAcase levels and nutrient metabolism and uptake. This would involve the coordinated regulation of the hexosamine biosynthetic pathway and play an important role in not only insulin resistance [103] but also myocardial apoptosis in the diet-induced insulin resistant rat [104] which in turn conversely depends critically on an adequate dark-phase. Any stress could increase flux through the HBP, leading to detrimental effects on the level of the cardiomyocyte [29, 104]. As the O-GlcNAcylation of proteins show clear circadian patterns and is high during the active phase and low during the inactive phase, it is thus proposed to have major consequences in the rat model of insulin resistance [93]. Any stress in the rodents during the inactive phase or at the transition from the active to inactive phase, as frequently is the case due to overnight starvation and early morning sampling, would lead to an increase in glucocorticoid levels which not only causes increased lipolysis and FFA levels, but also leads to inappropriately increased O-GlcNAcylation via direct recruitment of OGT [105]. Peak levels of corticosteroids occur at the start of the dark phase, and then fall during the light phase reaching the lowest level just before dark-light transition. Early morning sampling would thus possibly induce bias, due to the stress associated with starving and experimental procedures imposed on the animal.

A remedy for the deleterious introduction of bias, due to researcher convenience-of-sampling time, is to reverse the light-dark cycle, so that all animal handling and procedures are carried out during the animal's active phase. This constitutes the most effective scenario, but is exclusively dependent on the absence of dark-phase light contamination. Even dim light during the dark phase causes the inhibition of the circadian rhythms in blood glucose, lactic acid, insulin and corticosteroid levels [29] and would compromise or alter the outcome of scientific investigations.

6. Conclusions

In summary, this chapter described the importance of the dietary fatty acid profile, with particular reference to the ratio of omega-6:omega-3 essential fatty acids, and the role it plays in insulin-resistance with reference specifically to the utilization of animal research models. Fatty acids are well-known to play a cardinal role in lipid and glucose homeostasis, and there is now compelling evidence that a reduction in the intake of omega-6 fatty acids in the diet is crucial to prevent disease states such as insulin resistance, obesity and cardiovascular disease. The majority of studies in the field of diet-induced obesity are performed using the high fat rodent model, but consistency and comparability is severely lacking/compromised due to incomplete disclosure of dietary fat components, and in many cases uncontrolled variation in the diet due to rat chow manufacturers using different fat sources according to availability or personal preference. In addition, the importance of the circadian rhythm in fatty acid and glucose metabolism and metabolic disturbances in the rodent experimental model is underemphasized, and in many cases not taken into account. This too, is of concern in the accuracy of results expressed in such studies, especially those investigating dietary interventions in insulin resistance, as seen in the regulative role that the humoral factors and the hexosamine biosynthetic pathway plays the circadian clock of insulin, glucose and fatty acid metabolism. These points highlight some frequently overlooked aspects in the experimental use of the diet-induced rodent model for insulin resistance, T2D and CHD research. In order to utilize the model to its full potential, attention to the exact dietary composition and experimental conditions are of critical importance.

Author details

Annadie Krygsman
Department of Physiological Sciences, Stellenbosch University, Stellenbosch, South Africa

Acknowledgement

The author wishes to thank Prof Eugene Cloete, Dean of the Faculty of Science (now Vice-Rector Research and Innovation), Stellenbosch University, for funding of the publishing costs, and also Mr Danzil Joseph for review and expert input in the HBP section.

7. References

[1] Alberti, KG, P Zimmet, and J Shaw, Metabolic syndrome--a new world-wide definition. A Consensus Statement from the International Diabetes Federation. Diabet Med, 2006; 23(5) p 469-80.

[2] Flegal, KM, et al., Prevalence and trends in obesity among US adults, 1999-2008. JAMA, 2010; 303(3) p 235-41.

[3] Grundy, SM, The changing face of cardiovascular risk. J Am Coll Cardiol, 2005; 46(1) p 173-5.

[4] Nguyen, DM and HB El-Serag, The epidemiology of obesity. Gastroenterol Clin North Am, 2010; 39(1) p 1-7.

[5] Klimentidis, YC, et al., Canaries in the coal mine: a cross-species analysis of the plurality of obesity epidemics. Proc Biol Sci, 2011; 278(1712) p 1626-32.

[6] Bjorntorp, P, Metabolic implications of body fat distribution. Diabetes Care, 1991; 14(12) p 1132-43.

[7] Jakobsen, MU, et al., Major types of dietary fat and risk of coronary heart disease: a pooled analysis of 11 cohort studies. Am J Clin Nutr, 2009; 89(5) p 1425-32.

[8] Siri-Tarino, PW, et al., Saturated fat, carbohydrate, and cardiovascular disease. Am J Clin Nutr, 2010; 91(3) p 502-9.

[9] McNamara, DJ, Dietary cholesterol and blood cholesterolemia: a healthy relationship. World Rev Nutr Diet, 2009; 100 p 55-62.

[10] Simopoulos, AP, Evolutionary aspects of the dietary omega-6:omega-3 fatty acid ratio: medical implications. World Rev Nutr Diet, 2009; 100 p 1-21.

[11] Griffin, BA, How relevant is the ratio of dietary n-6 to n-3 polyunsaturated fatty acids to cardiovascular disease risk? Evidence from the OPTILIP study. Curr Opin Lipidol, 2008; 19(1) p 57-62.

[12] Ramsden, CE, et al., n-6 fatty acid-specific and mixed polyunsaturate dietary interventions have different effects on CHD risk: a meta-analysis of randomised controlled trials. Br J Nutr, 2010; 104(11) p 1586-600.

[13] Wijendran, V and KC Hayes, Dietary n-6 and n-3 fatty acid balance and cardiovascular health. Annu Rev Nutr, 2004; 24 p 597-615.

[14] Makowski, L and GS Hotamisligil, The role of fatty acid binding proteins in metabolic syndrome and atherosclerosis. Curr Opin Lipidol, 2005; 16(5) p 543-8.

[15] Chapkin, RS, et al., Dietary docosahexaenoic and eicosapentaenoic acid: emerging mediators of inflammation. Prostaglandins Leukot Essent Fatty Acids, 2009; 81(2-3) p 187-91.

[16] Storlien, LH, AJ Hulbert, and PL Else, Polyunsaturated fatty acids, membrane function and metabolic diseases such as diabetes and obesity. Curr Opin Clin Nutr Metab Care, 1998; 1(6) p 559-63.

[17] Mori, Y, et al., Effect of highly purified eicosapentaenoic acid ethyl ester on insulin resistance and hypertension in Dahl salt-sensitive rats. Metabolism, 1999; 48(9) p 1089-95.

[18] Kuda, O, et al., n-3 fatty acids and rosiglitazone improve insulin sensitivity through additive stimulatory effects on muscle glycogen synthesis in mice fed a high-fat diet. Diabetologia, 2009; 52(5) p 941-51.

[19] Lands, B, A critique of paradoxes in current advice on dietary lipids. Prog Lipid Res, 2008; 47(2) p 77-106.

[20] Griffin, MD, et al., Effects of altering the ratio of dietary n-6 to n-3 fatty acids on insulin sensitivity, lipoprotein size, and postprandial lipemia in men and postmenopausal women aged 45-70 y: the OPTILIP Study. Am J Clin Nutr, 2006; 84(6) p 1290-8.

[21] Giacco, R, et al., Insulin sensitivity is increased and fat oxidation after a high-fat meal is reduced in normal-weight healthy men with strong familial predisposition to overweight. Int J Obes Relat Metab Disord, 2004; 28(2) p 342-8.

[22] Giacco, R, et al., Fish oil, insulin sensitivity, insulin secretion and glucose tolerance in healthy people: is there any effect of fish oil supplementation in relation to the type of background diet and habitual dietary intake of n-6 and n-3 fatty acids? Nutr Metab Cardiovasc Dis, 2007; 17(8) p 572-80.

[23] Kagawa, Y, et al., Eicosapolyenoic acids of serum lipids of Japanese islanders with low incidence of cardiovascular diseases. J Nutr Sci Vitaminol (Tokyo), 1982; 28(4) p 441-53.

[24] Schraer, CD, et al., The Alaska Native diabetes program. Int J Circumpolar Health, 2001; 60(4) p 487-94.

[25] Thorsdottir, I, J Hill, and A Ramel, Omega-3 fatty acid supply from milk associates with lower type 2 diabetes in men and coronary heart disease in women. Prev Med, 2004; 39(3) p 630-4.

[26] Strandvik, B, The omega-6/omega-3 ratio is of importance! Prostaglandins Leukot Essent Fatty Acids, 2011; 85(6) p 405-6.

[27] Cerf, ME and J Louw, High fat programming induces glucose intolerance in weanling Wistar rats. Horm Metab Res, 2010; 42(5) p 307-10.

[28] Larue-Achagiotis, C and J Le Magnen, Fast-induced changes in plasma glucose, insulin and free fatty acid concentration compared in rats during the night and day. Physiol Behav, 1983; 30(1) p 93-6.

[29] Dauchy, RT, et al., Dark-phase light contamination disrupts circadian rhythms in plasma measures of endocrine physiology and metabolism in rats. Comp Med, 2010; 60(5) p 348-56.

[30] Kemppainen, J, et al., Myocardial and skeletal muscle glucose uptake during exercise in humans. J Physiol, 2002; 542(Pt 2) p 403-12.

[31] Harizi, H, JB Corcuff, and N Gualde, Arachidonic-acid-derived eicosanoids: roles in biology and immunopathology. Trends Mol Med, 2008; 14(10) p 461-9.

[32] Horrillo, R, et al., 5-lipoxygenase activating protein signals adipose tissue inflammation and lipid dysfunction in experimental obesity. J Immunol, 2010; 184(7) p 3978-87.

[33] Oliver, E, et al., The role of inflammation and macrophage accumulation in the development of obesity-induced type 2 diabetes mellitus and the possible therapeutic effects of long-chain n-3 PUFA. Proc Nutr Soc, 2010; 69(2) p 232-43.

[34] Blok, WL, et al., Dietary fish-oil supplementation in experimental gram-negative infection and in cerebral malaria in mice. J Infect Dis, 1992; 165(5) p 898-903.

[35] Tai, ES, et al., Insulin resistance is associated with a metabolic profile of altered protein metabolism in Chinese and Asian-Indian men. Diabetologia, 2010; 53(4) p 757-67.

[36] Keys, A, Mediterranean diet and public health: personal reflections. Am J Clin Nutr, 1995; 61(6 Suppl) p 1321S-1323S.

[37] Dolecek, TA and G Granditis, Dietary polyunsaturated fatty acids and mortality in the Multiple Risk Factor Intervention Trial (MRFIT). World Rev Nutr Diet, 1991; 66 p 205-16.
[38] Ravnskov, U, Cholesterol was healthy in the end. World Rev Nutr Diet, 2009; 100 p 90-109.
[39] Garemo, M, RA Lenner, and B Strandvik, Swedish pre-school children eat too much junk food and sucrose. Acta Paediatr, 2007; 96(2) p 266-72.
[40] Tierney, AC, et al., Effects of dietary fat modification on insulin sensitivity and on other risk factors of the metabolic syndrome--LIPGENE: a European randomized dietary intervention study. Int J Obes (Lond), 2011; 35(6) p 800-9.
[41] Jebb, SA, et al., Effect of changing the amount and type of fat and carbohydrate on insulin sensitivity and cardiovascular risk: the RISCK (Reading, Imperial, Surrey, Cambridge, and Kings) trial. Am J Clin Nutr, 2010; 92(4) p 748-58.
[42] Lands, B, Measuring blood fatty acids as a surrogate indicator for coronary heart disease risk in population studies. World Rev Nutr Diet, 2009; 100 p 22-34.
[43] Gibson, RA, et al., Docosahexaenoic acid synthesis from alpha-linolenic acid is inhibited by diets high in polyunsaturated fatty acids. Prostaglandins Leukot Essent Fatty Acids, 2012.
[44] Verschuren, WM, et al., Serum total cholesterol and long-term coronary heart disease mortality in different cultures. Twenty-five-year follow-up of the seven countries study. JAMA, 1995; 274(2) p 131-6.
[45] Robinson, JG and NJ Stone, Antiatherosclerotic and antithrombotic effects of omega-3 fatty acids. Am J Cardiol, 2006; 98(4A) p 39i-49i.
[46] Savva, SC, et al., Association of adipose tissue arachidonic acid content with BMI and overweight status in children from Cyprus and Crete. Br J Nutr, 2004; 91(4) p 643-9.
[47] Kalupahana, NS, et al., Eicosapentaenoic acid prevents and reverses insulin resistance in high-fat diet-induced obese mice via modulation of adipose tissue inflammation. J Nutr, 2010; 140(11) p 1915-22.
[48] Fedor, D and DS Kelley, Prevention of insulin resistance by n-3 polyunsaturated fatty acids. Curr Opin Clin Nutr Metab Care, 2009; 12(2) p 138-46.
[49] Kashiyama, T, et al., Relationship between coronary plaque vulnerability and serum n-3/n-6 polyunsaturated fatty acid ratio. Circ J, 2011; 75(10) p 2432-8.
[50] Yoshimoto, M, et al., In vivo SPECT imaging with 111In-DOTA-c(RGDfK) to detect early pancreatic cancer in a hamster pancreatic carcinogenesis model. J Nucl Med, 2012; 53(5) p 765-71.
[51] Harlan Laboratories. Teklad Research Diets. http://www.harlan.com/products_and_services/research_models_and_services/laboratory_animal_diets[accessed 12 July 2012]
[52] Khan, S, et al., Dietary long-chain n-3 PUFAs increase LPL gene expression in adipose tissue of subjects with an atherogenic lipoprotein phenotype. J Lipid Res, 2002; 43(6) p 979-85.

[53] Lindeberg, S, [Paleolithic diet and evolution medicine: the key to diseases of the western world]. Lakartidningen, 2005; 102(26-27) p 1976-8.

[54] Cordain, L, et al., Origins and evolution of the Western diet: health implications for the 21st century. Am J Clin Nutr, 2005; 81(2) p 341-54.

[55] Qureshi, AI, et al., Regular egg consumption does not increase the risk of stroke and cardiovascular diseases. Med Sci Monit, 2007; 13(1) p CR1-8.

[56] Eaton, SB, The ancestral human diet: what was it and should it be a paradigm for contemporary nutrition? Proc Nutr Soc, 2006; 65(1) p 1-6.

[57] Milton, K, Diet and primate evolution. Sci Am, 1993; 269(2) p 86-93.

[58] Eaton, SB, M Konner, and M Shostak, Stone agers in the fast lane: chronic degenerative diseases in evolutionary perspective. Am J Med, 1988; 84(4) p 739-49.

[59] Johnson, J. Health benefits of grass farming. www.americangrassfedbeef.com/grass-fed-natural-beef.asp[accessed 12 July 2012]

[60] Kirschenbauer, HG, Fats and oils : an outline of their chemistry and technology. 2nd ed. ed. 1960, New York: Reinhold ; London : Chapman and Hall.

[61] Blasbalg, TL, et al., Changes in consumption of omega-3 and omega-6 fatty acids in the United States during the 20th century. Am J Clin Nutr, 2011; 93(5) p 950-62.

[62] Korotkova, M, et al., Maternal dietary intake of essential fatty acids affects adipose tissue growth and leptin mRNA expression in suckling rat pups. Pediatr Res, 2002; 52(1) p 78-84.

[63] Korotkova, M, et al., Gender-related long-term effects in adult rats by perinatal dietary ratio of n-6/n-3 fatty acids. Am J Physiol Regul Integr Comp Physiol, 2005; 288(3) p R575-9.

[64] Palsdottir, V, et al., Postnatal deficiency of essential fatty acids in mice results in resistance to diet-induced obesity and low plasma insulin during adulthood. Prostaglandins Leukot Essent Fatty Acids, 2011; 84(3-4) p 85-92.

[65] Cunha, TM, et al., A cascade of cytokines mediates mechanical inflammatory hypernociception in mice. Proc Natl Acad Sci U S A, 2005; 102(5) p 1755-60.

[66] Daley, CA, et al., A review of fatty acid profiles and antioxidant content in grass-fed and grain-fed beef. Nutr J, 2010; 9 p 10.

[67] Dietary Reference Intakes: The Essential Guide to Nutrient Requirements, ed. JJ Otten, JP Hellwig, and LD Meyers. 2006: The National Academies Press.

[68] van der Schalie, WH, et al., Animals as sentinels of human health hazards of environmental chemicals. Environ Health Perspect, 1999; 107(4) p 309-15.

[69] Hannah, JS, et al., Changes in lipoprotein concentrations during the development of noninsulin-dependent diabetes mellitus in obese rhesus monkeys (Macaca mulatta). J Clin Endocrinol Metab, 1991; 72(5) p 1067-72.

[70] Russell, JC and SD Proctor, Small animal models of cardiovascular disease: tools for the study of the roles of metabolic syndrome, dyslipidemia, and atherosclerosis. Cardiovasc Pathol, 2006; 15(6) p 318-30.

[71] Orr, MW and WH McNeill, Plagues and peoples, William H. McNeill. Touchstone (Nashv), 1988;(12) p 3-5.

[72] Panchal, SK and L Brown, Rodent models for metabolic syndrome research. J Biomed Biotechnol, 2011; 2011 p 351982.

[73] Buettner, R, et al., Defining high-fat-diet rat models: metabolic and molecular effects of different fat types. J Mol Endocrinol, 2006; 36(3) p 485-501.

[74] Lomba, A, et al., Obesity induced by a pair-fed high fat sucrose diet: methylation and expression pattern of genes related to energy homeostasis. Lipids Health Dis, 2010; 9 p 60.

[75] Chun, MR, et al., Differential effects of high-carbohydrate and high-fat diet composition on muscle insulin resistance in rats. J Korean Med Sci, 2010; 25(7) p 1053-9.

[76] Sweazea, KL, M Lekic, and BR Walker, Comparison of mechanisms involved in impaired vascular reactivity between high sucrose and high fat diets in rats. Nutr Metab (Lond), 2010; 7 p 48.

[77] Krygsman, A, et al., Development of glucose intolerance in Wistar rats fed low and moderate fat diets differing in fatty acid profile. Exp Clin Endocrinol Diabetes, 2010; 118(7) p 434-41.

[78] Ouwens, DM, et al., The role of epicardial and perivascular adipose tissue in the pathophysiology of cardiovascular disease. J Cell Mol Med, 2010; 14(9) p 2223-34.

[79] Rennison, JH, et al., Enhanced acyl-CoA dehydrogenase activity is associated with improved mitochondrial and contractile function in heart failure. Cardiovasc Res, 2008; 79(2) p 331-40.

[80] Rennison, JH, et al., Prolonged exposure to high dietary lipids is not associated with lipotoxicity in heart failure. J Mol Cell Cardiol, 2009; 46(6) p 883-90.

[81] Nishina, PM, et al., Atherosclerosis and plasma and liver lipids in nine inbred strains of mice. Lipids, 1993; 28(7) p 599-605.

[82] Guyenet, SJ. The Diet-Heart Hypothesis: Oxidized LDL, Part I http://wholehealthsource.blogspot.com/2009/07/diet-heart-hypothesis-oxidized-ldl-part.html[accessed 12 July 2012]

[83] Reiter, RJ, Potential biological consequences of excessive light exposure: melatonin suppression, DNA damage, cancer and neurodegenerative diseases. Neuro Endocrinol Lett, 2002; 23 Suppl 2 p 9-13.

[84] Vorona, RD, et al., Overweight and obese patients in a primary care population report less sleep than patients with a normal body mass index. Arch Intern Med, 2005; 165(1) p 25-30.

[85] Damiola, F, et al., Restricted feeding uncouples circadian oscillators in peripheral tissues from the central pacemaker in the suprachiasmatic nucleus. Genes Dev, 2000; 14(23) p 2950-61.

[86] Zvonic, S, et al., Characterization of peripheral circadian clocks in adipose tissues. Diabetes, 2006; 55(4) p 962-70.

[87] Loboda, A, et al., Diurnal variation of the human adipose transcriptome and the link to metabolic disease. BMC Med Genomics, 2009; 2 p 7.

[88] Bolli, GB and JE Gerich, The "dawn phenomenon"--a common occurrence in both non-insulin-dependent and insulin-dependent diabetes mellitus. N Engl J Med, 1984; 310(12) p 746-50.

[89] Shih, KC, et al., Effect of reversing dark-light cycles on normal diurnal variation and related metabolic disturbance in rats. Chin J Physiol, 2007; 50(2) p 69-76.

[90] Stavinoha, MA, et al., Diurnal variations in the responsiveness of cardiac and skeletal muscle to fatty acids. Am J Physiol Endocrinol Metab, 2004; 287(5) p E878-87.

[91] Miles, JM, et al., Nocturnal and postprandial free fatty acid kinetics in normal and type 2 diabetic subjects: effects of insulin sensitization therapy. Diabetes, 2003; 52(3) p 675-81.

[92] Hoffmann, P, et al., Circadian rhythm of eicosanoid formation as affected by dietary linoleate. Prostaglandins Leukot Med, 1986; 25(2-3) p 91-103.

[93] Durgan, DJ, et al., O-GlcNAcylation, novel post-translational modification linking myocardial metabolism and cardiomyocyte circadian clock. J Biol Chem, 2011; 286(52) p 44606-19.

[94] Cornelissen, G, Galli, C., Halberg, F., De Meester, F., Rise, P., Circadian time structure of fatty acids and vascular monitoring. J Appl Biomed, 2010; 8 p 93-109.

[95] Randle, PJ, et al., The glucose fatty-acid cycle. Its role in insulin sensitivity and the metabolic disturbances of diabetes mellitus. Lancet, 1963; 1(7285) p 785-9.

[96] Randle, PJ, et al., The glucose fatty acid cycle in obesity and maturity onset diabetes mellitus. Ann N Y Acad Sci, 1965; 131(1) p 324-33.

[97] Cooksey, RC, et al., Mechanism of hexosamine-induced insulin resistance in transgenic mice overexpressing glutamine:fructose-6-phosphate amidotransferase: decreased glucose transporter GLUT4 translocation and reversal by treatment with thiazolidinedione. Endocrinology, 1999; 140(3) p 1151-7.

[98] Hazel, M, et al., Activation of the hexosamine signaling pathway in adipose tissue results in decreased serum adiponectin and skeletal muscle insulin resistance. Endocrinology, 2004; 145(5) p 2118-28.

[99] Buse, MG, Hexosamines, insulin resistance, and the complications of diabetes: current status. Am J Physiol Endocrinol Metab, 2006; 290(1) p E1-E8.

[100] Choi, CS, FN Lee, and JH Youn, Free fatty acids induce peripheral insulin resistance without increasing muscle hexosamine pathway product levels in rats. Diabetes, 2001; 50(2) p 418-24.

[101] Innis, SM, Effect of total parenteral nutrition with linoleic acid-rich emulsions on tissue omega 6 and omega 3 fatty acids in the rat. Lipids, 1986; 21(2) p 132-8.

[102] Boden, G, Obesity and free fatty acids. Endocrinol Metab Clin North Am, 2008; 37(3) p 635-46, viii-ix.

[103] Cooksey, RC and DA McClain, Increased hexosamine pathway flux and high fat feeding are not additive in inducing insulin resistance: evidence for a shared pathway. Amino Acids, 2011; 40(3) p 841-6.

[104] Rajamani, U, et al., The hexosamine biosynthetic pathway can mediate myocardial apoptosis in a rat model of diet-induced insulin resistance. Acta Physiol (Oxf), 2011; 202(2) p 151-7.

[105] Li, MD, et al., O-GlcNAc transferase is involved in glucocorticoid receptor-mediated transrepression. J Biol Chem, 2012; 287(16) p 12904-12.

Chapter 9

Intestinal Disaccharidase Activity and Uptake of Glucose from Sucrose

Kia Halschou Hansen, Klaus Bukhave and Jens Rikardt Andersen

Additional information is available at the end of the chapter

http://dx.doi.org/10.5772/53099

1. Introduction

Postprandial hyperglycemia is now established as an independent risk factor for the development of at least macro vascular complications in diabetes mellitus (1), as it is a widely accepted experience that it is more difficult to normalize postprandial blood glucose than the fasting concentrations. Furthermore, it is well known that impaired glucose tolerance (IGT) is related to increased cardiovascular morbidity and mortality (2) and that postprandial hyperglycemia plays a central role in progression from IGT to type 2 diabetes (3). It is possible to delay the appearance of type 2 diabetes and cardiovascular diseases in IGT patients by good glycemic control (4-8). The glycemic load as well as peak concentrations of glucose in the blood depend on many factors including gastric emptying, the nature of ingested food, intraluminal glucose concentration, and enzymatic activity in the brush border. On top of this several gut hormones play a role as well as the ability of the liver to reduce endogenous glucose production, being a special problem in patients with type 2 diabetes. This phenomenon increases the importance of reducing postprandial glucose uptake in type 2 diabetics. In addition, it seems possible to modify the insulin secretion after meals by addition of arabinose to the ingested sucrose (9). Sucrose contains equal amounts of glucose and fructose molecules. The absorption and metabolism of the two molecules is different. The absorbed glucose is utilized in an insulin dependent manner primarily in the peripheral tissues. Fructose is utilized in the liver in the glycolytic pathway with products like glucose, glycogen, lactate and pyruvate. Fructose is more lipogenic than glucose, an effect that might contribute to the development of cardiovascular diseases (CVD), insulin resistance and type 2 diabetes (10). Fructose does not stimulate insulin secretion as glucose why a modest intake of fructose is recomended in diabetes and heart patients due to the lipogenicity (10;11). Recently, a metaanalysis stated that fructose intake at a level of ≤ 36g/d, which is equivalent to daily intake of fruit, could have beneficial effects by decreasing endogenous glucose production and increasing glycogen synthesis, and thereby improve glycaemic control. This benefit is seen without the adverse cardiometabolic effects reported when fructose is ingested in high doses or as excess energy (12).

2. Disaccharidase activity *in vitro*

The digestive enzymes, α-amylase and α-glucosidase are the key enzymes responsible for the digestion of carbohydrates to glucose. In search for modulators and/or inhibitors of disaccharidases various *in vitro* models for determination have been described in the literature. These represent quick and cheap screening procedures and include among others intestinal mucosa homogenates (13;14), intestinal brush border preparations (15) from different experimental animals, and homogenates of human intestinal cell line Caco-2 (9). The Caco-2 cells were originally derived from a human colon adenocarcinoma. In culture they proliferate and differentiate to cells resembling mature jejunocytes with high levels of brush-border enzyme activity including alkaline phosphatase, amino-peptidase, and sucrase-isomaltase (16). Although the Caco-2 cells are derived from colonic cells they represent human tissue and are thereby superior to animal tissue in relation to human studies. For kinetic studies on disaccharidase activity an *in vitro* model with homogenates of Caco-2 cells was established. Caco-2 cells from passage number 38 and 39 were seeded onto polycarbonate membranes (Fisher Scientific, Transwell®membrane, 75mm) and cultured at 37°C and 5/95% CO_2/air. At day 20-22, when the transepithelial electrical resistance (TEER) has reached a steady state level of 3-400 Ω*cm^2, the Caco-2 cells were rinsed with phosphate buffered saline, scraped off the membranes, and homogenized by sonication. Homogenates

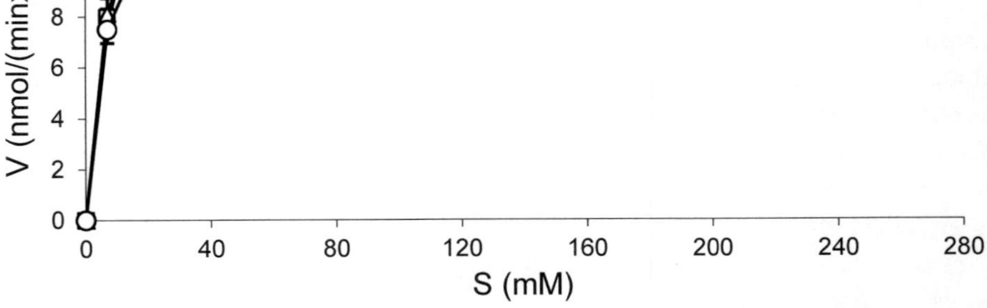

Figure 1. Michaelis-Menten curves for the substrate (sucrose) concentrations 0 – 280 mM with and without L-arabinose as inhibitor of sucrase (0.0mM (x), 0.84mM (□), 1.4mM (Δ) and 2.8mM (○)). Data are mean±SEM (n=6). S is the substrate concentration and V is the velocity of the reaction. (Reproduced from Krog-Mikkelsen et al (2) with permission).

corresponding to 2.2 mg protein/mL and disaccharide solutions at final concentrations of 7, 14, 28, 140, and 280 mM in 0.1 M maleate buffer, pH=6.0 were used. The amount of glucose released by the enzymatic reaction was linear with time up to 60 min, so a 30 min reaction time was used and glucose measured with a Cobas Mira Plus Spectrophotometer (Roche Diagnostic Systems, F Hoffmann-La Roche, Basel, Switzerland). Pentoses like L-arabinose and D-xylose were used as inhibitors at final concentrations of 0.84, 1.4, and 2.8 mM as exemplified with Michaelis-Menten curves for L-arabinose in fig 1 and Lineweaver-Burk plots in fig 2 (9).

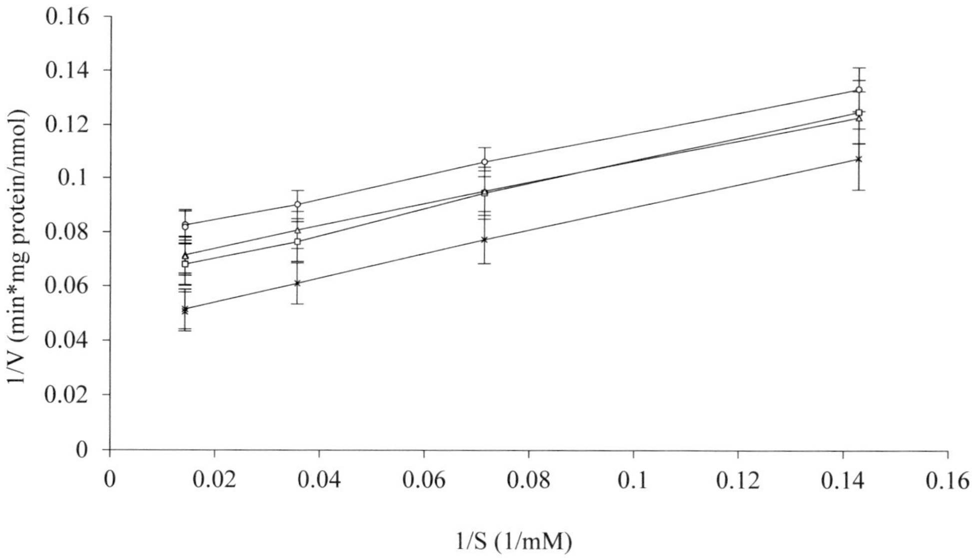

Figure 2. Lineweaver-Burk plots with and without L-arabinose as inhibitor of sucrase (0.0mM (x), 0.84mM (□), 1.4mM (Δ) and 2.8mM (○)). Data are mean±SEM (n=6). (Reproduced from Krog-Mikkelsen et al (2) with permission.)

Reaction velocity (v) plotted against substrate concentration (s) revealed classical Michaelis-Menten kinetics and demonstrated significant inhibition by increasing amounts of L-arabinose (fig 1) Lineweaver-Burke analysis (fig 2) indicated uncompetitive inhibition since V_{max} decreased from 19.8 over 14.7 and 14.1 to 12.2 nmol/(min*mg protein), and K_m decreased from 9.8 over 7.3 and 6.1 to 5.3 mmol/L when the inhibitor concentrations increased from zero over 0.84 and 1.4 to 2.8 mM L-arabinose (data not shown). Thus, addition of 0.84, 1.4, and 2.8 mM L-arabinose resulted in 25, 29 and 38% inhibition of the sucrase activity, respectively at V_{max}. The apparent K_i was calculated to 2.8±0.3 mM (mean±SEM, n=3) from the Lineweaver-Burke plots (2).

Similar results were obtained with sucrose as substrate and D-xylose as inhibitor, and with maltose as substrate and L-arabinose as inhibitor (data not shown).

The validity of the *in vitro* model was confirmed in a human intervention study with 15 healthy volunteers in a randomized double-blinded cross-over study. Sucrose beverages (75 g in 300 mL) supplemented with 0, 1, 2, or 3 g (0, 1.3, 2.7 and 4 w/w%, respectively) L-arabinose were tested (2). Blood was collected fasting and for 3-h postprandial with 15 minute intervals, and plasma glucose and serum insulin measured (fig 3 and 4).

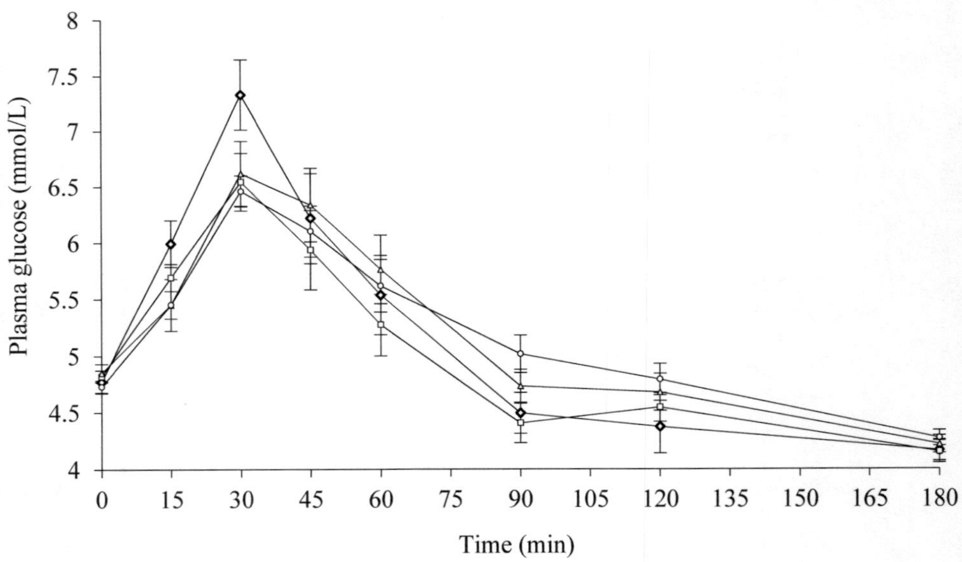

Figure 3. Plasma glucose in 15 normal male subjects after intake of sucrose drinks supplemented with 0 (x), 1(□), 2 (Δ), or 3 (○) grams of L-arabinose. Data are mean (± SEM). iAUC = incremental area under the curve. Statistical differences Peak, P=0.001. Time to peak, P=0.133. iAUC, P=0.245. (Reproduced from Krog-Mikkelsen et al (9) with permission.)

The present *in vivo* results in man strongly indicate that the Caco-2 cell model is useful in screening procedures in search for compounds which may lower the glycemic and insulimic responses in man. Importantly, because the Caco-2 cell line is of human origin, the results are more relevant for human physiology than studies with experimental animals.

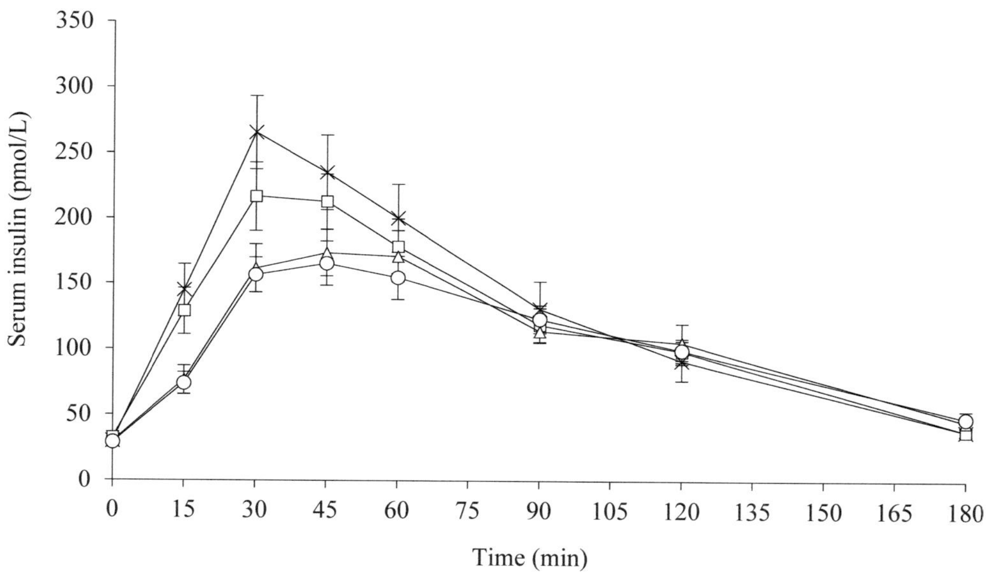

Figure 4. Serum insulin in 15 normal male subjects after intake of sucrose drinks supplemented with 0 (x), 1 (□), 2 (Δ), or 3 (○) grams of L-arabinose. Data are mean (± SEM). Statistical differences Peak, P<0.0001. Time to peak, P=0.002. iAUC, P=0.017. (Reproduced from Krog-Mikkelsen et al (9) with permission.)

3. The inhibition of the uptake of maltose and sucrose by food components

In addition to the pentoses L-arabinose and D-xylose growing evidence indicates that various dietary polyphenols may influence carbohydrate metabolism. Several efforts are made to identify new possible α-glucosidase inhibitors and interest in replacement of synthetic foods by natural ones has fostered research on vegetable sources and screening of raw materials to identify these α-glucosidase inhibitors (17-20). Polyphenols are abundant micronutrients in our diet, found in plants foods like fruits, vegetables, tea, coffee, red wine, and cacao. Studies with polyphenolic compounds, polyphenolic extracts of foods including berries, vegetables and colored grains such as black rice, green and black tea, and red wine have been shown to inhibit α-glucosidase activities and there by suppress the elevation of blood glucose concentrations when tested in especially small rodents (18). Additionally, different cell lines like Caco 2 cells mentioned above have been used *in vitro*. The inhibitory polyphenols includes flavonoids, phenolic acids, tannins (18). For example gallic acid and tannic acid have showed to be potential inhibitors of sucrase and other brush border enzymes in mice and rat (15;21;22). Extracts of acerola fruit have been studied and shows reduced plasma glucose level after oral administration of maltose or sucrose in mice, indicating inhibition of α-glucosidase effects on both sucrase and maltase in mice intestines (23-25). A hot water extract of leaves of *Nerium Indicum*, a bush from Pakistan, was found to reduce the rise in postprandial blood glucose when maltose and sucrose was given orally in rats. It was found that the extract inhibited α-glycosidase, suggesting the isolated polyphenols from the leaves extract, chlorogenic acid, to be the inhibitor of maltase and sucrose (26).

4. Sugar beets

The nutritional value of sucrose is to provide calories; nevertheless some studies have found that in the process of refining sugar from sugar beets and sugar cane some of the by products like pulp and molasses are important sources of bioactive compounds (polyphenols and pentoses). A study with sugar beet pulp revealed that the pulp contained polyphenolic compounds and had antioxidant properties (27;28). The same has been shown in studies with sugar cane products (29). The sugar beet molasses contains a variety of different phenolic acids mostly vanillic acid, syringic acid, p-coumaric acid, gallic acid, protocatechuic acid and ferulic acid the most abundant.

For kinetic studies of sucrase activity, we used the aforementioned assay (2). As inhibitors two different polyphenol-rich fractions from chromatographic separation of molasses from sugar beets and pure ferulic acid were used. Results from the kinetic studies of EDC molasses, fraction III-2 molasses and pure ferulic acid (obtained from Nordic Sugar Denmark) are represented in figure 5-7.

There were no inhibitory effects of EDC molasses or fraction III-2. Ferulic acid showed a week inhibition of 1.9 % for the concentration of 1 mM (Unpublished data). The variability of polyphenol content in foods is pronounced and in most cases, foods contain complex mixtures of polyphenols. The content is influenced by numerous factors such as variety, production practices at a particular processing plant, environmental factors and by storage variables. Even though, molasses contain a variety of different phenolic acids and pure ferulic acid inhibition of sucrose activity was weak at a relatively low concentration. This indicates that there are still much to learn about the potential bioactivities and the bioavailabilities of polyphenolic compounds (30).

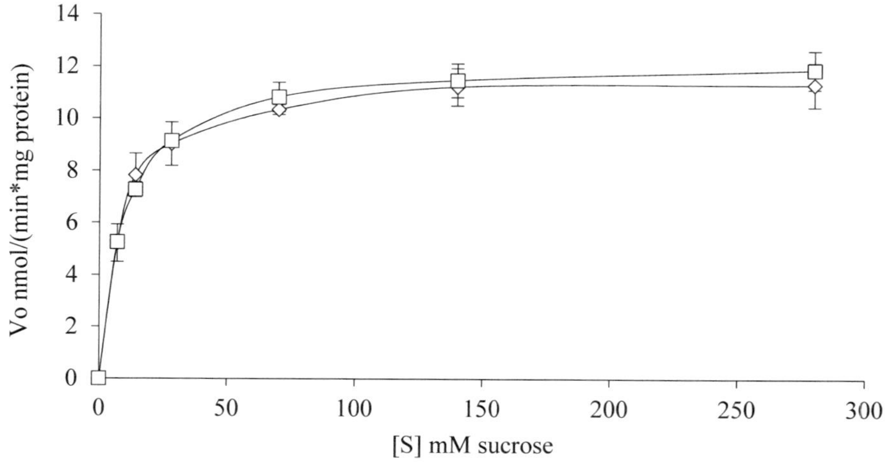

Figure 5. Michaelis-Menten curves for the substrate (sucrose) concentrations 0 – 280 mM with and without fraction III-2 molasses as inhibitor of sucrose (n=4). [sucrose (◊) Fraktion III-2 molasses (□)]

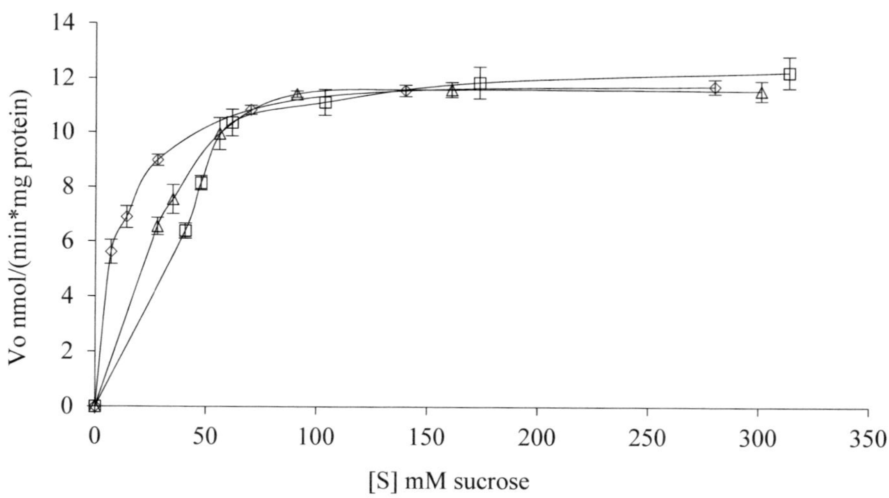

Figure 6. Michaelis-Menten curves for the substrate (sucrose) concentrations 0 – 280 mM with and without 3 % EDC molasses as inhibitor of sucrose (n=4). Sucrose placebo represents the amount of sucrose in the EDC molasses.[sucrose (◊) 3% EDC molasses (□), Sucrose placebo (Δ)]

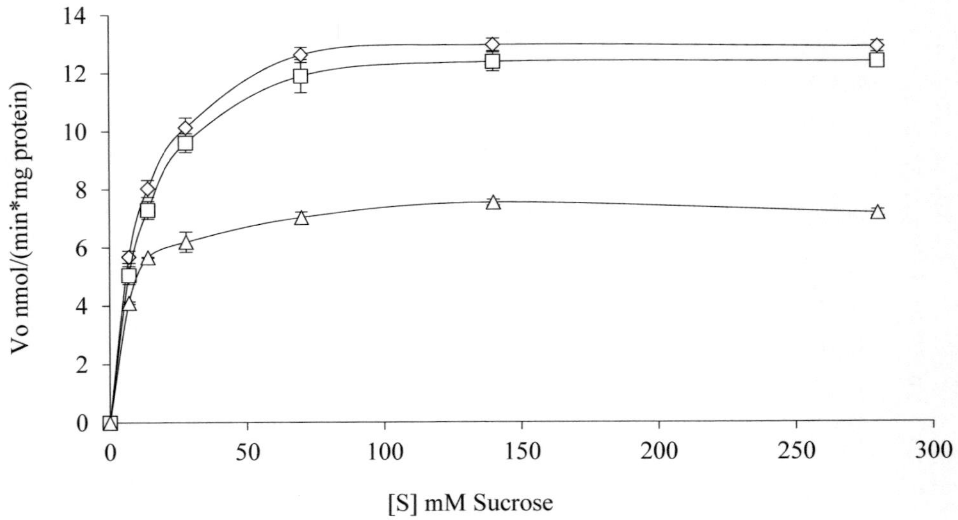

Figure 7. Michaelis-Menten curves for the substrate (sucrose) concentrations 0 – 280 mM with and without 1mM ferulic acid as inhibitor of sucrase and 5,6 mM arabinose as inhibitor of sucrase. [sucrose (◊) 1 mM ferulic acid (□), 5,6 mM arabinose (Δ)]

5. Intraluminal factors related to uptake of glucose

It has been known for many years that dietary fibers reduce postprandial glucose concentrations in the blood, insulin response and delay gastric emptying. These effects have been established for a variety of fibers, but most markedly for soluble fibers. The character of chemical binding to the fibers are not well elucidated, neither the questions of existing physical binding mechanisms. The different processing methods of carbohydrates such as parboiling have verified effects on the glycemic response.

One could ask whether the fiber-effects are due to the fibers, or can be explained by compensatory effects on the diet. That means if intake of fibers in the relevant amounts decreases appetite for fat and short chain carbohydrates, and thereby induces early satiety or changes food preferences towards other kinds of nutrients. These questions have only been addressed in very few publications and deserve to be discussed further. It has been very difficult to show that changes by fibers on appetite and food intake last more than around three weeks. This could be due to adaptation both to the direct effect of fibers, but also to adaption to the secondary effects such as food composition.

An additional question is the significance of formation of resistant starch during the preparation and production of food items.

During the 1980`s it was well documented that dietary fibers have beneficial effects on blood glucose levels, the postprandial values in particular. The mechanisms, however, were not clear, and chemical bindings of glucose to elements in the fibers were hypothesized. Such bindings have never been convincingly proven, and at an early point these hypothesis were questioned. A study used pectin in the glucose solution and modulated gastric emptying with propantheline (31) which demonstrated that pectin significantly reduced blood-glucose, but propantheline had a more pronounced effect. In an additional investigation in the same paper they demonstrated that both gastric emptying and paracetamol absorption were slower after inclusion of gel fiber (guar gum and pectin), but the total absorption of the drug, reflected in urinary recovery, was not significantly reduced. These results indicated that gastric emptying could be the dominating factor in the delay of glucose absorption. Later a long list of authors has contributed. Lavin and Read (32) found no difference in gastric emptying time when comparing fluent meal of 30 % glucose with or without guar gum, and speculated in an unknown mucosal receptor mechanism to explain the effects on postprandial blood glucose and insulin concentrations as well as satiety. In contradiction Horowitz et al (33) found convincing correlations between gastric emptying and peak plasma glucose as well as the total amount of glucose absorbed using a scintigraphic technique, but with almost twice the concentration of glucose in the fluent meal and a 40 % larger volume compared to Lavin and Read (32). Horowitz et al (33) calculated that gastric emptying accounts for about 34 % of the variance in postprandial peak plasma glucose. The difference between these results could be explained by the techniques used, but also by the concentrations of glucose in the test meals. A study investigated the rehydration ability of 2 and 10 % glucose-electrolyte solutions with osmolality of 189 and 654 mOsm/kg, respectively. Gastric volumes were determined via gastric aspiration at 15 min intervals. They showed that the reduced overall rate of fluid uptake following ingestion of the 10 % glucose solution was due largely to a relatively slow rate of gastric emptying (34). Hence the influence of gastric emptying on glucose uptake may only be relevant for solutions with very high concentrations of glucose, which is not relevant in relation to the human diet neither in normal persons nor in diabetic patients. This is in accordance with the hypothesis, that gastric content is only allowed access to the duodenum when iso-osmotic. Part of the delay in gastric emptying may well to allow a dilution with secreted water and sodium.

All these results indicate that gastric emptying is probably the dominating factor, but not the only one. Blackburn et al (35) had the same results as others concerning the lowering of blood glucose and insulin, but there was no correlation between the changes in the individual blood glucose responses and changes in gastric emptying rates induced by guar. By a steady-state perfusion technique, glucose absorption was found to be significantly reduced during perfusion of the jejunum with solutions containing guar. They estimated the thickness of unstirred layer in addition, and concluded that guar improves glucose tolerance predominantly by reducing glucose absorption in the small intestine. These were very elegant experiments, but has not been reproduced. However, another important influence on glucose uptake may be the rate of perfusion of the small intestine which can be modulated both by hormonal effects and meal composition (36).

After glucose meals it seems like gastric emptying is a dominant intraluminal factor for glucose absorption. However, glucose is rarely ingested as glucose, and production of glucose in the stomach due to acid hydrolysis is not a predominant mechanism of glucose production. For these reasons it would be valuable to look at starch and sucrose as well.

the hypothesis was investigated In another study with focus on particle size and structural features of the food. An extract from barley was used to modify the granules and the particle size, and found a decrease in the in-vitro starch digestion and accordingly release of glucose (37). Also starch-entrapped microspheres have been used with similar beneficial effects on the postprandial blood glucose response for different starch fractions (38). In addition it would be relevant to investigate the effects on brush border sucrose activity related to the different forms of glucose suppliers.

In animal studies promising results are emerging. Kett et al (39) found that starch gelatinized with α-casein resulted in lower postprandial glucose uptake than starch gelatinized with β-casein. In rats a study found indications of an effect of addition of resistant starch to bread, but different effects for maize and wheat based bread (40).

Besides from the more or less well described factors mentioned above, we see an emerging and probably very important field of intestinal sensing of nutrients, recently reviewed by Tolhurst et al (41). Of special interest in the glucose aspect are the documented effects of psyllium fibers in the diet prolonging pancreatic polypeptide (PYY) secretion and suppressing postprandial glucagon-like peptide-1(GLP-1) concentration (42).

6. Conclusions

All together, these findings imply that there must be many possible ways of modifying food components to reduce the postprandial glucose levels in the blood. These modifications can be made both by induction of physical changes in the carbohydrates (gelatinization), additives and addition of food components already existing in nature. Arabinose is present in considerable amounts in the sugar beet along with sucrose, but the components are separated during the manufacturing process. Modifications of food components generally cost money, so it will partly be the consciousness of the consumers that will determine whether such products have a future on the market.

The simplest way of getting an effect is still to increase the amount of dietary fibers in the diet, and hypothetically the largest effects would result from a change in eating habits in the total population. The results presented are from normal volunteers, and the same effects can be measured in diabetics, whereas results are lacking from persons/patients with insulin resistance but not yet diabetic.

Author details

Kia Halschou Hansen and Klaus Bukhave
Department of Human Nutrition, University of Copenhagen, Denmark

Jens Rikardt Andersen*
Department of Human Nutrition, University of Copenhagen, Denmark
Nutrition Unit 5711, Rigshospitalet, Copenhagen, Denmark

Conflicts of interest

Kia Halschou Hansen, MSc in clinical nutrition, is a PhD candidate, partly financed by Nordic Sugar Denmark.

7. References

[1] Gin H, Rigalleau V. Post-prandial hyperglycemia. post-prandial hyperglycemia and diabetes. Diabetes Metab 2000;26:265-72.
[2] Haffner SM, Stern MP, Hazuda HP, Mitchell BD, Patterson JK. Cardiovascular risk factors in confirmed prediabetic individuals. Does the clock for coronary heart disease start ticking before the onset of clinical diabetes? JAMA 1990;263:2893-8.
[3] Lindstrom J, Ilanne-Parikka P, Peltonen M et al. Sustained reduction in the incidence of type 2 diabetes by lifestyle intervention: follow-up of the Finnish Diabetes Prevention Study. Lancet 2006;368:1673-9.
[4] Knowler WC, Hamman RF, Edelstein SL et al. Prevention of type 2 diabetes with troglitazone in the Diabetes Prevention Program. Diabetes 2005;54:1150-6.
[5] Knowler WC, Barrett-Connor E, Fowler SE et al. Reduction in the incidence of type 2 diabetes with lifestyle intervention or metformin. N Engl J Med 2002;346:393-403.
[6] Gerstein HC, Yusuf S, Bosch J et al. Effect of rosiglitazone on the frequency of diabetes in patients with impaired glucose tolerance or impaired fasting glucose: a randomised controlled trial. Lancet 2006;368:1096-105.
[7] Pan XR, Li GW, Hu YH et al. Effects of diet and exercise in preventing NIDDM in people with impaired glucose tolerance. The Da Qing IGT and Diabetes Study. Diabetes Care 1997;20:537-44.
[8] Tuomilehto J, Lindstrom J, Eriksson JG et al. Prevention of type 2 diabetes mellitus by changes in lifestyle among subjects with impaired glucose tolerance. N Engl J Med 2001;344:1343-50.
[9] Krog-Mikkelsen I, Hels O, Tetens I, Holst JJ, Andersen JR, Bukhave K. The effects of l-arabinose on intestinal sucrase activity: dose-response studies in vitro and in humans. The American Journal of Clinical Nutrition 2011;94:472-8.

* Corresponding Author

[10] Elliott SS, Keim NL, Stern JS, Teff K, Havel PJ. Fructose, weight gain, and the insulin resistance syndrome. Am J Clin Nutr 2002;76:911-22.
[11] Sievenpiper JL, Carleton AJ, Chatha S et al. Heterogeneous effects of fructose on blood lipids in individuals with type 2 diabetes: systematic review and meta-analysis of experimental trials in humans. Diabetes Care 2009;32:1930-7.
[12] Sievenpiper JL, Chiavaroli L, de Souza RJ et al. 'Catalytic' doses of fructose may benefit glycaemic control without harming cardiometabolic risk factors: a small meta-analysis of randomised controlled feeding trials. Br J Nutr 2012;108:418-23.
[13] Seri K, Sanai K, Matsuo N, Kawakubo K, Xue C, Inoue S. L-arabinose selectively inhibits intestinal sucrase in an uncompetitive manner and suppresses glycemic response after sucrose ingestion in animals. Metabolism 1996;45:1368-74.
[14] Semenza G, von Balthazar AK. Steady-state kinetics of rabbit-intestinal sucrase. Kinetic mechanism, Na+ activation, inhibition by tris(hydroxymethyl)aminomethane at the glucose subsite. Eur J Biochem 1974;41:149-62.
[15] Welsch CA, Lachance PA, Wasserman BP. Effects of native and oxidized phenolic compounds on sucrase activity in rat brush border membrane vesicles. J Nutr 1989;119:1737-40.
[16] Delie F, Rubas W. A human colonic cell line sharing similarities with enterocytes as a model to examine oral absorption: advantages and limitations of the Caco-2 model. Crit Rev Ther Drug Carrier Syst 1997;14:221-86.
[17] Keen CL, Holt RR, Oteiza PI, Fraga CG, Schmitz HH. Cocoa antioxidants and cardiovascular health. Am J Clin Nutr 2005;81(suppl):298-303.
[18] Hanhineva K, Torronen R, Bondia-Pons I et al. Impact of Dietary Polyphenols on Carbohydrate Metabolism. Int J Mol Sci 2010;11:1365-402.
[19] Sies H, Schewe T, Heiss C, Kelm M. Cocoa polyphenols and inflammatory mediators. Am J Clin Nutr 2005;81(suppl):304-12.
[20] Vita JA. Polyphenols and cardiovascular disease: effects on endothelial and platelet function. Am J Clin Nutr 2005;81(suppl):292-7.
[21] Gupta S, Mahmood S, Khan RH, Mahmood A. Inhibition of brush border sucrase by polyphenols in mouse intestine. Biosci Rep 2010;30:111-7.
[22] Navita G, Shiffalli G, Akhtar MN. Gallic acid inhibits brush border disaccharidases in mammalian intestine. Nutrition Research 2007;27:230-5.
[23] Ani V, Varadaraj MC, Naidu KA. Antioxidant and antibacterial activities of polyphenolic compounds from bitter cumin (Cuminum nigrum L.). Eur Food Res Techn 2006;224:109-15.
[24] Hanamura T, Mayama C, Aoki H, Hirayama Y, Shimizu M. Antihyperglycemic effect of polyphenols from Acerola (Malpighia emarginata DC.) fruit. Biosci Biotechnol Biochem 2006;70:1813-20.
[25] Matsui T, Ogunwande IA, Abesundara KJ, Matsumoto K. Anti-hyperglycemic Potential of Natural Products. Mini Rev Med Chem 2006;6:349-56.

[26] Ishikawa A, Yamashita H, Hiemori M et al. Characterization of inhibitors of postprandial hyperglycemia from the leaves of Nerium indicum. J Nutr Sci Vitaminol 2007;53:166-73.
[27] Mohdaly AA, Sarhan MA, Smetanska I, Mahmoud A. Antioxidant properties of various solvent extracts of potato peel, sugar beet pulp and sesame cake. J Sci Food Agric 2010;90:218-26.
[28] Sakac MB, Gyura JF, Misan AC, Seres ZI. Antioxidant properties of sugarbeet fibers. Zuckerindustrie 2009;134:418-25.
[29] Ranilla LG, Kwon YI, Genovese MI, Lajolo FM, Shetty K. Antidiabetes and antihypertension potential of commonly consumed carbohydrate sweeteners using in vitro models. J Med Food 2008;11:337-48.
[30] Manach C, Scalbert A, Morand C, Remesy C, Jimenez L. Polyphenols: food sources and bioavailability. Am J Clin Nutr 2004;79:727-47.
[31] Holt S, Heading RC, Carter DC, Prescott LF, Tothill P. Effect of gel fibre on gastric emptying and absorption of glucose and paracetamol. Lancet 1979;1:636-9.
[32] Lavin JH, Read NW. The effect on hunger and satiety of slowing the absorption of glucose: relationship with gastric emptying and postprandial blood glucose and insulin responses. Appetite 1995;25:89-96.
[33] Horowitz M, Edelbroek MA, Wishart JM, Straathof JW. Relationship between oral glucose tolerance and gastric emptying in normal healthy subjects. Diabetologia 1993;36:857-62.
[34] Evans GH, Shirreffs SM, Maughan RJ. The effects of repeated ingestion of high and low glucose-electrolyte solutions on gastric emptying and blood 2H2O concentration after an overnight fast. Br J Nutr 2011;106:1732-9.
[35] Blackburn NA, Redfern JS, Jarjis H et al. The mechanism of action of guar gum in improving glucose tolerance in man. Clin Sci 1984;66:329-36.
[36] Macdonald IA. Physiological regulation of gastric emptying and glucose absorption. Diabet Med 1996;13:11-5.
[37] Razzaq HA, Sutton KH, Motoi L. Modifying glucose release from high carbohydrate foods with natural polymers extracted from cereals. J Sci Food Agric 2011;91:2621-7.
[38] Venkatachalam M, Kushnick MR, Zhang G, Hamaker BR. Starch-entrapped biopolymer microspheres as a novel approach to vary blood glucose profiles. J Am Coll Nutr 2009;28:583-90.
[39] Kett AP, Bruen CM, O'Halloran F et al. The effect of alpha- or beta-casein addition to waxy maize starch on postprandial levels of glucose, insulin, and incretin hormones in pigs as a model for humans. Food Nutr Res 2012;56.
[40] Brites CM, Trigo MJ, Carrapico B, Alvina M, Bessa RJ. Maize and resistant starch enriched breads reduce postprandial glycemic responses in rats. Nutr Res 2011;31:302-8.
[41] Tolhurst G, Reimann F, Gribble FM. Intestinal sensing of nutrients. Handb Exp Pharmacol 2012;309-35.

[42] Karhunen LJ, Juvonen KR, Flander SM et al. A psyllium fiber-enriched meal strongly attenuates postprandial gastrointestinal peptide release in healthy young adults. J Nutr 2010;140:737-44.

Section 4

Novel Therapeutic Targets and Pharmacologic Compounds with Antidiabetic Potential

Chapter 10

Glucose Tolerance Factor – Insulin Mimetic and Potentiating Agent – A Source for a Novel Anti Diabetic Medication

Nitsa Mirsky

Additional information is available at the end of the chapter

http://dx.doi.org/10.5772/54350

1. Introduction

Diabetes is the world's most common metabolic disease and one of the leading causes of morbidity and mortality. The medications currently in use are limited in their potency, have many side effects, and cannot be tolerated by many patients. As a result of the global epidemic of diabetes, the need for new diabetes therapies is expected to grow dramatically during the next decade. An intense research has been conducted to identify new therapeutic targets and pharmacologic compounds that might correct the impaired glucose tolerance. Materials that mimic insulin action or augment the effect of residual endogenous insulin are likely to be beneficial for both type 1 and 2 diabetic patients. During the recent years many investigators have shown that natural products are a potential source for new drug candidates for many diseases in general, and diabetes in particular. A research aimed at revealing new natural sources to treat diabetes is of high importance.

A variety of traditional anti diabetic plants are known in the folk medicine. Although some of them have been studied for their anti diabetic effects, the knowledge on their efficacy and mechanism of action is very limited.

The Glucose Tolerance Factor (GTF) is a dietary agent first extracted from Brewer's yeast [1]. GTF reversed the impaired glucose tolerance of both diabetic rats and diabetic patients. In vitro studies with GTF showed remarkable increase in glucose transport into adipocytes, and cardiomyocytes. An increase in glucose incorporation into glycogen in rat hepatocytes was also found for GTF preparations [2].

Despite the high anti diabetic activity of this natural compound, GTF has not been fully characterized or identified, mainly due to the instability of the purified fractions. Our laboratory succeeded in extraction and partial purification of an active and stable GTF preparation from brewer's yeast. We examined GTF effects in animal models for both types of diabetes, and found high and rapid anti diabetic activity. We also examined GTF effects on the cellular level and found high insulin mimetic and insulin potentiating activity for GTF. The mechanism of action of GTF along insulin signaling pathway was also studied.

2. Prevalence of diabetes mellitus

Diabetes is the world's most common metabolic disease and one of the leading causes of morbidity and mortality. According to WHO (World Health Organization) report [3], **346** million people worldwide are diabetic. The number is expected to grow to **438** million until 2030 [8% of the world population!) [4]. Diabetes is the greatest healthcare threat in both developed countries and the third world: diabetes is the third leading cause of death in most developed countries; moreover, it is epidemic in many third world nations. Diabetes imposes an increasing economic burden on national health care systems worldwide [5]. The global health expenditure on diabetes in 2010 was 376$ billion and is expected to grow to 490$ billion by 2030 [6].

3. Diabetes mellitus and its complications

Diabetes mellitus is a complex syndrome involving severe insulin dysfunction along with gross abnormalities in glucose homeostasis and lipid and protein metabolism. The disease is generally divided into two major types: Insulin Dependent Diabetes Mellitus (IDDM, or type 1], and Non Insulin Dependent Diabetes Mellitus (NIDDM, or type 2 DM). Both forms are devastating with respect to their latter complications. People with diabetes have a 25-fold increase in the risk of blindness, a 20-fold increase in the risk of renal failure, a 20-fold increase in the risk of amputation as a result of gangrene and a 2 to 6-fold increase in the risk of coronary heart disease and ischemic brain damage. In general, life expectancy for a person with diabetes is decreased by one-third [5].

4. Diabetes mellitus and oxidative stress

Oxidative stress and non enzymatic glycation play a major role in the pathogenesis of diabetes mellitus [7, 8]. During diabetes, persistent high concentrations of blood glucose increase the production of oxygen free radicals – OFRs. through auto oxidation of glucose Hunt et al., 1990, and also by non enzymatic lipid and protein glycation [9]. OFRs react with membrane phospholipids forming malondialdehyde (MDA) [10, 11]. Lipid peroxide levels, and especially oxidized LDL, are significantly higher in diabetic patients than in healthy individuals. [12-14]. These Major changes in lipid metabolism cause lipid peroxidation in plasma and cellular membranes which lead to micro and macro vascular pathologies [15].

The natural protective system of antioxidant enzymes like superoxide dismutase, glutathione peroxidase and catalase that provides the detoxification steps for the oxidative products, cannot overcome massive production of free radicals to prevent oxidative damage. [16]. It was shown that the activity of the antioxidant systems is decreased in diabetic patients. [17, 18]. This leads to oxidative stress and to the development of diabetes complications.

5. Diabetes mellitus and aldose reductase

The reduction of glucose by the aldose reductase (AR) catalyzed polyol pathway has been linked to the development of secondary diabetic complications like cataract, nephropathy, retinopathy and neuropathy. Accumulation of sorbitol in the organs, due to AR-catalyzed reduction of glucose, causes osmotic swelling resulting in ionic imbalance and protein insolubilization leading to diabetes complications. [19]. Although treatment with AR inhibitors has been shown to prevent tissue injury in animal models of diabetes, the clinical efficacy of these drugs remains to be established. [20].

6. Treatment of diabetes mellitus

Daily injections of insulin are the only treatment for type 1 diabetes. The treatment for type 2 ranges from diet, to classical oral drugs (Sulfonyl urea and biguanides), and to Thiazolidinediones and the new GLP1 analogues. About 40% of type 2 diabetics use insulin in addition to oral drugs.

Although the pathogenesis of diabetes and its long-term complications are well known, optimal treatment remains elusive. The medications currently in use are limited in their potency, have many side effects, and cannot be tolerated by many patients. Only half of the patients achieve the recommended hemoglobin A1c target using conventional treatment [21]. As a result of the global epidemic of diabetes, the need for new diabetes therapies is expected to grow dramatically during the next years. [22]. Pharmaceutical research conducted over the past decades has shown that natural sources like herbs, medicinal plants and yeast extract, are potential sources for new drug candidates for many diseases in general [23], and diabetes in particular [24].

7. Anti diabetic medicinal plants

Several reviews published in recent years screen many plant sources with anti-diabetic properties [24, 25, 26, 27, 28, 29]. Among these plants: Trigonella foenum, graecum, Allium cepa. & Allim sativum, Silybum marianum, Mordica charantia, Camellia sinensis, Morus nigra, Gymnema sylvestre L., Ginkgo biloba L., and many others. Anti-diabetic health effects include increasing serum insulin, decreasing blood glucose, increasing glucose metabolism, and/or stimulating pancreatic function. Adverse effects, contraindications, and interactions between herbal medicines and synthetic drugs exist and may cause clinical consequences.

We shall briefly screen here some of the most potent anti diabetic sources.

Fenugreek (Trigonella Foenum Graecum), is one of the safest and most effective plants in treating diabetes. Clinical studies showed that fenugreek seeds have anti diabetic effects

[30]. "Bitter melon" (Momordica Charantia) fruit extract reduced blood glucose and was found effective in treating diabetes [31]. Garlic has been reported to possess a variety of medicinal properties including hypoglycemic, hypocholesterolemic and hypolipidemic activities [32]. Raw garlic extract reversed proteinuria in diabetic rats in addition to reducing blood glucose, cholesterol and triglyceride in diabetic rats [33]. Silybum Extract (Silybum Marianum) increases the cellular sensitivity to insulin and thus reduces blood glucose total cholesterol and LDL levels in diabetic patients [34]. Bitter cucumber plant fruit (Mamordica Charantia) reduced blood glucose in patients with type 1 diabetes [35]. Green tea (Camellia Sinensis) can reduce blood sugar in diabetic patients. Studies show that the consumption of one and a half gram dry powder of green tea, improved the metabolism of blood sugar in diabetic patients [36]. Ginkgo biloba plant is capable of lowering glucose, fat, and lipid peroxide in diabetic patients [37]. The ethanolic extract of Allium porrum leaves had hypoglycemic effects on diabetic animals probably through the increase of insulin release [38].

Some nutritional factors, such as polyphenols, counteract insulin resistance and therefore may be beneficial for patients with type 2 diabetes mellitus through their insulin-potentiating, antioxidant, and anti-inflammatory properties. The common cinnamon (CN) has a long history of use as a spice, preservative, and pharmacological agent; CN is also a source of polyphenols. Several studies demonstrated that in animals and humans, CN and aqueous extracts of cinnamon improved the level of blood glucose, lipids and insulin, and may be beneficial to counteract the features of insulin resistance, metabolic syndrome, and the onset of type 2 diabetes mellitus [39, 40, 41, 42].

Although many medicinal plants have been traditionally used for treating diabetes [43, 44, 45], the influence of most of them has only rarely been scientifically tested and validated, and the knowledge on their efficacy and mechanisms of action is very limited.

7.1. Yeast as a natural source for anti diabetic material

Brewers' yeast is also included among the anti diabetic natural sources [46, 47]. Schwartz and Mertz were the first to discover the natural anti diabetic agent present in yeast and called it "Glucose Tolerance Factor" (GTF) [1].

8. Glucose Tolerance Factor (GTF) a natural anti diabetic agent

The Glucose Tolerance Factor (GTF) is a dietary agent first extracted from Brewer's yeast [1]. This natural compound reversed the impaired glucose tolerance of diabetic rats [48, 49], and of diabetic patients [50]. GTF can be extracted from several sources, among them: liver [51], black pepper, and kidneys. Especially rich source for GTF are brewers' yeast [52, 53, 54, 55].

Addition of partially purified GTF to the diet of glucose intolerant rats rapidly returned them to normal [56]. Doisy and his group found an improvement in glucose tolerance in elderly people who were treated for two months with GTF. In 50% of the patients, glucose tolerance was restored to normal values. [57].

Offenbacher and Pi Sunyer [46], examined 24 elderly subjects, who were fed daily for 8 weeks with brewers' yeast as a sorce for GTF. They found a considerable improvement in glucose tolerance and insulin sensitivity, and a reduction of total lipids in these patients.

Grant and McMullen [50] treated 37 type 2 diabetics for 7 weeks, in a double blind study, with either brewers' yeast as a source of GTF, or placebo. Supplementation of brewers' yeast significantly decreased HbA1c and increased HDL cholesterol in the treated group. Elwood [58] supplemented 11 normolipidemic and 16 hyperlipidemic subjects with brewers' yeast. They found that total circulating cholesterol was significantly reduced and the HDL levels were significantly increased in both the normo and hyperlipidemic subjects supplemented with brewers' yeast. Riales [59] reported that human subjects receiving 7g of brewers' yeast for 6 weeks had a significant decrease in serum LDL and an increase in HDL cholesterol.

In vitro studies with partially purified preparations of GTF, showed stimulation of glucose metabolism in several tissues. GTF potentiated glucose oxidation to CO_2 in adipose tissue [54, 60], or adipocytes [53, 61]. In those studies the enhancement was shown only in the presence of insulin, and the stimulation of CO_2 production by GTF in the absence of insulin was negligible [53, 54, 60, 61].

In contrast to the findings above, showing GTF activity only in the presence of insulin, other groups found an increase of glucose metabolism by adding GTF in the absence of insulin. Tokuda et al, [62] examined GTF obtained from yeast extract powder on glucose uptake in adipocytes. They found a stimulation of glucose uptake (5.6 times greater than the basal level) in the absence of insulin. Our group also showed an increase in glucose transport both to yeast cells [63, 64], and to animal cells [65].

Since GTF is supposed to be essential for normal glucose tolerance in mammals, and as muscle tissue consumes a major part of blood glucose in the post prandial state, it is most important to assess the effect of GTF on muscle tissue. Fischer and his group [66] examined the effect of GTF obtained by partial purification of yeast extract, on glucose transport in isolated cardiomyocytes. They found that GTF samples increased the rate of glucose transport in the isolated cells, 2 to 2.5 fold, in the absence of insulin. Hwang et al [67] showed enhancement of ^{14}C -glucose oxidation into CO_2 in rat adipocytes by the addition of several fractions extracted from yeast. The authors found only insulin like activity and not insulin potentiating activity for the fractions examined.

The exact composition and structure of GTF are still obscure. Mertz and his group suggested that GTF is probably a small organic molecule comprising one trivalent chromium ion, two molecules of nicotinic acid, and three amino acids: glycine, cystein and glutamic acid [54, 68, 69]. Its molecular weight is estimated to be around 500 daltons [54, 69], It is cationic, soluble in water, and stable in physiological solutions [54, 68].

Several groups who tried to identify the active components present in brewers' yeast, claimed that they are quinoline derivatives [70], or phosphatidylinositol glycans [71]. Other investigators tried to further purify and identify the exact structure and composition of GTF. There is no standard accepted method to isolate GTF, and this fact can probably explain the diversity of the results reported in the literature. In addition, a major problem related to GTF purification, is the instability of the partially purified fractions. This lability, can partially explain the complexity of the subject, and the fact that in spite of the long time since the material was discovered, its exact composition and structure have not been determined.

Tuman [48] who presented the activity of GTF and several synthetic complexes on lowering blood glucose found that in 10 days both the natural compound and the synthetic complexes lost their activity. Mertz reported that highly purified preparations of GTF from yeast or pork kidney tend to be unstable, and lost their activity very quickly [52]. Yamamoto [51] found that GTF like activity of the purified LMCr (low molecular weight chromium binding substance) reduced gradually, and finally there could not be detected any activity. Even at -20 °C, no recovery of the active material could be achieved. We can explain the instability of the purified fractions of GTF by a loss of a co-factor(s) which is probably responsible for the stability of the complex.

Most of the groups who tried to purify GTF from brewers' yeast agree that the GTF is a cationic compound. Only several researchers claimed that the GTF is an anionic compound: Votava and his group [72] reported that GTF is an anionic chromium complex of molecular weight 400-600, containing at least six amino acids. Since the authors measured only the absorption of the complex by rats, and no biological activity assay was done on it, it is hard to compare Votava's compound to other extracts exhibiting GTF activity.

A low molecular weight chromium binding substance (LMCr), was isolated from mouse or rabbit liver and bovine colostrum by Yamamoto and his group [51, 73]. LMCr appears as anionic organic Cr compound, with a relative molecular mass of 1500 daltons. It is composed of glutamic acid, glycine, cysteine and aspartic acid in a ratio of Cr: Amino acid 1:4. The purified LMCr enhanced glucose conversion to CO_2 in rat epididymal adipocytes in the presence of insulin. The rate of glucose incorporation into lipid was stimulated by 30-40% with insulin, or by 15-23% without insulin [51]. Yamamoto and his colleagues were not able to detect nicotinic acid in the extract of LMCr, but some UV absorption was present [73]. This substance appeared to posses properties similar to GTF extracted from yeast.

Another question is related to the nature of the amino acids present in the GTF complex. Urumow & Wieland [74], suggested that GTF activity in stimulating ^{14}C-glucose oxidation is attributable to the combined action of certain amino acids (aspartate, cystein) and nucleosides (adenosine). Fischer [66] came to a conclusion that GTF activity is attributed to the presence of alanine. Hwang and his group [70] suggested that the GTF obtained was a quinoline derivative, which easily binds chromium.

While many research groups in the past agreed with the concept suggested by Mertz that GTF contains chromium [51, 55, 73, 75], accumulating data during the years indicates that there is no chromium present in the GTF preparation. Haylock and his group, who tried to purify and identify GTF for many years, did not find a correlation between chromium content and the biologic activity. They came to the conclusion that: "GTF from brewers' yeast can no longer be regarded as a chromium complex" [76] . Shepherd [77] also came to a similar conclusion.

Stearns [78] summarized the purification research that had been done on GTF and discussed the relation of the active component to chromium. She did not find a correlation between chromium and GTF activity. Stearns also investigated the issue of the essentiality of chromium to human health, and found that "no chromium-containing glucose tolerance factor has been characterized, the purpose of the low-molecular-weight chromium-binding protein is questionable, and no direct interaction between chromium and insulin has been found" [79]. Moreover, she criticized the dietary supplementation of chromium: "Chromium+3 may act clinically by decreasing the iron stores that are linked to diabetes and heart disease. This would make chromium+3 a pharmacological agent, not an essential metal" [79].

Eddens and his colleagues [47], isolated three separate fractions by eluting yeast extract from C18 column and found diverse activities in increasing glucose metabolism and inhibiting lipolysis for the different fractions, not connected to their chromium content.

Recently, our group also measured the chromium concentrations in the active fractions isolated from yeast extract and did not find any correlation between the chromium content and the biologic activity (Mirsky et al, unpublished data).

To summarize the chromium issue: Although the active material isolated from yeast (GTF) has been known for years to be a chromium complex, accumulating evidence during recent years show that the active anti diabetic fractions in GTF do not contain chromium.

Our laboratory succeeded in extraction and partial purification of an active and stable GTF preparation from brewer's yeast. We used several separation techniques including membranes with different molecular cut off, ion exchange columns and reversed phase HPLC. Our GTF preparation has a molecular weight below 1000 dalton. It was found to be very stable: it is stable to high and low pH and it keeps its activity up to 12 months in 4°C. Moreover, GTF is also stable to proteolytic enzymes. This finding enables an oral treatment with GTF, in contrast to insulin, which is a protein and has to be injected [49, 80, 81].

In the following paragraphs we shall present several of our findings on GTF both in vivo and in vitro. We examined GTF effects in animal models for both types of diabetes, and found high and rapid anti diabetic, hypolipidemic and antioxidant activity. We also found a remarkable reduction in the complications of diabetes: nephropathy and retinopathy, by treating the diabetic animals with oral doses of GTF [81].

In vitro studies done in our laboratory showed insulin mimetic and insulin potentiating activity for GTF [65].

9. In vivo effects of GTF

9.1. GTF decreases blood glucose in diabetic rat models

A single oral dose of GTF, orally administered to both types of diabetic animals, decreased immediately and remarkably glucose and lipid levels in their blood [49, 80]. Glucose reduction appeared immediately after the administration of GTF, reached a maximum within 2 hours, and lasted for several hours. When GTF was administered in concert with marginal insulin doses, the reduction in blood glucose was much higher than for each agent alone, demonstrating a synergy between GTF and insulin [80].

9.1.1. GTF improves oral glucose tolerance test (OGTT) in diabetic rats

We examined GTF effects in two rat models exhibiting insulin deficiency: the streptozotocin (STZ) diabetic rat, which is characterized by the damage induced to beta cells by the drug, and the hyperglycemic Cohen diabetic-sensitive ((hyp-CDs) rat, which is characterized by beta cell dysfunction and decreased glucose stimulated insulin secretion (from Wexler-Zangen et al, [65].

Control-vehicle treated hyp-CDs and STZ rats exhibited an abnormal glucose-tolerance curve, characterized by elevated blood glucose levels (Figs 1A and B) Administration of an oral dose of GTF (at zero time) lowered the blood glucose area under the curve (BG-AUC) of both hyp-CDs and STZ rats compared to vehicle treated rats. The decrease in BG-AUC depended on the dose of GTF administered. Insulin secretion in response to glucose stimulation did not change significantly in GTF treated hyp-CDs rats (From Wexler-Zangen et al, [65], indicating that the glucose lowering effect of GTF is not related to stimulation of insulin secretion.

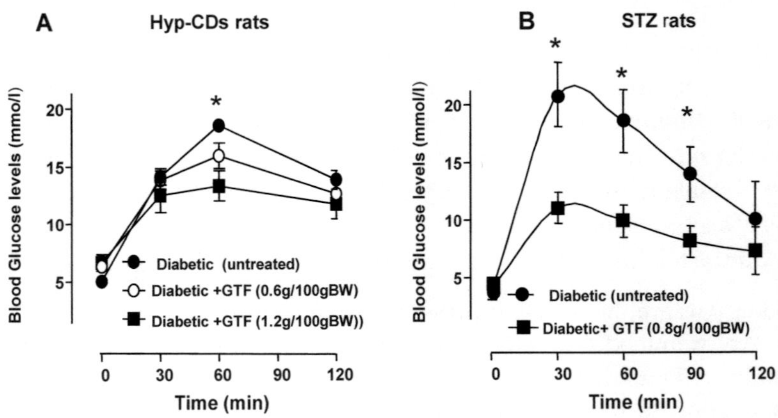

A: OGTT profiles of diabetic untreated Hyp-CDs rats (black circles), GTF (0.6g/100g BW) treated Hyp-CDs rats (white circles) and GTF (1.2g/100g BW) treated Hyp-CDs rats (black squares). B: OGTT profiles of diabetic untreated STZ rats (black circles) and GTF (0.8g/100g BW) treated STZ rats (black squares). GTF was administered at time 0. BG levels were measured after an overnight fast [0], and at 30, 60 and 120 min period after glucose (3.5g/kg for Hyp-CDs and 2g/kg for STZ rats) administration. Data are means ± SE for 5 or 6 rats per group. * P< 0.001, Diabetic vs. respective untreated control. (From Wexler-Zangen et al, [65]

Figure 1. Oral Glucose Tolerance Test (OGTT) of GTF treated diabetic rats

9.2. GTF reduces postprandial blood glucose concentration in diabetic rats

Post prandial (PP) blood glucose level is very high in both hyp-CDs and STZ diabetic rats. In the vehicle treated hyp-CDs and STZ rats, the markedly elevated BG concentrations remained high for more than 120 min (Figs 2A and B). A single oral dose of GTF administered at zero time significantly reduced (P<0.001) the high BG concentrations in both hyp-CDs [33%) and STZ rats [38%).

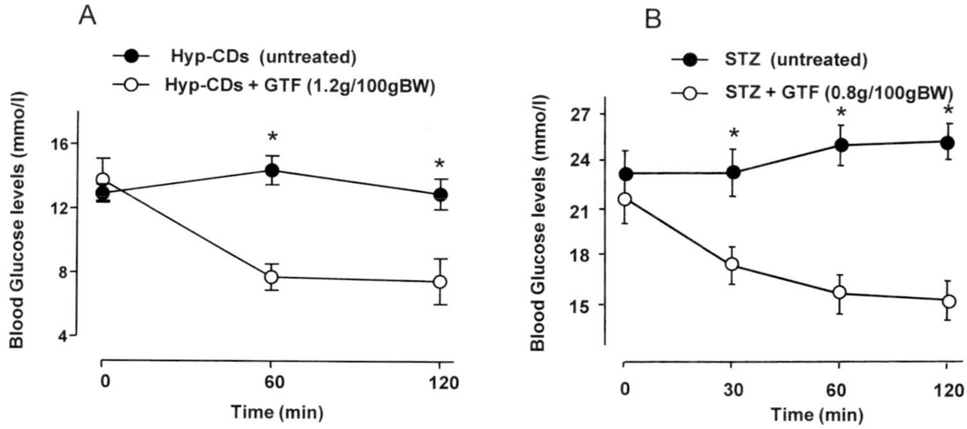

A: PP glucose levels of control untreated Hyp-CDs rats (black circles), GTF treated (1.2g/100g BW) Hyp-CDs rats (white circles). At time 0 GTF was administered to the indicated groups. **B:** Postprandial glucose levels of untreated STZ rats (black circles) and GTF treated (0.8g/100g BW) STZ rats (white circles). At time 0 GTF was administered to the indicated groups. Data are means ± SE for 5 or 6 rats per group. * P< 0.001, Diabetic vs. respective untreated control. (From Wexler-Zangen et al, [65]

Figure 2. GTF decreases Postprandial (PP) glucose levels in diabetic rats

9.3. GTF decreases tri glyceride and LDL cholesterol and increases HDL cholesterol

A remarkable decrease in triglyceride level was observed in diabetic animals administered with 5 daily oral doses of GTF (Figure 3). The treatment with GTF also remarkably decreased the level of LDL cholesterol (Figure 4A), and increased the level of HDL cholesterol (Figure 4B), (Ampel et al., unpublished data). The reduction in LDL cholesterol was also demonstrated in healthy animals treated with GTF, indicating a potential preventive effect of GTF in healthy subjects.

9.4. GTF reduces lipid peroxidation in the plasma, both in vivo and in vitro

GTF can inhibit the deleterious elevation in lipid peroxides induced by diabetes. Type 1 diabetic rats were treated with 5 daily oral doses of GTF. The animals were killed and the levels of lipid peroxidation products - malondialdehyde (measured as TBARS – thiobarbituric acid reactive substances), in healthy, diabetic and diabetic rats treated with GTF were determined. Figure 5 demonstrates the level of lipid peroxidation products detected in the plasma of healthy, diabetic, and diabetic rats treated with GTF, showing a major decrease in the level of plasma peroxides in diabetic animals treated with GTF. These results indicate high antioxidant activity of the GTF preparation (From Ampel et al., unpublished data).

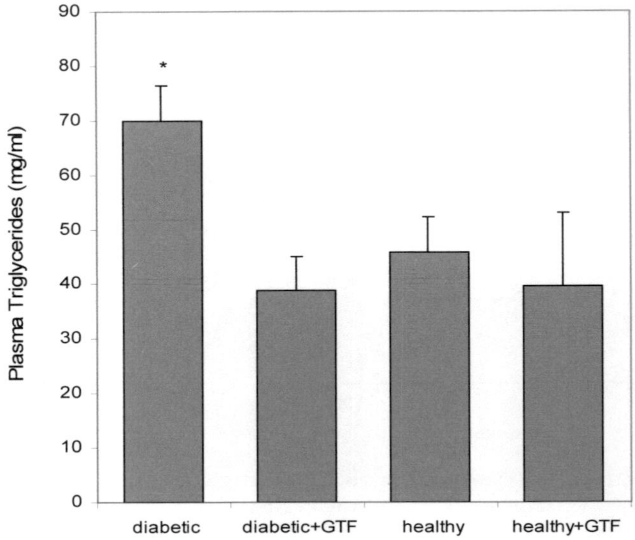

Figure 3. Effect of GTF on plasma triglycerides. Plasma triglyceride concentration in healthy rats, diabetic rats and diabetic rats treated with 5 daily oral doses of GTF [1,64g /rat). All animals were 15 weeks old, diabetic animals were 10 weeks after onset of diabetes. (from Ampel et al., unpublished data).

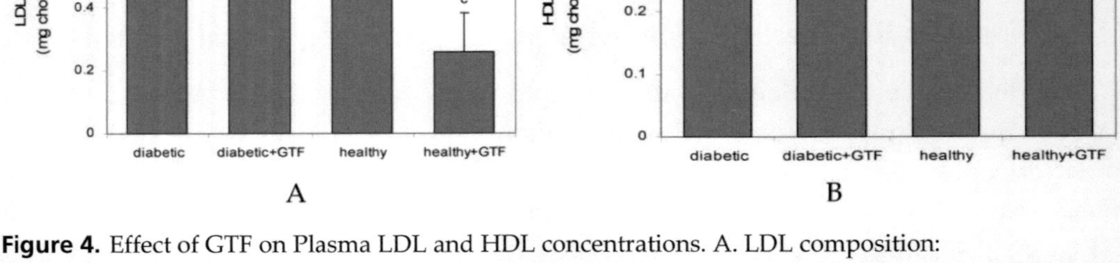

Figure 4. Effect of GTF on Plasma LDL and HDL concentrations. A. LDL composition: cholesterol/protein ratio in healthy rats, diabetic rats and diabetic rats treated with 5 daily oral doses of GTF [1,64g /rat). All animals were 15 weeks old, diabetic animals were 10 weeks after onset of diabetes. B. HDL composition: cholesterol/protein ratio in healthy rats, diabetic rats and diabetic rats treated with 5 daily oral doses of GTF [1,64g /rat). All animals were 15 weeks old, diabetic animals were 10 weeks after onset of diabetes. (from Ampel et al., unpublished data).

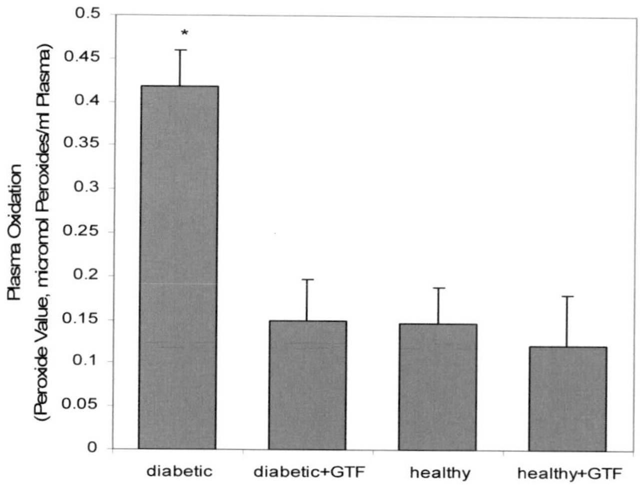

Figure 5. Effect of GTF on plasma peroxides. Plasma oxidation level, measured as peroxide concentration, in healthy rats, diabetic rats and diabetic rats treated with 5 daily oral doses of GTF (1,64g /rat). All Animals were 15 weeks old, diabetic animals were 10 weeks after onset of diabetes (From Ampel et al., 2000).

In vitro studies with GTF added to tubes containing human LDL, indicated a protective effect of GTF against LDL oxidation (Ampel et al., unpublished data).

9.5. GTF reduces lipid peroxidation in the heart and kidneys of diabetic rats

The levels of lipid peroxidation products, TBARS, in the kidneys and hearts removed from healthy, diabetic, and diabetic rats treated with GTF are shown in figures 6 & 7 (From Nakhoul et al., [81] Figure 6 presents the level of lipid peroxidation products determined in the hearts of the various experimental groups. The value of lipid peroxides in untreated diabetic rats was significantly higher than the value detected for healthy animals. The level of lipid peroxides in the hearts of diabetic rats treated with 5 oral doses of GTF was very low - a higher effect seen for the higher dose of GTF, similar to the level found in healthy animals. A remarkable decrease in lipid peroxidation level is shown also in kidneys removed from diabetic rats treated with GTF (Figure 7). Peroxide values found in the animals treated with GTF were very similar to those found in healthy controls. The above assays show the remarkable effect of GTF treatment on lipid peroxidation level in diabetic animals, both in plasma and in cardinal organs.

9.6. GTF decreases aldose reductase activity

Elevated activity of aldose reductase (AR) in the organs is one of the events occurring in hyperglycemic conditions. We measured aldose reductase activity in the hearts of healthy, diabetic and diabetic treated with GTF (Figure 8). AR activity in the hearts of diabetic rats was much higher than that found in healthy rats. 5 oral doses of GTF remarkably reduced the activity of the enzyme in the hearts of the treated diabetic animals in a dose dependent mode, indicating a potent aldose reductase inhibition activity in GTF preparation.

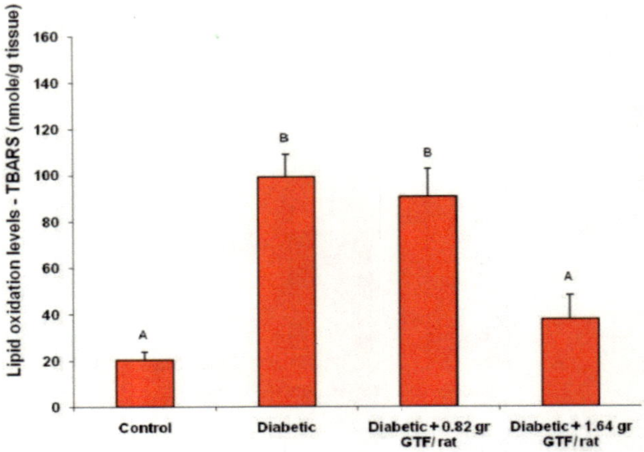

Effect of treatment with GTF on lipid peroxidation products measured as TBARS in the heart of control, untreated diabetic rats and diabetic rats treated with two different doses of GTF: 0,82 and 1,64 g/rat. The rats were treated with repeated doses for 5 days. The age of the rats was 9 weeks. Diabetes was induced with STZ injection (60mg/Kg BW) at the age of 5 weeks. Every group represents 8-11 animals. One way ANOVA test showed significant differences between groups (P<0,001). Different letters above bars indicate significant differences between groups. (From Nakhoul et al., [81].

Figure 6. Effect of GTF on lipid peroxidation in the heart

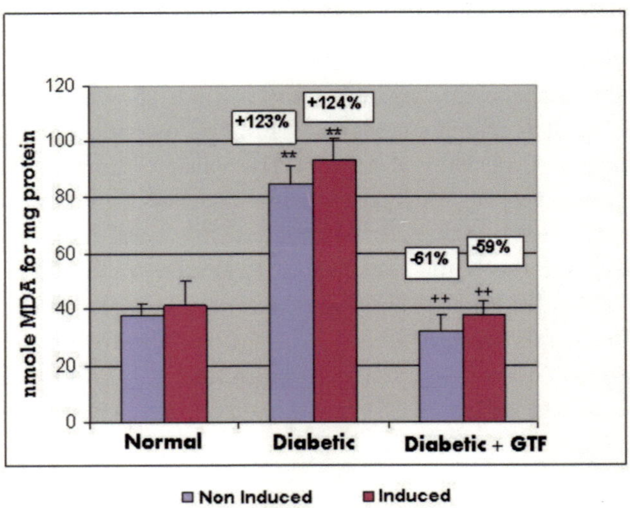

GTF reduces the level of lipid peroxidation products in renal cortex of diabetic rats. Streptozotocin diabetic rats were administered with 5 repeated oral doses of GTF (1.64 g/rat).The level of lipid peroxidation products (TBARS nmole/g tissue) was determined in control rats (n=5], untreated diabetic rats (n=8], and diabetic rats treated with GTF (n=8). Products of lipid peroxidation were measured in the presence (induced) and absence (non-induced) of $FeSO_4$. P < 0.01 compared with untreated diabetic animals. ** P < 0.01 compared with healthy controls. From Nakhoul et al., [81]

Figure 7. Effect of GTF on lipid peroxidation in renal cortex

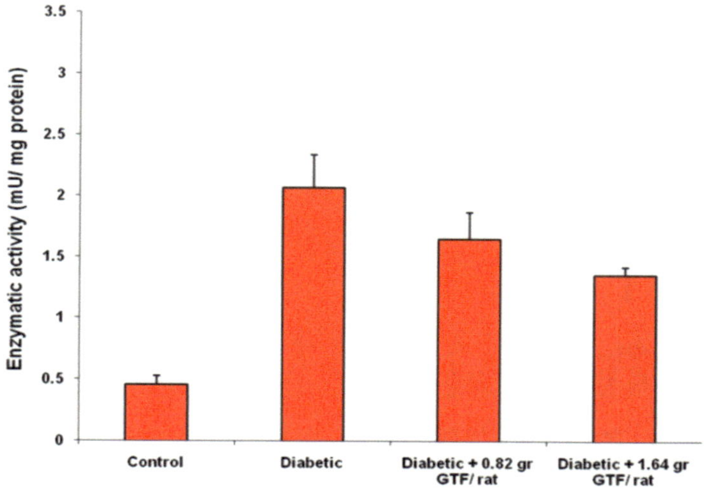

Effect of treatment with GTF on aldose reductase activity in the hearts of control, untreated diabetic rats and diabetic rats treated with two different doses of GTF: 0,82 and 1,64 g/rat. The rats were treated with repeated doses for 5 days. The age of the rats was 9 weeks. Diabetes was induced with STZ injection (60mg/Kg BW) at the age of 5 weeks. Every group represents 8-11 animals. (From Mirsky et al unpublished data).

Figure 8. Effect of GTF on aldose reductase activity in the heart

9.7. GTF decreases nephropathy in diabetic rats

9.7.1. Decreased urine volume and urine protein in diabetic rats treated with GTF

We measured the urine volume and urine protein of healthy, diabetic, and diabetic rats treated for two weeks with oral doses of GTF. Diabetes was induced at zero time. The group of diabetic animals treated with GTF received daily doses of GTF mixed in their food immediately with the induction of diabetes. The animals were kept in metabolic cages, and urine was collected daily. Fig. 9 presents the urine volume and Fig 10 presents urine protein of the different groups, indicating a significant reduction both in urine volume and in urine protein of diabetic rats treated with GTF (from Nakhoul et al., [81]).

9.8. GTF decreases retinopathy in diabetic rats

9.8.1. GFAP expression in healthy, diabetic and Diabetic rats treated with GTF

Glial Fibrillary Acidic Protein (GFAP) is normally expressed in retinal astrocytes. Under pathologic conditions like hyperglycemia or ischemia, GFAP can be detected in other retina's areas like Muller cells layer. GFAP has been widely used as a cellular marker for retinal pathology.

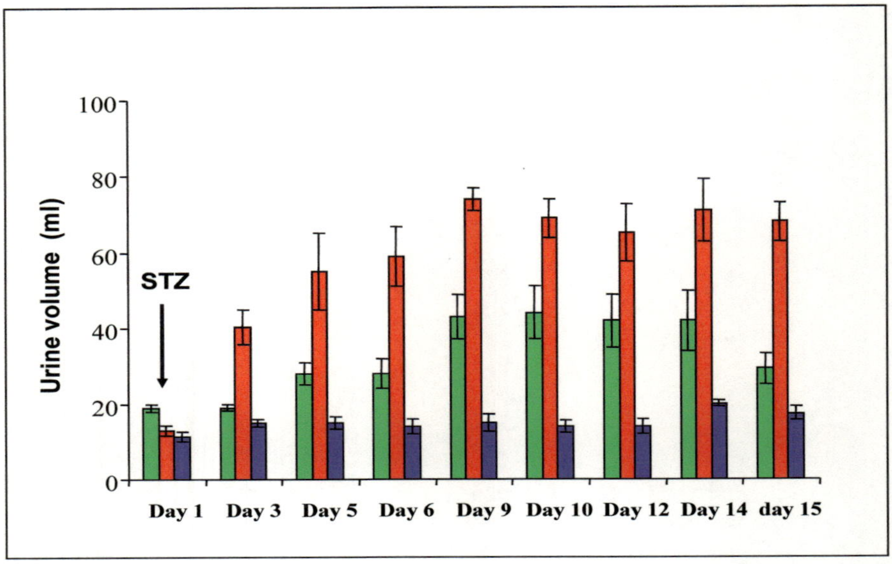

Daily urinary volume of healthy rats (n=5], diabetic rats (n=8] and diabetic rats treated with daily doses of GTF [4g/day) for 2 weeks. (From Nakhoul et al., [81].

Figure 9. Effect of GTF on urine volume

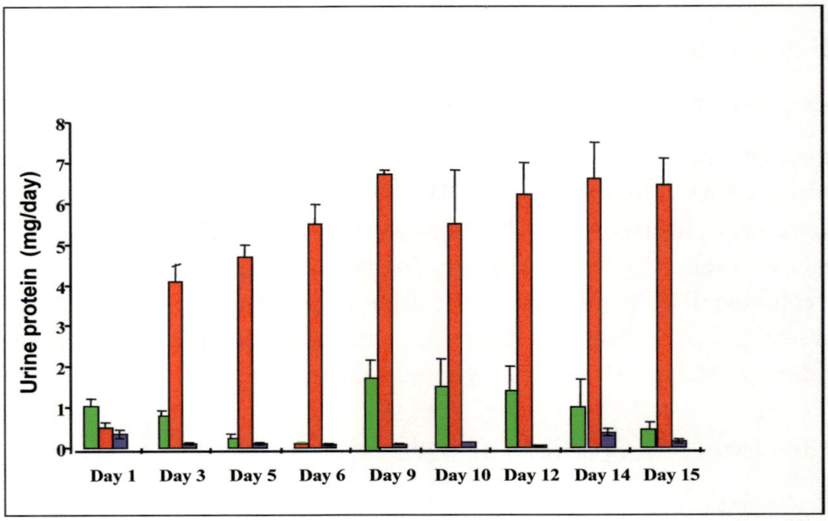

Urine protein (mg protein / day) excreted by healthy (N=5), diabetic (N=8) and diabetic rats treated with GTF (N=8) (4g/day) for 2 weeks. (From Nakhoul et al., [81].

Figure 10. Effect of GTF on urine protein

In a study done in our laboratory on healthy, diabetic, and diabetic rats treated for two weeks with GTF, a large amount of GFAP staining in Muller cell layer was demonstrated in diabetic untreated retinas (Fig. 11). (Mirsky et al., unpublished data). A remarkable reduction in GFAP expression was demonstrated in retinas derived from diabetic animals treated with GTF, where GFAP could be seen only in the glial astrocytes layer, very similar to what was found in the healthy retinas.

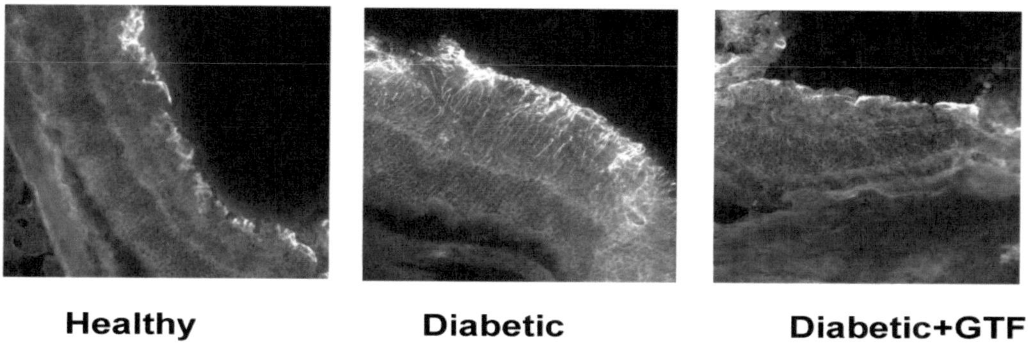

GFAP Immuno histochemistry in neural retina of healthy, diabetic and diabetic rats treated with GTF (4g/day) for 2 weeks (healthy, diabetic, and diabetic treated with GTF). Magnification X400 (Mirsky et al., unpublished data)

Figure 11. Effect of GTF on GFAP in the retina

9.8.2. GTF prevents the diabetic damage to Na/K ATPase in retinas

Sodium / Potassium ATPase is located in the pigment epithelial layer of the retina. In healthy retinas stained histochemically for Sodium / Potassium ATPase, the activity of the enzyme can easily be detected, whereas it was remarkably reduced in diabetic retinas. A prevention of the damage could be detected in retinas isolated from diabetic animals treated for two weeks with GTF, where the activity of the pump is similar to the activity shown for healthy controls. (Figure 12) (Mirsky et al., unpublished data).

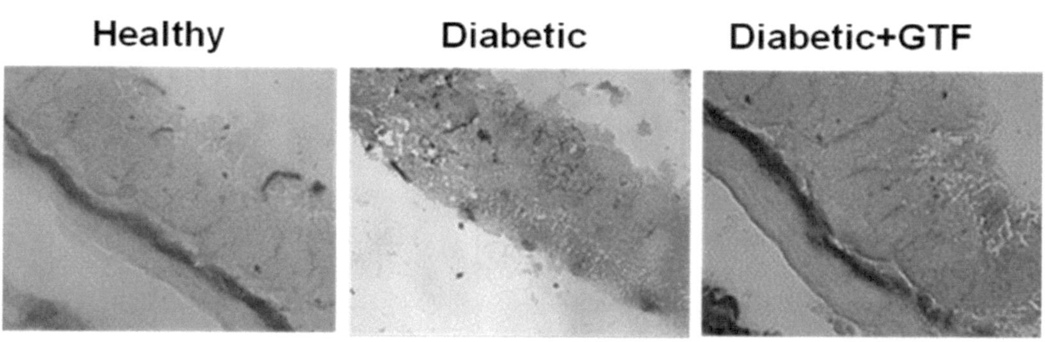

Histochemical localization of Sodium / Potassium ATPase in retinas of healthy, diabetic and diabetic rats treated for two weeks with GTF(4g/day) for 2 weeks. Magnification X400 (From Mirsky et al., unpublished data).

Figure 12. Effect of GTF on Sodium/Potassium ATPase in the retina.

10. Mechanism of action of GTF: Insulin mimetic activity

Binding of insulin to its receptor initiates a cascade of phosphorylations of several substrates, including insulin receptor substrate (IRS) proteins. IRS-1 is widely expressed in insulin-sensitive tissues, and it transmits the signal from insulin receptor to biological endpoints, such as glucose transport, protein, lipid, and glycogen synthesis. Phosphorylation of IRS-1 subsequently triggers the activation of downstream signal molecules such as phosphatidylinositol 3-kinase (PI3K), protein kinase B (PKB/AKT), several isoforms of protein kinase C (PKC), and mitogen-activated protein kinase (MAPK).

Studies done in our laboratory on L6 myoblasts and 3T3-L1 adipocytes presented a marked increase in 2-deoxy-glucose [2-DG) uptake induced by GTF, in a rate similar to insulin, indicating a high positive effect on glucose uptake (Figure 13) (From Weksler-Zangen et al., [65].

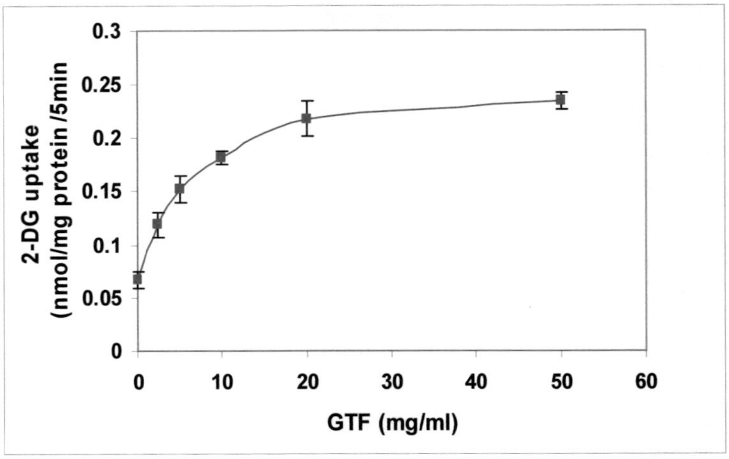

Glucose transport was measured in 3T3-L1 adipocytes in PBS (pH 7.4), at 37°C, with the addition of 0.05mmol/L (3H) 2-deoxyglucose. Different concentrations of GTF (0-20mg/ml) were assayed. Incubation time was 1 hour. Cells were dissolved in 1N NaOH, and aliquots were taken for scintillation counting and protein determination. Data are means ± SE n=3-4 plates in all experiments ($P<0.05$). (From Weksler-Zangen et al., [65].

Figure 13. GTF increases 2-Deoxy glucose uptake to 3T3-L1 adipocytes.

We also found that the increased glucose transport induced by GTF is dose dependent (Weksler-Zangen et al., [65]. A similar synergy between GTF and insulin that was demonstrated in diabetic animals in vivo was also found in vitro: The increase in 2-DG transport detected for the combination of GTF and insulin was much higher than for each agent alone. The rate of 2-DG transport found for the combined treatment exceeded the sum of the two separate treatments, indicating a synergy between GTF and insulin (Weksler-Zangen et al., [65]. We also found increased phosphorylation of key proteins along insulin signaling pathway, like IRS1, AKT, ccbl and MAPK, by the addition of GTF to the medium (Figures 14-16). GTF induced phophorylation of key proteins was dose and time dependent. The phosphorylation obtained by GTF was similar to that induced by insulin. However, we did not find any augmented phosphorylation of the insulin receptor following GTF addition, indicating a possible "by pass" of the insulin receptor by GTF.

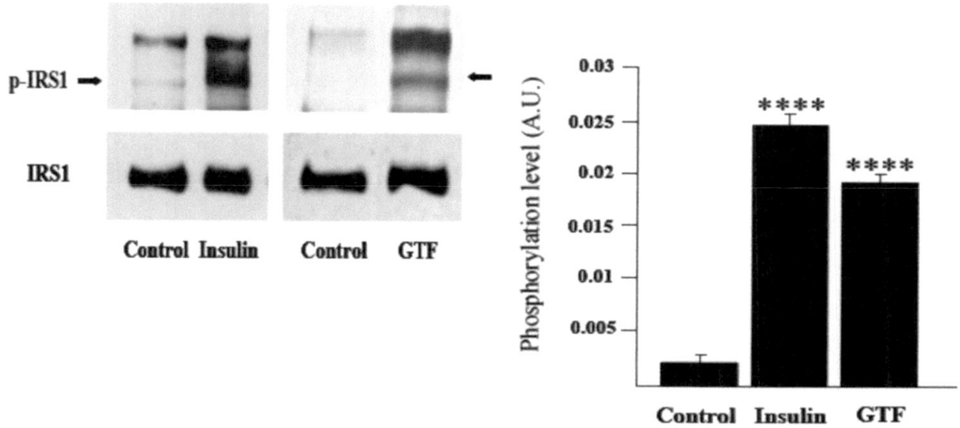

Differentiated 3T3-L1 adipocytes were serum starved for 18 hr. Cells were treated with 100nM insulin for 1 min or with 20 mg/ml GTF for 15 min. Cells were lysed and western blot analysis was performed with antibodies for phosphotyrosine followed by stripping and reblotting with antibodies for total IRS1 as a loading control. Quantification of the bands of P-IRS1 (mean ± SE) based on scanning densitometry of three independent immunoblots is represented by the bar graph (From Weksler-Zangen et al., [65].

Figure 14. GTF stimulates tyrosine phosphorylation on IRS1.

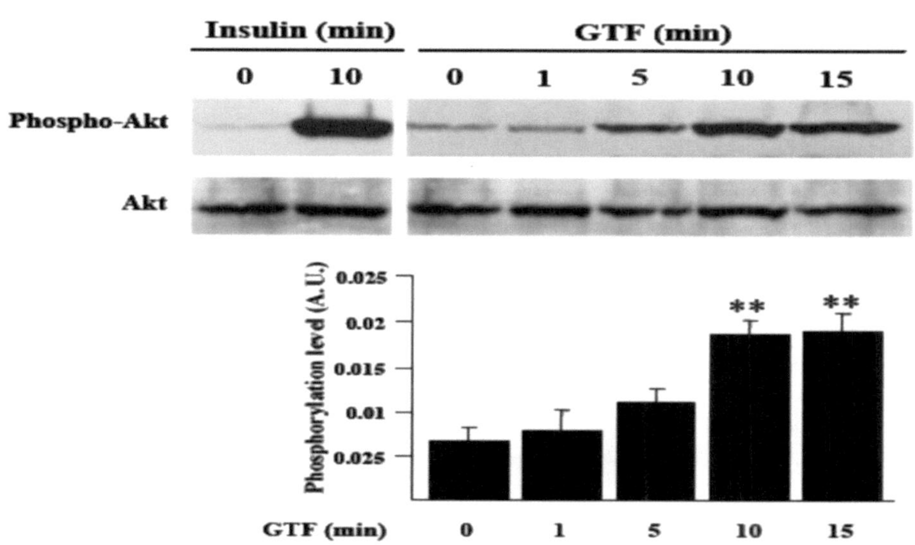

Differentiated 3T3-L1 adipocytes were serum starved for 18 hr. Cells were treated with 100nM insulin for 10 min or with 20 mg/ml GTF for 1, 5, 10 or 15 min. Cells were lysed and western blot analysis was performed with antibodies for phospho-Akt followed by stripping and reblotting with antibodies for total Akt as a loading control. Quantification of the bands of P-AKT (mean ± SE) based on scanning densitometry of three independent immunoblots is represented by the bar graph (From Weksler-Zangen et al., [65].

Figure 15. GTF stimulates AKT phosphorylation.

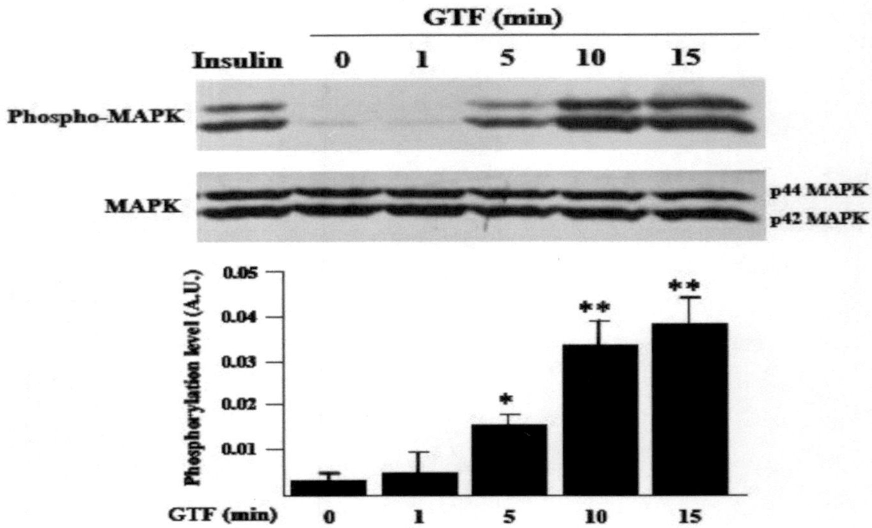

Differentiated 3T3-L1 adipocytes were serum starved for 18 hr. Cells were treated with 100nM insulin for 10 min or with 20 mg/ml GTF for 1, 5, 10 or 15 min. Cells were lysed and western blot analysis was performed with antibodies for phospho-p42/44 MAPK followed by stripping and reblotting with antibodies for total p42/44 MAPK as a loading control. Quantification of the bands of p42/44 MAPK (mean ± SE) based on scanning densitometry of three independent immunoblots is represented by the bar graph (From Weksler-Zangen et al., [65].

Figure 16. GTF stimulates MAPK phosphorylation.

11. Conclusions

In a search for new and effective medications for diabetes mellitus, there is a growing interest in natural derived hypoglycemic agents such as medicinal plants, herbs, and yeast. The Glucose Tolerance Factor (GTF), which is an active anti diabetic material extracted from yeast, is presented in the current manuscript.

GTF effectively decreased the elevated blood glucose in diabetic animals and humans. It also decreased triglycerides and LDL cholestrerol and increased HDL cholesterol in diabetic subjects. GTF treatment also prevented diabetes complications like nephropathy and retinopathy.

Not being a protein, GTF can be taken orally. GTF is both insulin mimicker and insulin potentiator: It can decrease glucose and lipids in the blood when given without any additional medication, but can also activate insulin effect: a small dose of insulin becomes more effective when administered with a dose of GTF.

GTF exerts insulin-mimetic and insulin-potentiating activity also in-vitro: glucose transport is increased by the addition of GTF. When GTF is added with insulin - an augmented glucose transport is detected.

In vitro studies shed light on the mechanism of action of GTF: GTF produces insulin-like effect by acting on cellular signals downstream of insulin receptor, regulating glucose transport, glycogen, and protein synthesis and modulating nuclear activity in the same manner as insulin. These results demonstrate GTF as a potential natural source for a novel oral anti diabetic drug in the future.

Author details

Nitsa Mirsky
Department of Biology, University of Haifa at Oranim, Tivon, Israel

12. References

[1] Schwarz, K., Mertz, W. (1959) Chromium III and the glucose tolerance factor. *Arch Biochem Biophys,* Vol. 85 pp. 292-295.
[2] Holdsworth, E.S., & Neville, E. (1990). Effects of extracts of high- and low-chromium brewer's yeast on. metabolism of glucose by hepatocytes from rats fed on high- or low-Cr diets. Br. J. Nutr. 63: pp 623-630
[3] WHO - World Health Organization report August 2011
[4] Shaw, J.E., Sicree, R.A., Zimmet, P.Z. (2010) Global estimates of the prevalence of diabetes for 2010 and 2030. *Diabetes Res Clin Pract.,* Vol. 87 pp.4-14
[5] Amos, A.F., McCarty, D.J., & Zimmet, P. (2010). The rising global burden of diabetes and its complications: estimates and projections to the year 2010. *Diabet Med.,* Vol 14, Issue S5, pp. S7–S85.
[6] Zhang , P., Zhang, X., Brown, J., Vistisen, D., Sicree, R., Shaw, J., & Nichols, G. (2010). Global healthcare expenditure on diabetes for 2010 and 2030 *Diab. Res. Clin. Pract.,* Vol 87, pp. 293-301.
[7] Baynes J.W., Thorpe S.R. (1999). Role of oxidative stress in diabetic complications. A new perspective on an old paradigm. *Diabetes.,* Vol 48, pp. 1-9.
[8] Brownlee, M. (2001). Biochemistry and molecular cell biology of diabetic complications. *Nature.,* Vol 414 pp. 813-820.
[9] Wolff, S.P., Dean, R.T. (1987). Glucose autoxidation and protein modification: the potential role of autoxidative glycosylation in diabetes. *Biochem. J.,* Vol. 245, pp. 243-250.
[10] Halliwell, B., Gutteridge, J.M.C. (1984). Lipid peroxidation, oxygen radicals, cell damage and antioxidant therapy. *Lancet* Vol. 1, pp. 1396-1397.
[11] Meerson, F.Z., Kagan, V.E., Kozlov, Y.P., Belkina, L.M., & Arkhipenko. Y.V. (1982). The role of lipid peroxidation in pathogenesis of ischemic damage and antioxidant protection in the heart. *Basic Res Cardiol,* Vol. 77, pp. 465-468.
[12] Kakkar, R., Kalra, J., Mantha, S.V., & Prasad, K. (1995). Lipid peroxidation and activity of antioxidant enzymes in diabetic rats. *Mol. Cell. Biochem,* Vol. 151, pp. 113- 119.
[13] Oberley, L.W. (1988). Free radicals and diabetes. Free Rad. Biol. Med, Vol. 5 pp. 111-124.
[14] Wolff, S.P. (1993). Diabetes mellitus and free radicals. *Brit. Med. Bull.,* Vol. 49, pp. 642-652.

[15] Hunt J.V., Smith, C.C.T., & Wolf, S.P. (1990). Autoxidative glycosylation and possible involvement of peroxides and free radicals in LDL modification by glucose. *Diabetes,* Vol. 39, pp. 1420-1424.

[16] Fridovich, I. (1998). Oxygen toxicity: a radical explanation J. Exp. Biol. 201: pp 1203–1209.

[17] Matkovics, B., Varga, S.I., Szabo, L., & Witas, H. (1983). The effect of diabetes on the activities of the peroxides metabolizing enzymes. *Horm Metab Res* 14, pp. 77-79.

[18] Baynes J.W., Thorpe S.R. (1996). The role of oxidative stress in diabetic complications. *Curr Opin Endocrinol.*, Vol 3, pp. 277-284.

[19] Srivastava, S.K., Ramana, K.V., & Bhatnagar, A. (2005). Role of aldose reductase and oxidative damage in diabetes and the consequent potential for therapeutic options. *Endocrine Reviews,* Vol. 26 No, 3, pp. 380–392.

[20] Miyamoto, S. (2002). Recent advances in aldose reductase inhibitors: Potential agents for the treatment of diabetic complications. *Expert Opin Ther Patents,* Vol. 12, pp. 621–631.

[21] Nyenwe, E.A., Jerkins T.W., Umpierrez G.E., & Kitabchi, A.E. (2011). Management of type 2 diabetes: evolving strategies for the treatment of patients with type 2 diabetes. *Metabolism,* Vol. 60, pp. 1-23.

[22] Chaturvedi, N. (2007). The burden of diabetes and its complications. trends and implications for intervention. *Diabetes Res. Clin. Pract.*, Vol 76, No. 1, pp. S3–12.

[23] Farnsworth, N.R. (1994). Ethnopharmacology and drug development. In: Chadwick DJ, Marsh J (eds). *Ethnobotany and the search for new drugs.* Ciba Foundation Symposium 185. John Wiley & sons. Chichester NY,pp 42-51.

[24] Marles R.J, Fransworth, N.R. (1995). Antidiabetic plants and their active constituents. *Phytomedicine* Vol. 2, pp. 137-189.

[25] Platel, K., Srinivasan K. (1997). Plant foods in the management of diabetes mellitus: vegetables as potential hypoglycaemic agents. *Food/Nahrung,* Vol. 41, No, 2, pp. 68-74.

[26] Tanira, M.O.M. (1994). Antidiabetic medicinal plants: a review of the present status and future directions. *Int J Diabetes,* Vol. 2, No.1, pp. 15-22.

[27] Zareba, G., Serradell, N., Castañer, R., Davies, S.L., Prous, J., & Mealy, N. (2005). Phytotherapies for diabetes. *Drugs of the Future,* Vol. 30, No. 12 pp. 1253-1282.

[28] Malviya, N., Jain, S. (2010). Anti diabetic potential of medicinal plants. *Acta Poloniae Pharmaceutica & Drug Research.* Vol. 67 No. 2, pp. 113-118.

[29] Bakhtiuary, Z. (2011). Herbal Medicines in Diabetes. *Iranian J. Diabetes & Obesity.*, Vol 3, No. 2, pp. 88-95.

[30] Madar. Z., Abel R., Samish, S., & Arad, J. (1988). Glucose lowering effect of fenugreek in non-insulin dependent diabetics. *Eur J. Clin. Nutr* Vol. 42, No.1, pp. 51-54.

[31] Basch, E., Gabardi, S., & Ulbricht, C. (2003). Bitter melon (Momordica charantia): a review of efficacy and safety. *Am. J. Health System.*, Vol 60, No. 4, pp. 356-359.

[32] Thomson, M., Al-Amin, Z.M., Al-Qattan, K.K., Shaban, L.H., & Ali, M. (2007). Anti-diabetic and hypolipidaemic properties of garlic (Allium sativum) in stereptozotocin-induced diabetic rats. *Int J Diabetes Metabol* , Vol.15, pp.108-115.

[33] Sheela, C.G., Augusti, K.T. (1992). Antidiabetic effects of Sallyl cysteine sulphoxide isolated from garlic Allium sativum Linn. *Indian J. Exp. biol,* Vol. 30 No. 6, pp. 523-526.

[34] Ramezani, M., Azar, A.M., Hosseini, H., Abdi, H., Baher, G.H., & Hosseini M.A.S. (2008). The effects of Silybum marianum (L.) Gaertn. seed extract on glycemic control in type II diabetic patient's candidate for insulin therapy visiting endocrinology clinic in Baqiyatallah Hospital in the years of 2006. *J. Med. Plants,* Vol. 7 No 26, pp. 79-84.

[35] Welihinda, J., Arvidson, G., Gylfe, E., Hellman, B., & Karlsson, E. (1982). The insulin-releasing activity of the tropical plant Momordica charantia. *Acta Bio., Med. Germ. Band,* Vol. 41, pp. 1229-1240.

[36] Tsuneki H, Ishizuka M, Terasawa M, Wu JB, Sasaoka T, Kimura I. (2004). Effect of green tea on blood glucose levels and serum proteomic patterns in diabetic (db/db) mice and on glucose metabolism in healthy humans. *BMC pharmacology,* Vol. 4, No.1, pp. 18-21.

[37] Zhou, L., Meng, Q., Qian, T., & Yang, Z., (2011). Ginkgo biloba extract enhances glucose tolerance in hyperinsulinism-induced hepatic cells. J, Nat, Med. Vol. 65, No. 1, pp. 50-6.

[38] Eydi, M., Solymani, F., & Ebrahimi, S. (2007). Hypolipidemic Effects of Allium porrum L. Leaves in Healthy and Streptozotocin-Induced Diabetic Mice. *J. Med Plants.* Vol. 6 No. 24, pp. 85-91.

[39] Anderson, R.A. (2008). Chromium and polyphenols from cinnamon improve insulin sensitivity. *Proc Nutr Soc.,* Vol 67, pp. 48-53

[40] Anderson, R.A., Roussel A.M. (2008). Cinnamon, glucose and insulin sensitivity. In: Pasupuleti V, Anderson JW, editors. *Nutraceuticals, glycemic health and type 2 diabetes.,* IFT press series. Wiley-Blackwell Publishing. pp. 127-140.

[41] Panickar, K.S., Cao, H., Qin, B., & Anderson, R.A. (2009). Molecular targets and health benefits of cinnamon. In: *Molecular targets and therapeutic uses of spices.*Aggarwal, B.B., Kunnumakkara, A.B., editors. pp. 87-116. World Scientific Publishing Co. Pte. Ltd., Hackensack, NJ.

[42] Qin, B., Panickar K.S., & Anderson R.A. (2010). Cinnamon: potential role in the prevention of insulin resistance, metabolic syndrome, and type 2 diabetes. *J. Diab. Sci Technol,* Vol. 4 pp. 685-693.

[43] Nahas, R., Moher, M. (2009). Complementary and alternative medicine for the treatment of type 2 diabetes. *Canadian Family Physician,* Vol. 55, pp. 591–596.

[44] Prabhakar, P.K., Doble, M. (2008). A target based therapeutic approach towards diabetes mellitus using medicinal plants. *Curr. Diab. Rev.,* Vol. 4, pp. 291–308.

[45] Samad, A., Shams, M.S., Ullah, Z., Wais, M., Nazish, I., Sultana, Y., & Aqil, M. (2009). Status of herbal medicines in the treatment of diabetes: a review. *Curr. Diab. Rev.,* Vol. 5, pp. 102–111.

[46] Offenbacher, E. G., Pi-Sunyer, F. X., (1980). Beneficial effect of chromium-rich yeast on glucose tolerance and blood lipids in elderly subjects. *Diabetes,* Vol. 29 pp. 919–925.

[47] Edens, N.K., Reaves, L.A,, Bergana, M.S., Reyzer, I.L., O'Mara, P., Baxter, J.H., & Snowden, M.K. (2002). Yeast extract stimulates glucose metabolism and inhibits lipolysis in rat adipocytes in vitro. *J. Nutr.* Vol. 132, No6, pp. 1141-1148.

[48] Tuman R.W., Bilbo, J.T., & Doisy, R.J. (1978) Comparison and effects of natural and synthetic Glucose Tolerance Factor in normal and genetically diabetic mice. *Diabetes,* Vol. 27 pp. 49-56.

[49] Mirsky, N. (1993) Glucose Tolerance Factor reduces blood glucose and free fatty acids levels in diabetic rats. *J Inorg Biochem,* Vol. 49, pp. 123-128.

[50] Grant A.P., McMullen J.K. (1982). The effect of brewer's yeast containing glucose tolerance factor on the response to treatment in type 2 diabetes, a short controlled study. *Ulster Med J,* Vol. 5, pp. 110-114.

[51] Yamamoto, A., Wada, O., & Ono, T. (1987). Isolation of a biologically active low molecular mass chromium compound from rabbit liver. *Eur. J. Biochem.,* Vol. 165, pp. 627-631.

[52] Mertz, W. (1975). Effects and metabolism of glucose tolerance factor. *Nutr. Rev,* Vol. 33, No. 5, pp. 129-135.

[53] Anderson, R.A., Brantner, J.H., & Polansky, M.M. (1978). An improved assay for biologically active chromium. *J. Agric Food Chem.*, Vol 26, pp. 1219-1221.

[54] Toepfer, E.W., Mertz, W., Polansky, M.M., & Wolf, W.R. (1977). Preparation of chromium containing material of glucose tolerance factor activity from brewer's yeast extracts and by synthesis. *J. Agric. Food Chem.,* Vol. 25, pp. 162-166.

[55] Mirsky, N., Weiss, A., & Dori, Z. (1980). Chromium in biological systems, I. Some observations on glucose tolerance factor in yeast. *J. Inorg. Biochem,* Vol. 13, pp. 11-21 (1980).

[56] Glinsmann, W. H., Feldman F. J. &. Mertz, W (1966). Plasma chromium after glucose administration. *Science,* Vol 152, pp. 1243-1245.

[57] Doisy, R.J., Streeten D.H.P. & Freiberg, J.M. (1976). Chromium metabolism in man and biochemical effects. In: *Trace elements in human health and disease,* edited by Prasad A.S. N.Y.: Academic Press, Vol. II, pp. 79-86.

[58] Elwood, J.C., Nash, D.T., & D. H. P. Streeton, D.H.P. (1982). Effect of high chromium brewer's yeast on human serum lipids, *J. Am. Coll. Nutr.,* Vol. 1, pp. 263-274.

[59] Riales, R. (1979). Influence of brewer's yeast on lipoprotein cholesterol concentrations. A preliminary report. In: *Chromium in nutrition and metabolism.* D. Shapcott, D., & Hubert, J. (eds), pp. 199-212, Amsterdam ; Elsvier / North Holland.

[60] Evans, G.W., Roginski, E.E., & W. Mertz, W. (1973). Interaction of the glucose tolerance factor (GTF) with insulin. *Biochem. Biophys. Res. Commun.* Vol. 50, pp. 718-722.

[61] Davies, D.M., Holdsworth, E.S., & J. L. Sherriff, J.L. (1985). The isolation of glucose tolerance factor from brewer's yeast and their relationship to chromium. *Biochem. Med.,* Vol 33, pp. 297-311.

[62] Tokuda, M., Kashiwagi, A., Wakamiya, E., Oguni, T., Mino, M., & Kagamiyama, H. (1987). Glucose Tolerance Factor stimulates 3-0 methylglucose transport into isolated rat adipocytes. *Biochem. Biophys. Res. Comm.,* Vol. 144 No. 3, pp. 1237-1242.

[63] Mirsky, N., Weiss, A., & Dori, Z. (1981). The effect of glucose tolerance factor on glucose uptake by yeast, *J. Inorg. Biochem,* Vol 15, pp. 275-279.

[64] Mirsky, N., Berdicevsky, I. (1994). Effects of insulin and glucose tolerance factor (GTF) on glucose uptake by yeast cells. *Biological Signals,* Vol. 3, pp. 271-277

[65] Weksler-Zangen, S., Mizrahi, T., Raz, I., & Mirsky, N. (2012). Glucose Tolerance Factor (GTF) extracted from yeast: oral insulin mimetic and insulin potentiating agent. In vivo and in vitro studies. *Br. J. Nutr.*, Vol. 108, pp. 875-882.

[66] Fischer, Y., Thomas, J., Rose, H., & Kammermeier, H. (1992). Alanine and hyperosmolarity are responsible for the stimulation of cardiomyocyte glucose transport by samples containing glucose tolerance factor. *Life Sciences,* Vol. 50, pp. 1963-1972.

[67] Hwang, D.L., Lev-Ran, A., Papoian, T., & Beech, W.K. (1987). Insulin like activity of chromium binding fractions from brewer's yeast, *J. Inorg. Biochem*, Vol. 30, pp. 219-225.

[68] Mertz, W., Toepfer, E.W., Roginski, E.E., & Anderson, R.A. (1974). Present knowledge of the role of chromium. *Fed. Proc,* Vol. 33, pp. 2275-2280.

[69] Anderson, R.A., Mertz, W. (1977). Glucose Tolerance Factor: an essential dietary agent. *Trends in Biochem., Sci.* Vol 2, pp. 277-279.

[70] Hwang, D., Lev-Ran, A., & Barseghian, K. (1991) U.S. Patent 4,985,439. Anheuser-Busch Companies, St. Louis MO.

[71] Muller, G., Wied, S., Crecelius, A., Kessler, A., & Eckel, J. (1997) Phosphoinositolglycan-peptides from yeast potently induce metabolic insulin actions in isolated rat adipocytes, cardiomyocytes, and diaphragms. *Endocrinology,* Vol. 138, pp. 3459–3475.

[72] Votava, H.J., Hahn, C.J., & Evans, G.W. (1973). Isolation and partial characterization of a 51Cr complex from brewer's yeast. *Biochem. Biophys. Res. Comm.,* Vol. 55, No. 2, pp. 312-319.

[73] Yamamoto, A., Wada, O., & Suzuki, H. (1988). Puurification and properties of biologically active chromium complex from bovine colostrums. *J.Nutr.,* Vol. 118, pp. 39-45.

[74] Urumow, T., Wieland, O.H. (1984). On the nature of the glucose tolerance factor from yeast. *Horm. Metabol. Res.,* Vol. 16, pp. 51-54 Suppl.

[75] Zetic,V.G., Stehlik-Tomas, V., Grba, S., Lutilsky, L., & Kozlek, D. (2001). Chromium uptake by Saccharomyces cerevisiae and isolation of glucose tolerance factor from yeast biomass. *J. Biosci.,* Vol. 26, No. 2 pp. 217–223.

[76] Haylock, S.J., Buckley, P.D., Blackwell, L.F. (1983). Separation of biologically active chromium-containing complexes from yeast extracts and other sources of glucose tolerance factor (GTF) activity. J. Inorg. Biochem. Vol 18 No 3. pp 195-211

[77] Shepherd, P.R., Elwood, C., Buckley, P.D., Blackwell, L.F. (1992). Glucose tolerance factor potentiation of insulin action in adipocytes from rats raised on a torula yeast diet cannot be attributed to a deficiency of chromium or glucose tolerance factor activity in the diet. *Biol Trace Elem Res,* Vol. 32, pp. 109-113.

[78] Stearns, D.M. (1996). Isolation and in vitro analysis of biologically active chromium. In: *Trace elements in laboratory rodents,* Watson, R. D., ed., vol. 1, pp. 3–37. CRC Press, Boca Raton, FL.

[79] Stearns, D.M. (2000). Is chromium a trace essential metal? *Bio Factors,* Vol. 11, No. 3, pp. 149–162.

[80] Mirsky, N., Aharoni, A., Rabinowitz, C., & Izhaki, I. (1999). Naturally occuring chromium compounds in brewer's yeast and saltbush plant. *J. Trace Elements Exp. Med,* Vol. 12, pp. 111-124.

[81] Nakhoul, F., Abassi, Z., Morgan, M., Sussan, S., & Mirsky N. (2006). Inhibition of diabetic nephropathy in rats by an oral anti diabetic material extracted from yeast. *J Am Soc Nephrol*, Vol. 17, pp. 127-131

Chapter 11

Medicinal Plants and Natural Compounds from the Genus *Morus* (Moraceae) with Hypoglycemic Activity: A Review

Jackson Roberto Guedes da Silva Almeida, Grasielly Rocha Souza, Edigênia Cavalcante da Cruz Araújo, Fabrício Souza Silva, Julianeli Tolentino de Lima, Luciano Augusto de Araújo Ribeiro, Xirley Pereira Nunes, José Maria Barbosa Filho, Lucindo José Quintans Júnior and Márcio Roberto Viana dos Santos

Additional information is available at the end of the chapter

http://dx.doi.org/10.5772/53145

1. Introduction

Diabetes mellitus (DM) is a metabolic disorder resulting from defects in insulin secretion or reduced sensitivity of the tissues to insulin action or both [1]. It is characterized by chronic high blood glucose that causes glycation of body proteins which could lead to severe complications. These complications are classified into acute, sub-acute and chronic.

Acute complications include hypoglycemia, diabetic ketoacidosis, hyperosmolar and hyperglycaemic non-ketotic syndrome while sub acute complications are thirst, polyuria, lack of energy, visual blurriness and weight loss. The chronic complications of diabetes mellitus include hypertension, neuropathy, nephropathy, retinopathy and diabetic foot ulcers which could result in amputation [2].

On the basis of aetiology and clinical presentation, diabetes mellitus can be grouped into type 1 known as insulin- dependent diabetes mellitus (IDDM) and type 2 also known as non insulin-dependent diabetes mellitus (NIDDM). The World Health Organization (WHO) recommends that the terms type 1 and type 2 should be reintroduced, because they classify the patients on the basis of the pathogenesis and not on the basis of treatment. Type 1 diabetes mellitus is caused by immunological destruction of pancreatic β cells leading to insulin deficiency [3], whereas type 2 diabetes results from defects in insulin secretion or rather insulin resistance. It is the most common type of diabetes, afflicting 85-95% of all diabetic individuals. It is a prevalent form of the disease and common in individuals over 40 years of age. The increasing number of ageing population, consumption of calorie-rich diet, obesity and sedentary life style have led to a tremendous increase in the number of diabetes mellitus world wide [2]. About 173 million people suffer with this disease. The number of people with diabetes mellitus will be more than double over the next 25 years to reach a total of 366 million by 2030 [4].

The only therapy of type 1 diabetes is the substitution of insulin. Many and diverse therapeutic strategies for the treatment of type 2 diabetes are known. Conventional treatments include the reduction of the demand for insulin, stimulation of endogenous insulin secretion, enhancement of the action of insulin at the target tissues and the inhibition of degradation of oligo- and disaccharides. One group of drugs introduced in the management of type 2 diabetes is represented by the inhibitors of α-glycosidase [4].

In a general manner DM is a group of metabolic disorders characterized by hyperglycemia. These metabolic disorders include alterations in carbohydrate, fat and protein metabolisms associated with absolute and relative deficiencies in insulin secretion and/or insulin action [5]. Insulin is a hormone needed to convert sugar, starch and other food into energy needed for daily life. The cause of diabetes continues to be a mystery, although both genetic and environmental factors such as obesity and lack of exercise appear to play a part [6]. The control of DM normally involves exercise, diet and drug therapy. In the last years there has been an increasing demand for natural products with antidiabetic activity, mainly due to the side effects associated with the use of insulin and oral hypoglycemic agents [7]. The available therapies for diabetes include insulin and oral antidiabetic agents such as sulfonylureas, biguanides and α-glycosidase inhibitors. Many of these oral antiabetic agents have a number of serious adverse effects [8]. Thus, the management of diabetes without any side effects is still a challenge.

Plants have always been an important source of drugs and many of the currently available drugs have been derived directly or indirectly from them. Ethnobotanical reports indicate about 1200 plants in the world with anti-diabetic potential [9], of which more than three hundred have been reported in the literature referring to a large variety of identified chemical substances. The discovery of the widely used hypoglycemic drug, metformin (*N,N*-dimethylguanylguanidine) came from the traditional approach through the use of *Galega officinalis* [10].

In this regard, several medicinal plants among which are those belonging to the genus *Morus* have been reported to be used in traditional medicine for the treatment of DM. Medicinal plants are one of the few therapeutic resources available to most population. According to this reality it is essential to search new alternatives for the treatment of DM. Several plant species have been studied as potential antidiabetic agents.

Considering the importance of species of the genus *Morus* in treatment of diabetes mellitus, this chapter is a review of medicinal plants and natural products with hypoglycaemic activity from genus *Morus* and the main methods used in the assessment of hypoglycemic potential of these plants.

2. Methods

With the objective of contributing to these studies, a literature search on the ethnomedical information and use of natural products (crude plant extracts, semi-purified fractions and chemically defined molecules) from the genus *Morus* which have already been evaluated particularly for hypoglycemic activity was carried out. The keywords used for the literature search for this review were *Morus*, Moraceae, hypoglycemic activity, antidiabetic activity, medicinal plants and natural products. The search was carried out using Biological Abstracts, Chemical Abstracts, and the data bank of the University of Illinois in Chicago NAPRALERT (Acronym for NAtural PRoducts ALERT), updated to December 2011. The references found in the search were then studied in detail. Only those plants whose extracts and/or isolated constituents that showed clear pharmacological effects with hypoglycemic activity in animal models were included in this review.

3. Results and discussion

In this section we present some considerations about the Moraceae family, the main species from the genus *Morus* and chemical constituents isolated from species of this genus with hypoglycemic activity as well as important methods for assessing the hypoglycemic potential of natural products and plant extracts.

Consultation of various literature sources resulted in the elaboration of a list of some active biomolecules of different *Morus* species and natural products evaluated for hypoglycemic activity (Tables 1, 2 and 3). It should be noted that most of the references cited are not first-hand observations, but compilations copied from other sources. For details on the models or mechanism-based bioassays utilized for selecting crude plant extracts, fractions and other preparations for hypoglycemic activity, the original references should be consulted.

3.1. The family Moraceae and the genus *Morus*

Moraceae is a family of flowering plants that comprises about 40 genera and over 1000 species [11]. The genus *Morus*, is widely distributed in Asia, Europe, North America, South America, and Africa, and is cultivated extensively in the eastern, central, and southern Asia for silk production. Mulberry (*Morus* sp.) has been domesticated over thousands of years and has been adapted to a wide area of tropical, subtropical, and temperate zones of the world [12].

Morus is a genus with species of deciduous trees [11]. There are 24 species of *Morus* and one subspecie, with at least 100 known varieties. Mulberry is found from temperate to subtropical regions of the Northern hemisphere to the tropics of the Southern hemisphere and they can grow in a wide range of climatic, topographic and soil conditions [13]. Some species of this genus are widely cultived in many countries, in particular in China and Japan, where mulberry is used for its foliage to feed the silkworm [14].

Species of this genus has also been used in folk medicine (especially in Chinese traditional medicine) as antiphlogistic, hepatoprotective, hypotensive, antipyretic, analgesic, diuretic, expectorant, antidiabetic [14, 15] as well as to treat anemia and arthritis [12]. The leaves of mulberry species are consumed in Korea and Japan as anti-hyperglycemic nutraceutical food for patients with diabetes mellitus because the leaves are rich in alkaloid components, including 1-deoxynojirymicin (**1**), which is known to be one of the most potent α-glycosidase inhibitors [16] that decreases blood sugar levels.

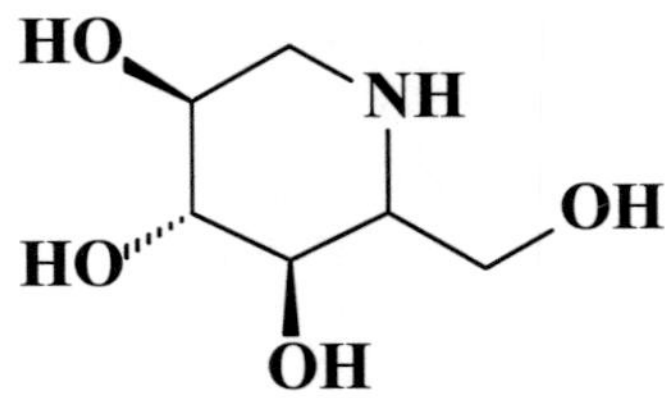

Figure 1. Chemical structure of compound (**1**) isolated from species of *Morus*.

This genus contains a variety of phenolic compounds including isoprenylated flavonoids, stilbenes, 2-arylbenzopyrans, coumarins, chromones, xanthones and a variety of Diels-Alder adduct compounds [14, 17]. Some of these compounds exhibit interesting biological properties such as antiphlogistic, antiinflammatory, diuretic, hypotensive effects and some are known as phytoalexins [18]. The antioxidant potential of some phenolic compounds of *Morus alba* also been reported in the literature [19].

The production of mulberry fruits in 2005 was 78,000 tonnes in Turkey and its cultivation in Turkey have been known for more than 400 years [20].

3.2. *Morus alba* L.

Morus alba, known as white mulberry, is a species native to China and now widely cultivated in other countries. It has white and purple fruits with a very sweet taste and low acidity. Its fruits are perishable and mostly used for fresh consumption. The fruit of white mulberry (which is also found in the Eastern United States) is white to pinkish, unlike the red or black berries of most other *Morus* species. According to sources, white mulberry is the species that has been used exclusively in Chinese medicine since A.D- 659. The Chinese Pharmacopoeia (1985) lists the leaves, root bark, branches, and fruits as ingredients in medicinal preparations, but other parts, including the sap and wood ash, are also widely used [21].

The different parts of this plant have been used in the traditional Chinese medicine for many purposes. The white mulberry leaves, an important food for silkworm, are used to treat hypertension, arthritis, and the fruit is a diuretic and a tonic agent. The root bark of the plant is considered as an important medicine to treat cough, inflammation, diabetes, cancer, hepatitis and heart diseases. Previous studies showed that *M. alba* mainly contained polyphenolic constituents including prenylated flavonoids, benzofurans and Diels–Alder type adducts with various biological activities such as cytotoxicity, antioxidant, inhibition of NF-κB, LOX-1, cancer cell invasion and migration, and hepatoprotection. The glycosidase inhibitory activity of several alkaloids in *M. alba* has also been reported [22]. The root is astringent and bark is anti-helmintic. Root is one of the constituents of the Chinese drug named "Sohaku-hi" which reduces the plasma sugar level in mice. Decorked bark is used against chronic bronchitis and emphysema [23].

The root bark also contain an alkaloid, 1-deoxynojirimycin (**1**) that inhibited glycogenolyses, glycoprotein, processing and saccharide hydrolysis enzymes whereas its derivatives have great therapeutic potential for the treatment of viral infections, diabetes, obesity and cancer [21]. *Morus alba* leaves containing many nutritional components are the best feed for silkworms and they have been used in traditional Chinese medicine as an antihyperglycemic to treat and to prevent diabetes mellitus. The components are flavones, steroids, triterpenes, amino acids, vitamins and other trace minerals. Among the 6 N-containing sugars isolated, 2-*O*-α-D-galactopyranosyl-DNJ (GAL-DNJ) and fagomine have the most potent antihyperglycemic effects [24]. Table 1 lists some active biomolecules of different *Morus* species with their medicinal properties.

3.3. *Morus bombycis*

This plant is found in China, Japan, Korea and Southern Sakhaline. Root bark contains quinones named as Kwanons G and H with hypotensive activity, phytoalexins like Moracin A-Z and Albanins A-H with antimicrobial activity. The leaves also contain *N*-methyl-1-deoxynojirimycin which is used against diabetes mellitus. This compound is also inhibits the infectivity of human immunodeficiency virus [21].

3.4. *Morus indica* L.

Over the years, medicinal plants and their extracts are gaining importance in the treatment of hyperglycemia and diabetes. The extracts of *Morus indica,* commonly known as mulberry, have been reported to possess medicinal properties, including hypoglycemic, hypotensive and diuretic activities. The hypoglycemic effect of mulberry leaves or shoot culture extract has been demonstrated using streptozotocin-induced diabetic animals [25]. The ethanol extract from the leaves of *Morus indica* showed antiinflammatory activity on carragenan-induced edema in rats and cotton pellet granuloma models [26].

3.5. *Morus insignis*

Ethyl acetate and n-butanol-soluble fractions of the leaves of *Morus insignis* showed a significant hypoglycemic activity on streptozotocin (STZ)-induced hyperglycemic rats. From these hypoglycemic activity-showing fractions, two new compounds, mulberrofuran U and moracin M-3-*O*-β-*D*-glucopyranoside were isolated, along with six known compounds (β-sitosterol, β-sitosterol-3-*O*-β-glucopyranoside, ursolic acid, moracin M, kaempferol-3-*O*-β-glucopyranoside and quercetin-3-*O*-β-glucopyranoside) [27]. The fungicidal, bactericidal and hypoglycemic activities of leaves of *M. insignis* have been attributed to benzofurans Mulberrofuran U and Moracin M-3'-*O*-β-*D*-glucopyranoside [28].

Name of Morus species	Active constituents	Plant part used	Medicinal properties
Morus alba	Kwanon I; Kwanon I hexamethyl ether; Kwanon I octamethyl ether; 2′-Hydroxy-2,4,4′-trimethoxychalcone; 2′-Hydroxy-3′-prenyl-2,4,4′-trimethoxychalcone III; Mulberrofuran T; Kwanon E; Morusin, Mulberrofuran D, G, K; Kwanon G, H; Mulberroside A; *Cis*-mulberrosideA; Oxyresveratrol; Isoquercetin; Kwanon G; Moracin E, F, G and H; Kwanon D, E, F; Deoxynojirimycin-1	Root, stem, leaves, fruit	Astringent, anti-helmintic, HIV, cough, antiinflammatory, exudative, high blood pressure, diaphoretic, purgative, emollient, diarhoea, **diabetes**, atherosclerosis, anti-tumor, hypoglycemia
Morus australis	Australone A; triterpenoid 3β-[(*m*-methoxybenzoyl) oxy]-urs-12-en-28-oic acid; morusin; Kwanon C; betulinic acid; β-amyrin; quercetin; ursolic acid; Mulberrofuran D; sanggenols N and O	Root, leaves, fruits	Astringent, anti-helmintic, purgative, antiplatelet
Morus bombycis	*N*-methyl-1-Deoxynojirimycin; Kwanon G, H; Moracin A-Z; Albanins A-H; γ-aminobutyric acid; *L*-asparagine; *L*-arginine; *L*- lysine; choline; Mulberrofuran I	Root, leaves	Hypotensive, antimicrobial, **diabetes**, HIV, antiphlogistic, diuretic
Morus laevigata	Citrulline; hydroxyproline; free amino acids	Fruit	Plaster for sores, cools the blood
Morus nigra	Deoxynojirimycin	Root, leaves, fruits	**Diabetes**, AIDS, purgative, arterial pressure, vermifuge, cancer
Morus serrata	β-Amyrin acetate; betulinic acid; cerylalcohol; quercetin; morin	Root	-----
Morus rubra	Rubraflavones A, B, C, D	Root	Anti-dysenteric, laxative, purgative, vermifuge, urinary problems, weakness
Morus macroura	Guangsangons A-N; albafuran C; Kwanon J, X, Y; Mulberrofuran G, K, J	Stem	Antiinflammatory, antioxidative
Morus cathayana	Sanggenols F, G, H, I, J, K; cathayanon A, B	Root	Antiinflammatory, hypertension

Adapted from reference [21].

Table 1. Active biomolecules of different *Morus* species

3.6. *Morus nigra* L.

Morus nigra, known as black mulberry, is one of the most important species of the genus *Morus*. It has juicy fruits with extraordinary color and a unique, slightly acidic flavor. The fruits are 2-3 cm long [12].

A medium or small sized tree 6-9 m high, native to West Asia. It is also cultivated in Kashmir, Darjeeling, leaves are ovate-cordate, flower dioecious or monoecious, fruits are syncarp, ovoid, purple to black, juicy, edible. The root bark is purgative and vermifuge. Root has and effect on pancreas and glycogenolysis while its juice reduces the blood sugar level in diabetic patient. The root bark extract contains deoxynojirimycin (DNJ), an alkaloid which said to be active against AIDS virus. An infusion of leaves causes a drop in blood sugar, sometimes diuresis and a reduction of arterial pressure [21].

DNJ is a potent source α-glycosidase inhibitor and helpful to establish greater glycemic control in type 2 diabetes. Young mulberry leaves taken from top part of branches in summer contains the highest amount of DNJ. In a human study, DNJ enriched powder of mulberry leaves significantly suppressed elevation of post-prandial glucose. Newly developed DNJ enriched powder can be used as a dietary supplement for preventing diabetes mellitus [21].

Morus nigra and other members of its genus can be grown without protection in many countries. The berries, bark and leaves of the black mulberry are all used medicinally, the berries for inflammation and to stop bleeding, the bark for toothache, and the leaves for snake bites and as an antidote to action poisoning. In Europe, black mulberry leaves have been used recently to stimulate insulin production in diabetes. Mulberry contains soluble plant chemicals known as bioflavonoids. These powerful antioxidants may be responsible for their medicinal properties [29].

Morus nigra has been used in folk medicine as an analgesic, diuretic, antitussive, sedative, anxiolytic and hypotensive, in addition to its uses in the treatment of a variety of ailments, including inflammatory disorders [17]. There are few studies involving the chemical composition and evaluation of biological and pharmacological properties of *Morus nigra*. Morusin, the main prenylflavonoid present in the root bark of this specie have been investigated in classical models of pain in mice and exhibits a promising antinociceptive or analgesic profile [30]. In recent studies, Naderi et al. [29] demonstrated that extracts of *Morus nigra* fruits have a protective action against peroxidative damage to biomembranes and biomolecules. Antiinflammatory properties of methylene chloride extract from leaves [31] as well as antinociceptive effects [32] were reported. Three new compounds including two flavonoids and a new 2-phenylbenzofuran, named morunigrols A-C, together with three known compounds albafuran A, albafuran B and mulberrofuran L were isolated from the barks of Morus nigra [33]. Two new prenylflavonoids, mornigrol E and mornigrol F were isolated from the barks of this specie [34], as well as germanicol, betulinic acid and β-sitosterol [31]. Figure 2 shows the chemical structures of some chemical constituents isolated from species of the genus *Morus*.

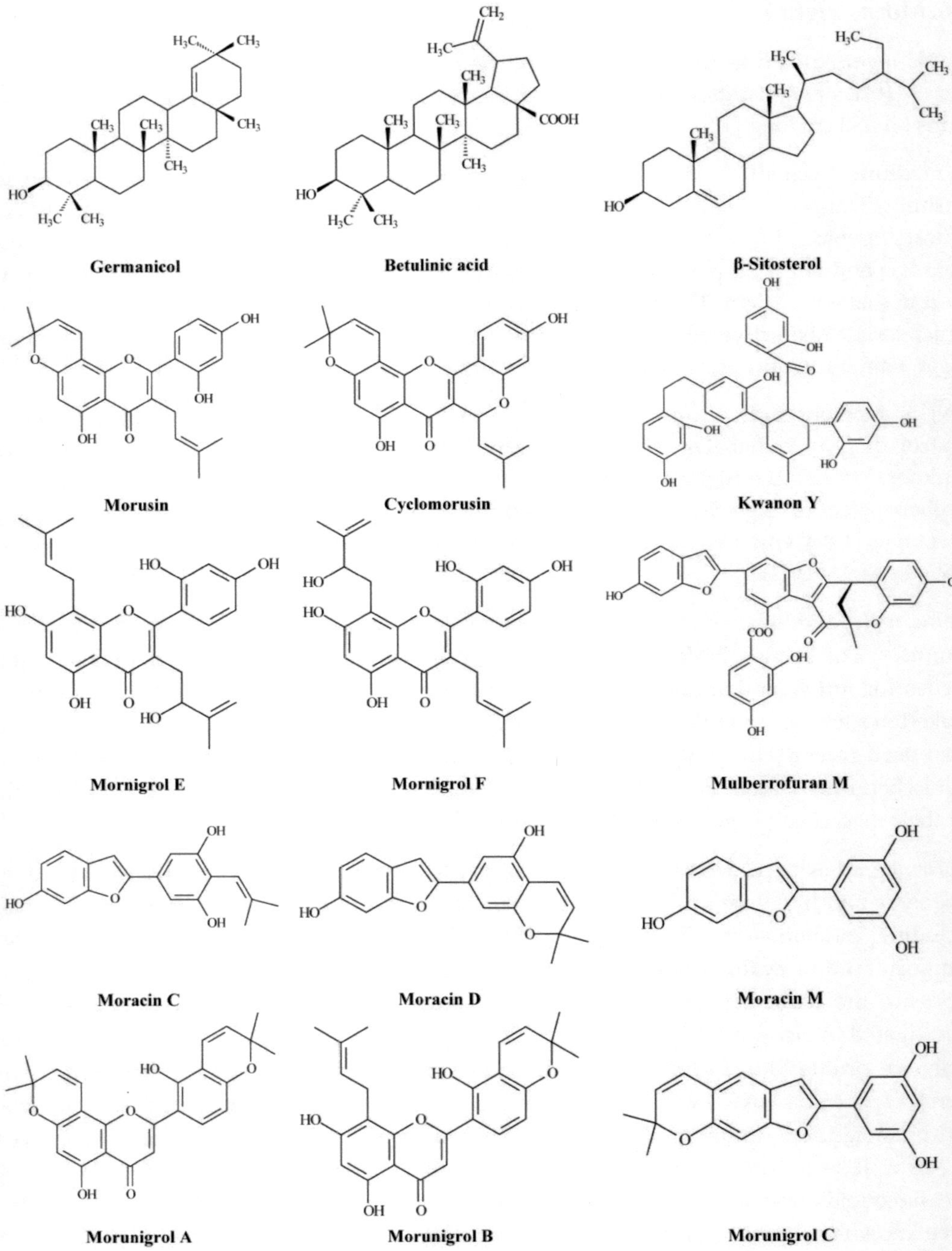

Figure 2. Chemical structures of some natural compounds isolated from species of the genus *Morus*.

Botanical name	Origin (Part used)	Use	Preparation	Via	Organism	References
Morus alba	Japan (B)	Used for diabetes	Decoction	Oral	Human adult	[42]
	Japan (C)	Used as an antidiabetic	Bark	Oral	Human adult	[43]
	Chile (L)	Used to treat diabetes	Infusion	Oral	Human adult	[44]
	Spain (L)	Used as a hypoglycemic	Hot H_2O extract	Oral	Human adult	[45]
	Turkey (L)	Used for diabetes	Decoction	Oral	Human adult	[46]
	Yugoslavia (L)	Used for diabetes	Hot H_2O extract	Oral	Human adult	[47]
	Peru (L + S)	Used as an antidiabetic	Hot H_2O extract	Oral	Human adult	[48]
	France (L)	Used for diabetes	Hot H_2O extract	Oral	Human adult	[49]
Morus lhou	Italy (L)	Used as an antidiabetic	Infusion	Oral	Human adult	[50]
Morus nigra	Canary Islands (FL)	Used as a hypoglycemic	Infusion	Oral	Human adult	[51]
	Iran (L)	Used in diabetes	Decoction	Oral	Human adult	[52]
	Yugoslavia (L)	Used for diabetes	Hot H_2O extract	Oral	Human adult	[53]
	Puerto Rico (NS)	Used for diabetes	Hot H_2O extract	Oral	Human adult	[54]
	Iran (RB)	Used in diabetes	Decoction	Oral	Human adult	[52]
Morus species	USSR (L)	Used for diabetes mellitus	Hot H_2O extract	Oral	Human adult	[55]

B= barks; C= cortex; F= fruit; FL= flowers; L= leaf; NS= not specified; RB= root bark; S= stem

Table 2. Ethnomedical information of *Morus*.

The leaves of *M. nigra* are commonly used by women in menopause as a substitute for the conventional hormonal replacement therapy, with a similar effect to that obtained after estrogen use. Moreover, the leaves are also used by younger women as a reliever of the symptoms of the premenstrual tension. The use of *M. nigra* usually involves the preparation of a "tea" (i.e. through decoction or infusion of the leaves) and is reported to ameliorate the symptoms of menopause, particularly hot flashes, which are related to the sudden vasodilatation that causes the feeling of intense heat and redness of the skin, namely the face [35].

In Brazil, the cultivation of *M. nigra* began with the Japanese migration into the country, adapting well to conditions of climate and soil. In a recent study realized by our research group [36], we evaluated the hypoglycemic potential and acute toxicity of the crude ethanol extract of the leaves, and we observed that the extract may be considered of low toxicity since it did not cause death or alterations on hematological and biochemical parameters in animals.

Botanical name	Origin (Part used)	Activity	Extract	Dose/concent.	Result	References
Morus alba	Iran (B)	Antihyperglycemic	Decoction	500.0 mg/kg	Inactive	[56]
	Japan (B)	α-Glycosidase inhibition	Hot H_2O extract	80.0 mg/kg	Active	[57]
	South Korea (B)	Hypoglycemic activity	MeOH extract	2.0 mg/kg	Inactive	[58]
	China (BR)	Antihyperglycemic	Hot H_2O extract	1.25 mg/kg	Active	[59]
	China (BR)	Hypoglycemic activity	Hot H_2O extract	1.25 mg/kg	Active	[59]
	China (BR)	Antihyperglycemic	H_2O extract	2.1 mg/kg	Active	[59]
	Japan (C)	Glucose transport stimulation	MeOH extract	5.0 mcg/ml	Weak activity	[43]
	Iran (F)	Antihyperglycemic	Decoction	500.0 mg/kg	Inactive	[56]
	Chile (L)	Antihyperglycemic	Infusion	0.40 g/animal	Active	[44]
	Chile (L)	Antihyperglycemic	Infusion	0.40 g/animal	Inactive	[44]
	China (L)	Antihyperglycemic	Hot H_2O extract	200.0 mg/kg	Active	[60]
	Egypt (L)	Hypoglycemic activity	EtOH (100%) extract	Dose not stated	Active	[61]
	Egypt (L)	Antihyperglycemic	EtOH (100%) extract	Dose not stated	Active	[61]
	Egypt (L)	Antihyperglycemic	Leaf	Dose not stated	Active	[61]
	Egypt (L)	Antihyperglycemic	EtOH (100%) extract	Dose not stated	Inactive	[61]
	Iran (L)	Antihyperglycemic	Decoction	500.0 mg/kg	Inactive	[56]
	Iran (L)	Hypoglycemic activity	Decoction	500.0 mg/kg	Inactive	[56]
	Japan (L)	Antihyperglycemic	Hot H_2O extract	80.0 mg/kg	Active	[57]

Botanical name	Origin (Part used)	Activity	Extract	Dose/concent.	Result	References
	Japan (L)	Antihyperglycemic	Hot H_2O extract	200.0 mg/kg	Active	[60]
	Roumania (L)	Antihyperglycemic	Infusion	150.0 ml/person	Active	[62]
	South Korea (L)	Antihyperglycemic	Not specified	Dose not stated	Active	[63]
	Zimbabwe (L)	Hypoglycemic activity	EtOH (80%) extract	200.0 mg/kg	Active	[64]
	Zimbabwe (L)	Antihyperglycemic	EtOH (80%) extract	200.0 mg/kg	Active	[64]
	Zimbabwe (L)	Insulin level increase	EtOH (80%) extract	200.0 mg/kg	Inactive	[64]
	Japan (L)	Antihyperglycemic	EtOH (5%) extract	200.0 mg/kg	Active	[65]
	Japan (P)	Antihyperglycemic	Lyophilized extract	200.0 mg/kg	Active	[65]
	Iran (R)	Antihyperglycemic	Decoction	500.0 mg/kg	Inactive	[56]
	China (RB)	Hypoglycemic activity	EtOH:H_2O (1:1) extract	20.0 mg/kg	Active	[66]
	Egypt (RB)	Antihyperglycemic	EtOH (70%) extract	600.0 mg/kg	Active	[67]
	South Korea (RB)	Antihyperglycemic	H_2O extract	1.0 mg/kg	Strong activity	[68]
	China (R)	Antihyperglycemic	Hot H_2O extract	200.0 mg/kg	Active	[60]
Morus bombycis	China (NS)	Hypoglycemic activity	EtOH (95%) extract	Dose not stated	Active	[69]
Morus indica	India (L)	Antihyperglycemic	H_2O extract	250.0 mg/animal	Active	[70]
	India (SC)	Antihyperglycemic	H_2O extract	130.0 mg/animal	Active	[70]
Morus insignis	Argentina (L)	Antihyperglycemic	EtOH (70%) extract	100.0 mg/kg	Active	[27]
	Argentina (L)	Hypoglycemic activity	EtOAc extract	50.0 mg/kg	Active	[27]
	Argentina (L)	Hypoglycemic activity	BuOH extract	50.0 mg/kg	Active	[27]
	Argentina (L)	Hypoglycemic activity	H_2O extract	50.0 mg/kg	Active	[27]
	Argentina (L)	Antihyperglycemic	EtOAc extract	100.0 mg/kg	Active	[27]
	Argentina (L)	Antihyperglycemic	BuOH extract	100.0 mg/kg	Active	[27]

Botanical name	Origin (Part used)	Activity	Extract	Dose/concent.	Result	References
Morus nigra	Iran (B)	Antihyperglycemic	Decoction	500.0 mg/kg	Active	[56]
	Iran (B)	Antihyperglycemic	Decoction	500.0 mg/kg	Inactive	[56]
	France (L)	Hypoglycemic activity	Hot H_2O extract	Dose not stated	Active	[49]
	France (L)	Hypoglycemic activity	Hot H_2O extract	Dose not stated	Active	[71]
	Iran (L)	Hypoglycemic activity	EtOH (95%) extract	0.25 mg/kg	Inactive	[72]
	Iran (L)	Hypoglycemic activity	EtOH (95%) extract	1.0 mg/kg	Inactive	[72]
	Iran (L)	Antihyperglycemic	EtOH (95%) extract	0.25 mg/kg	Active	[72]
	Iran (L)	Antihyperglycemic	EtOH (95%) extract	0.5 mg/kg	Active	[72]
	Iran (L)	Antihyperglycemic	Decoction	500.0 mg/kg	Active	[56]
	Iran (L)	Hypoglycemic activity	Decoction	500.0 mg/kg	Inactive	[56]
	Iran (L)	Antihyperglycemic	Decoction	500.0 mg/kg	Inactive	[56]
	Iran (RB)	Antihyperglycemic	Decoction	500.0 mg/kg	Inactive	[56]
Morus species	India (L)	Antihyperglycemic	EtOH (95%) extract	0.5 ml/animal	Inactive	[73]
	India (L)	Hypoglycemic activity	EtOH (95%) extract	0.5 ml/animal	Equivocal	[73]
	India (L)	Antihyperglycemic	EtOH (95%) extract	0.5 ml/animal	Equivocal	[73]
	USSR (L)	Antihyperglycemic	Tincture	Dose not stated	Active	[55]
	Japan (L)	Antihyperglycemic	Infusion	150.0 mg/kg	Active	[74]

B= barks; BR= branches; C= cortex; F= fruit; FL= flowers; L= leaf; NS= not specified; P= protoplasts; R= root; RB= rootbark; S= stem; SC= shoot culture

Table 3. Biological activities for extracts of *Morus*.

3.7. Methods for evaluation of hypoglycemic activity of medicinal plants

3.7.1. Oral glucose tolerance test

The oral glucose tolerance test is a fast and inexpensive technique and allows you to check the effects of drugs on glucose metabolism. In normoglycemic rats, the increase of post-prandial glucose level, after glucose load, and the consequent standardization to baseline levels after about 2 h, characterizes a normal metabolism of glucose. The oral glucose tolerance test is an acute methodology for evaluating the resistance of the body to absorb glucose and reduce blood glucose levels. Therefore, it's a method to perform a screening of drugs with potential hypoglycemic action, but with a profile in the absorption of glucose (type 2 DM) and not in the production of insulin (type 1 DM) [37].

In this experiment, normal Wistar rats are fasted overnight. They are divided into three groups containing six animals each.

Control rats (Group I) are given 1 ml distilled water orally. Extracts of plants in different concentrations (mg/kg body weight) are administered orally using a syringe to second and third groups. Glucose (2 g/kg b.wt.) is given orally using a syringe to all groups immediately after the extracts administration. Blood samples are collected from the tail vein just prior to and 30, 60, 120 and 240 min after the glucose loading and serum glucose levels are measured [38].

3.7.2. Alloxan-induced diabetic rats

Alloxan induces "chemical diabetes" in a wide variety of animal species by damaging the insulin secreting pancreatic β-cell, resulting in a decrease in endogenous insulin release [39]. Numerous studies demonstrated that a variety of plant extracts effectively lowered the glucose level in alloxan-induced diabetic animals. Alloxan produces oxygen radicals in the body, which cause pancreatic injury which is responsible for increased blood sugar seen in the animals. However, it is found that action is not specific to pancreas as other organs such as liver, kidney and haemopoietic system are also affected by alloxan administration as seen from the elevation of marker enzymes and reduction of hematological parameters [40].

In this experiment, diabetes is induced in male rats by single intraperitonial injection of 120 mg/kg b.wt. of alloxan monohydrate. Serum glucose level is checked after 72 h. Animals with serum glucose levels >250 mg/dl are considered diabetic and are used for the study. The rats are divided into four groups of six rats each. Both group I control normal rats (no alloxan treatment) and group II diabetic animals are given 1 ml of distilled water. Group III and IV are given the extracts orally in different doses on 3rd day after alloxan treatment. Overnight fasted blood samples are collected from the tail vein on 3rd day of alloxan treatment prior to and at 2, 4, 6 and 8 h intervals after the administration of the extract orally. Serum is separated and glucose levels are estimated as before [38].

3.7.3. Streptozotocin-induced diabetic rats

Streptozotocin (STZ) at low dose for Wistar rats induces light damage to islet cells, leading to glucose intolerance. Previous studies have showed that STZ-induced diabetic rats had low production of insulin and high levels of blood circulating glucose, which were similar to those found in diabetic humans. The precise mechanisms responsible for this defect remain unknown.

Male rats weighing 150-200 g are used in the study and type 2 diabetes is induced. The rats are fed with high fat diet (diet containing 74% carbohydrate, 22% protein and 4% fat, formulated as 60% total energy is derived from fat) for 15 days except normal control rats and then injected with streptozotocin (40 mg/kg). Five days after injection, the rats are fasted and the plasma glucose levels are estimated; rats having plasma glucose levels ≥300 mg/dl are taken for further studies with administration of plant extracts. The rats are fed with high fat diet throughout the experimental period [41].

4. Conclusion

Diabetes mellitus is a public health problem worldwide. Ethnomedical informations and the scientific knowledge of the hypoglycemic activity of species of *Morus* demonstrate the potential of these species in the treatment of diabetes. *In vivo* testing has become an important tool in the search for new antidiabetic agents. The present work showed that therapy with species from the genus *Morus* traditionally used in many countries could be a possibility to treat diabetes. On the other hand, medicinal plants contain an enormous potential for the development of new antidiabetic drugs. In conclusion, the present study provides data which suggest that therapy with mulberry is capable of enhancing glycemic control in patients with diabetes.

Author details

Jackson Roberto Guedes da Silva Almeida, Grasielly Rocha Souza,
Edigênia Cavalcante da Cruz Araújo, Fabrício Souza Silva,
Julianeli Tolentino de Lima, Luciano Augusto de Araújo Ribeiro and Xirley Pereira Nunes
1Nucleus of Studies and Research of Medicinal Plants, Federal University of San Francisco Valley, Petrolina, Pernambuco, Brazil

José Maria Barbosa Filho
Federal University of Paraíba, João Pessoa, Paraíba, Brazil

Lucindo José Quintans Júnior and Márcio Roberto Viana dos Santos
Department of Physiology, Federal University of Sergipe, São Cristóvão, Sergipe, Brazil

Acknowledgement

The authors wish to express their sincere thanks to the College of Pharmacy, The University of Illinois at Chicago, Chicago, Illinois 60612-7231, U.S.A., for helping with the computer-aided NAPRALERT search and Brazilian agencies CNPq and FACEPE for financial support.

5. References

[1] Lanza RP, Ecker DM, Kuhtreiber WM, Marsh JP, Ringelling J, Chink WL. Transplantation of islets using microencapsulation: studies in diabetic rodents and dogs. Journal of Molecular Medicine 1999;77(1), 206-210.

[2] Oyedemi SO, Bradley G, Afolayan AJ. Ethnobotanical survey of medicinal plants used for the management of diabetes mellitus in the Nkonkobe municipality of South Africa. Journal of Medicinal Plants Research 2009;3(12), 1040-1044.

[3] Notkins AL. Immunologic and genetic factors in type 1 diabetes. Journal of Biological Chemistry 2002;277(46), 43545-43548.

[4] Funke I, Melzig MF. Traditionally used plants in diabetes therapy - phytotherapeutics as inhibitors of α-amylase activity. Brazilian Journal of Pharmacognosy 2006;16(1), 1-5.

[5] Rao BK, Kesavulu MM, Apparao Ch. Antihyperglycemic activity of *Momordica cymbalaria* in alloxan diabetic rats. Journal of Ethnopharmacology 2001;78(1), 67-71.

[6] Barbosa-Filho JM, Vasconcelos THC, Alencar AA, Batista LM, Oliveira RAG, Guedes DN, Falcão HS, Moura MD, Diniz MFFM, Modesto-Filho J. Plants and their active constituents from South, Central, and North America with hypoglycemic activity. Brazilian Journal of Pharmacognosy 2005;15(4), 392-413.

[7] Cunha WR, Arantes GM, Ferreira DS, Lucarini R, Silva MLA, Furtado NAJC, Silva-Filho AA, Crotti AEM, Araújo ARB. Hypoglicemic effect of *Leandra lacunosa* in normal and alloxan-induced diabetic rats. Fitoterapia 2008;79(5), 356-360.

[8] Zhang BB, Moller DE. New approaches in the treatment of type 2 diabetes. Current Opinion in Chemical Biology 2000;4(4), 461-467.

[9] Alarcon-Aguilar FJ, Roman-Ramos R, Flores-Saenz JL, Aguirre-Garcia F. Investigation on the hypoglycaemic effects of extracts of four Mexican medicinal plants in normal and alloxan-diabetic mice. Phytotherapy Research 2002;16(4), 383-386.

[10] Grover JK, Yadav S, Vats V. Medicinal plants of India with anti-diabetic potential. Journal of Ethnopharmacology 2002;81(1), 81-100.

[11] Pawlowska AM, Oleszek W, Braca A. Quali-quantitative analyses of flavonoids of *Morus nigra* L. and *Morus alba* L. (Moraceae) fruits. Journal of Agricultural and Food Chemistry 2008;56, 3377-3380.

[12] Ozgen M, Serçe S, Kaya C. Phytochemical and antioxidant properties of anthocyanin-rich *Morus nigra* and *Morus rubra* fruits. Scientia Horticulturae 2009;119(3), 275-279.

[13] Ercisli S, Orhan E. Chemical composition of white (*Morus alba*), red (*Morus rubra*) and black (*Morus nigra*) mulberry fruits. Food Chemistry 2007;103(4), 1380-1384.

[14] Nomura T. Phenolic compounds of the mulberry tree and related plants. Progress in the Chemistry of Organic Natural Products 1988;53, 87-201.

[15] Chen FJ, Nakashima N, Kimura I, Kimura M. Hypoglicemic activity and mechanisms of extracts from mulberry leaves (folium mori) and cortex mori radicis in streptozotocin-induced diabetic mice. Yakugaku Zasshi 1995;115, 476-482.

[16] Kim JW, Kim SU, Lee HS, Kim I, Ahn MY, Ryu KS. Determination of 1-deoxynojirimycin in *Morus alba* L. leaves by derivatization with 9-fluorenylmethyl chloroformate followed by reversed-phase high-performance liquid chromatography. Journal of Chromatography A 2003;1002(1-2), 93-99.

[17] Nomura T, Hano Y. Isoprenoid-substituted phenolic compounds of moraceous plants. Natural Products Reports 1994; 11(2); 205-218.

[18] Syah YM, Achmad SA, Ghisalberti EL, Hakim EH, Iman MZN, Makmur L, Mujahiddin D. Andalasin A, a new stilbene dimmer from *Morus macroura*. Fitoterapia 2000;71(6), 630-635.

[19] Fukai T, Satoh K, Nomura T, Sakagami H. Antinephritis and radical scavenging activities of prenylflavonoids. Fitoterapia 2003;74(7-8), 720-724.

[20] Ercisli S, Orhan E. Some physico-chemical characteristics of black mulberry (*Morus nigra* L.) genotypes from Northeast Anatolia region of Turkey. Scientia Horticulturae 2008;116(1), 41-46.

[21] Kumar VR, Chauhan S. Mulberry: Life enhancer. Journal of Medicinal Plants Research 2008;2(10), 271-278.

[22] Dat NT, Binh PTX, Quynh LTP, Minh CV, Huong HT, Lee JJ. Cytotoxic prenylated flavonoids from *Morus alba*. Fitoterapia 2010;81(8), 1224-1227.

[23] Bhattarai NK. Folk anthelmintic drugs of central Nepal. International Journal of Pharmacognosy 1992;30(2), 145-150.

[24] Andallu B, Suryakantham V, Srikanthi BL, Reddy GK. Effect of mulberry (*Morus indica* L) therapy on plasma and erythrocyte membrane lipids in patients with type 2 diabetes. Clinica Chimica Acta 2001;314(1-2), 47-53.

[25] Andallu B, Varadacharyulu N.Ch. Antioxidant role of mulberry (*Morus indica* L. cv. *Anantha*) leaves in streptozotocin-diabetic rats. Clinica Chimica Acta 2003;338(1-2) 3-10.

[26] Balasubramanian A, Ramalingam K, Krishnan S, Ajm C. Antiinflammatory activity of *Morus indica* Linn. Iran Journal of Pharmacology 2005;4, 13-15.

[27] Basnet P, Kadota S, Terashima S, ShimizuM, Namba T. Two new 2-arylbenzofuran derivatives from hypoglycemic activity-bearing fractions of *Morus insignis*. Chemical and Pharmaceutical Bulletin 1993;41(7), 1238-1243.

[28] Azevedo MS, Alves APL, Alves GBC, Cardoso JN, Lopes RSC, Lopes CC. Uma nova síntese de α-bromoacetofenonas e sua aplicação na obtenção de 2-benzoil-benzofuranas. Química Nova 2006;29(6), 1259-1265.

[29] Naderi GA, Asgary1 S, Sarraf-Zadegan N, Oroojy H, Afshin-Nia F. Antioxidant activity of three extracts of *Morus nigra*. Phytotherapy Research 2004;18(5), 365-369.

[30] Souza MM, Bittar M, Cechinel-Filho V, Yunes RA, Messana I, Delle-Monache F, Ferrari F. Antinociceptive properties of morusin, a prenylflavonoid isolated from *Morus nigra* root bark. Zeitschrift für Naturforschung 2000;55c, 256-260.

[31] Padilha MM, Vilela FC, Rocha CQ, Dias MJ, Soncini R, Santos MH, Alves-da-Silva G, Giusti-Paiva A. Antiinflammatory properties of *Morus nigra* leaves. Phytotherapy Research 2010;24(10), 1496-1500.

[32] Padilha MM, Vilela FC, Silva MJD, Santos MH, Alves-da-Silva G, Giusti-Paiva A. Antinociceptive effect of *Morus nigra* leaves in mice. Journal of Medicinal Food 2009;12(6), 1381-1385.

[33] Wang L, Cui XQ, Gong T, Yan RY, Tan YX, Chen RY. Three new compounds from the barks of *Morus nigra*. Journal of Asian Natural Products Research 2008;10(9-10), 897-892.

[34] Wang L, Gong T, Chen RY. Two new prenylflavonoids from *Morus nigra* L. Chinese Chemical Letters 2009;20(12), 1469-1471.

[35] Queiroz GT, Santos TR, Macedo R, Peters VM, Leite MN, Sá RCS, Guerra MO. Efficacy of *Morus nigra* L. on reproduction in female Wistar rats. Food and Chemical Toxicology 2012;50(3-4), 816-822.

[36] Almeida JRGS, Guimarães AL, Oliveira AP, Araújo ECC, Silva FS, Neves LF, Oliveira RA, Sá PGS, Quintans-Júnior LJ. Evaluation of hypoglycemic potential and pre-clinical toxicology of *Morus nigra* L. (Moraceae). Latin American Journal of Pharmacy 2011;30(1), 96-100.

[37] Souza VH, Barbosa APO, Cardoso GC, Marreto RN, Barreto-Filho JAS, Antoniolli AR, Santos MRV. Avaliação do potencial antidiabético de cinco plantas medicinais em ratos. Latin American Journal of Pharmacy 2009;28(4), 609-612.

[38] Sabu MC, Smitha K, Kuttan R. Anti-diabetic activity of green tea polyphenols and their role in reducing oxidative stress in experimental diabetes. Journal of Ethnopharmacology 2002;83(1-2) 109-116.
[39] Oberley LW. Free radicals and diabetes. Free Radical Biology and Medicine 1988;5(2), 113-124.
[40] Kim JS, Ju JB , Choi CW, Kim SC. Hypoglycemic and antihyperlipidemic effect of four Korean medicinal plants in alloxan induced diabetic rats. American Journal of Biochemistry and Biotechnology 2006;2(4), 154-160.
[41] Sunila C, Ignacimuthua S, Agastian P. Antidiabetic effect of *Symplocos cochinchinensis* (Lour.) S. Moore. in type 2 diabetic rats. Journal of Ethnopharmacology 2011;134(2), 298-304.
[42] Murakami C, Myoga K, Kasai R, Ohtani K, Kurokawa T, Ishibashi S, Dayrit F, Padolina W G, Yamasaki K. Screening of plant constituents for effect on glucose transport activity in ehrlich ascites tumour cells. Chemical and Pharmaceutical Bulletin 1993;41(12): 2129-2131.
[43] Yamasaki K. Effect on some saponins on glucose transport system. Advances in Cirrhosis, Hyperammonemia, And Hepatic Encephalopathy 1996;404, 195-206.
[44] Lemus I, Garcia R, Delvillar E, Knop G. Hypoglycaemic activity of four plants used in Chilean Popular Medicine. Phytotherapy Research 1999;13(2), 91-94.
[45] Rios J L, Recio M C, Villar A. Antimicrobial activity of selected plants employed in the Spanish mediterranean area. Journal of Ethnopharmacology 1987;21(2), 139-152.
[46] Yazicioglu A, Tuzlac E. Folk Medicinal Plants of Trabzon (Turkey). Fitoterapia 1996;67(4), 307-318.
[47] Tucakov J. Ethnophytotherapy of diabetes: critical view on the use of medicinal plant extracts in our national medicine in the treatment of diabetes mellitus. Srpski Arhiv Celokupino Lekvarstvo 1978;106(2), 159-173.
[48] Ramirez VR, Mostacero LJ, Garcia AE, Mejia CF, Pelaez PF, Medina CD, Miranda CH. Vegetales empleados en medicina tradicional norperuana. Banco Agrario Del Peru & Nacl Univ Trujillo 1988; 54.
[49] Leclerc H. The blood sugar lowering action of the leaves of *Morus alba*. Presse Medicine 1934;42, 1522.
[50] De Feo V, Aquino R, Menghini A, Ramundo E, Senatoare F. Traditional phytotherapy in the Peninsula Sorrentina. Journal of Ethnopharmacology 1992;36(2), 113-125.
[51] Darias V, Abdala S, Martin D, Ramos F. Hypoglycaemic plants from the Canary Islands. Phytotherapy Research Suppl 1996;10, S3-S5.
[52] Zagari A. Medicinal plants. Tehran University Publications 1992;4(1810/4), 969.
[53] Tucakov J. Ethnophytotherapy of diabetes. Critical view on the use of medicinal plant extracts in our national medicine in the treatment of diabetes mellitus. Srpski Arhiv zav Celokupno Lekarstvo 1978;106(2),159-173.
[54] Rivera G. Preliminary chemical and pharmacological studies on "Cundeamor," *Momordica charantia* L. (Part I). American Journal of Pharmacy 1941;113 (7), 281-297.
[55] Kit SM, Boichuk RV, Khananayev LI, Ozarkiv TT. Experimental study of the hypoglycemic effect of some plants found near Carpathia. Farm Zh (Kiev) 1972;27(4), 61.
[56] Hosseinzadeh H, Sadeghi A. Antihyperglycemic effects of *Morus nigra* and *Morus alba* in mice. Pharmaceutical and Pharmacological Letters 1999;9(2), 63-65.

[57] Yamada H, Oya I, Nagai T, Matsumoto T, Kiyohara H, Omura S. Screening of alpha-glucosidase II inhibitor from Chinese Herbs and its application on the quality control of mulberry Bark. Shoyakugaku Zasshi 1993;47(1), 47-55.

[58] Kim OK, Lee EB. The screening of plants for hypoglycemic action in normal and alloxan-induced hyperglycemic rats. Korean Journal of Pharmacognosy 1992;23(2), 117-119.

[59] Ye F, Shen Z, Xie M. Alpha-glucosidase inhibition from a Chinese Medical Herb (*Ramulus mori*) in normal and diabetic rats and mice. Phytomedicine 2002;9(2), 161-166.

[60] Chen F, Nakashima N, Kimura I, Kimura M, Asano N, Koya S. Potentiating effects on pilocarpine-induced salvia secretion, by extracts and N-containing sugars derived from mulberry leaves, in streptozotocin-diabetic mice. Biological and Pharmaceutical Bulletin 1995;18(12), 1676-1680.

[61] Sharaf A, Mansour M Y. Pharmacological studies on the leaves of *Morus alba*, with special reference to its hypoglycemic activity. Planta Medica 1964;12(1), 71-76.

[62] Ionescu-Tirgoviste C, Popa E, Mirodon Z, Simionescu M, Mincu I. Effect of a mixture of plants on the metabolic equilibrium in patients with Diabetes Mellitus of the 2nd type. Revista de Medicina Interna 1989;41(2), 185-192.

[63] Kim SY, Ryu KS, Lee WC, Ku HO, Lee HS, Lee KR. Hypoglycemic effect of mulberry leaves with anaerobic treatment in alloxan-induced diabetic mice. Korean Journal of Pharmacognosy 1999;30(2), 123-129.

[64] Bwitti P, Musabayane CT. The effects of plant extracts on plasma glucose levels in rats. Acta Medical Biology 1997;45(4), 167-169.

[65] Kubo M, Ido Y, Matsuda H, Mikami H. Anti-diabetic effect of protoplast preparation from fresh leaves of mulberry (*Morus alba*). Natural Medicines 2001;55(4), 181-186.

[66] Hikino H, Mizuno T, Oshima Y, Konno C. Isolation and hypoglycemic activity of Moran A, a glycoprotein of *Morus alba* root barks. Planta Medica 1985;51(2), 159-160.

[67] Singab ANB, El-Beshbishy HA, Yonekawa M, Nomura T, Fukai T. Hypoglycemic effect of Egyptian *Morus alba* root bark extract: Effect on diabetes and lipid peroxidation of streptozotocin-induced diabetic rats. Journal of Ethnopharmacology 2005;100(3), 333-338.

[68] Kim CJ, Cho SK, Shin MS, Cho H, Ro DS, Park JS, Yook CS. Hypoglycemic activity of medicinal plants. Archives of Pharmacological Research 1990;13(4), 371-373.

[69] Min P. The drugs employed in Chinese Medicine as antidiabetic. Noriyuki sugihara. III. Experimental investigation on the influence of the drugs employed in Chinese Medicine as antidiabetic on the blood sugar of rabbits. Nippon Yakurigaku Zasshi 1930;11(2), 181-187.

[70] Kelkar SM, Bapat VA, Ganapathi TR, Kaklij GS, Rao PS, Heble MR. Determination of hypoglycemic activity in *Morus indica* L. (Mulberry) shoot cultures. Current Science 1996;71(1), 71-72.

[71] Bart C. Hypoglycemic action of mulberry leaves. Comptes Rendus des Seances de La Societe de Biologie Et de Ses Filiales 1932;109, 897.

[72] Oryan S, Eidi M, Yazdi E, Eidi A, Solati J. Hypoglycaemic effect of alcoholic extract of *Morus nigra* L. leaves in normal and diabetic rats. Journal of Medicinal Plants 2006;2(6), 27-32.

[73] Sharaf AA, Hussein AM, Mansour MY. The antidiabetic effect of some plants. Planta Medica 1963;11, 159.

[74] Lizuka Y, Sakurai E, Tanaka Y. Antidiabetic effect of Folium Mori in GK rats. Yakugaku Zasshi 2001;121(5), 365-369.

Chapter 12

Hypoglycaemic and Hypolipidaemic Effects of an Ethylacetate Fraction of *Artocarpus heterophyllus* Leaves

Sureka Chackrewarthy and M.I. Thabrew

Additional information is available at the end of the chapter

http://dx.doi.org/10.5772/52538

1. Introduction

1.1. Pharmacognosy of Diabetes Mellitus

Diabetes mellitus type II (T2DM) is a global public health crisis that threatens the economies of all nations, particularly developing countries. Fueled by rapid urbanization, nutrition transition, and increasingly sedentary lifestyles, the epidemic has grown in parallel with the worldwide rise in obesity. According to the International Diabetes Federation [1], diabetes affects at least 285 million people worldwide, and that number is expected to reach 438 million by the year 2030, with two-thirds of all diabetes cases occurring in low- to middle-income countries. The number of adults with impaired glucose tolerance will rise from 344 million in 2010 to an estimated 472 million by 2030. Several factors contribute to accelerated diabetes epidemic, including the "normal-weight metabolically obese" phenotype; high prevalence of smoking and heavy alcohol use; high intake of refined carbohydrates (e.g., white rice); and dramatically decreased physical activity levels [2].

In spite of the tremendous progress in the management of diabetes using synthetic drugs, potential new and inexpensive treatments should be used to reduce the global morbidity and mortality, as most of the people with T2DM lives in areas of the world, where existing treatments are unavailable or are too expensive. It is well documented that insulin sensitivity and glucose tolerance can be modulated by use of traditional medicines that are mainly derived from plants [3-5]. Natural antidiabetic agents with fewer side effects from readily available medicinal plants offer great potential in the discovery of new antidiabetic drugs.

Pharmacognosy (the study of the medicinal properties of materials of natural origin) has played an important role in the management of diabetes mellitus since ancient times.

Indeed, it has been estimated that more than 800 herbal or plant-derived products have been used for the management of T2DM across geographically and culturally diverse populations worldwide [6-9].

World Health Organization (WHO) recommendations [10] on the use of alternative medicines for treating diabetes mellitus provide an impetus for research in this area. Currently, the focus of research includes discovering newer antidiabetic agents as well as isolating the active compounds from herbal sources that have been documented to have antidiabetic properties as have been described in ancient texts. The active components of a number of plant-derived antidiabetic compounds have been identified, and amongst these are flavonoids, alkaloids, glycosides, polysaccharides, peptidoglycans, hypoglycans, guanidine, steroids, carbohydrates, glycopeptides, terpenoids and amino acids. Potentially beneficial effects on the rate of food digestion, glucose transport, potentiation of insulin release, inhibition of insulin clearance, insulin-mimetic effects, reduced gluconeogenesis, and β-cell protection have been attributed to these agents [11].

Type 2 diabetes (T2DM) is a disease characterized by a dual defect: 1) by insulin resistance which prevents cells from using insulin properly and 2) degrees of reduced pancreatic insulin secretion. It is a progressive disease that shows a consistent deterioration in glycemic control over time. While the pathophysiology and pathogenesis of the T2DM is not fully understood, it is clear that impaired glucose tolerance (IGT) often develops into T2DM. Interventions that may delay or prevent the progression of IGT to T2DM are desperately needed. Hyperlipidaemia is a secondary complication in diabetes and there is a growing interest in plants with both hypoglycaemic and hypolipidemic properties since they have a potential to be developed further for effective treatment for diabetes specially associated with a hyperlipidaemic state. Since *Artocarpus heterophyllus* is traditionally used for management of diabetes mellitus, it may hold promise in this regard and warrants pharmacognostical, pharmacological and clinical studies to investigate the therapeutic potential of this plant in the treatment of T2DM.

1.2. Overview of *Artocarpus heterophyllus*

Artocarpus heterophyllus Lam (family Moraceae), commonly known as jakfruit is one of the most significant trees in tropical homegardens and perhaps the most widespread tree in the genus *Artocarpus*. It is a medium-size evergreen tree typically reaching 8–25 m (26–82 ft) in height with evergreen, alternate, glossy and leathery leaves to 22.5 cm (9 in) in length. Jackfruit's place of origin is believed to be indigenous to the rainforests of the Western Ghats. Today, it is cultivated at low elevations throughout India, Sri Lanka, Myanmar, southern China, Malaya, East Indies, Queensland, Mauritius, Kenya, Uganda and former Zanzibar, Pacific islands and Brazil [12].

Many parts of the plant including the bark, roots, leaves, and fruit are attributed with medicinal properties. It is reported in Ayurveda (a traditional medicine system in Sri Lanka and India) to possess antibacterial, anti-inflammatory, antidiabetic, antioxidant and immunomodulatory properties. It is an important source of compounds like morin, dihydromorin, cynomacurin, artocarpin, isoartocarpin, cyloartocarpin, artocarpesin, oxydihydroartocarpesin, artocarpetin, norartocarpetin, cycloartinone, betulinic acid, artocarpanone and heterophylol which have therapeutic properties [13].

The root is a remedy for skin diseases and asthma and the extract is taken in cases of fever and diarrhea. The ashes of the leaves, burned together with corn and coconut shells are used alone or mixed with coconut oil to heal ulcers. Mixed with vinegar, the latex promotes healing of abscesses, snakebite and glandular swellings. Heated leaves alone are placed on wounds and the bark is made into poultices. The seed starch is given to relieve biliousness and the roasted seeds are regarded as aphrodisiac. In Chinese medicine the pulp and seeds are considered tonic and nutritious [12].

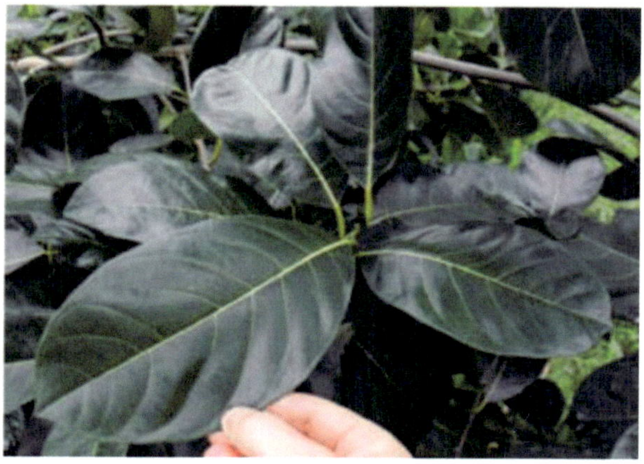

Figure 1. Mature leaves of *A. heterophyllus*

1.3. Aim of the chapter

Alternative systems of medicine such as Ayurveda is widely used in Sri Lanka and India.

In Ayurveda diabetes falls under the term *Madhumeha* [14]. Various types of herbal preparations such as decoctions (boiled extracts), *Swaras* (expressed juices), *Asav-Arisht* (fermented juices), and powders have been used for the treatment of *Madhumeha* [14].

Hot water extracts of *A. heterophyllus* leaves are used in the treatment of T2DM by traditional medical practioners in Sri lanka and India [15,16]. This traditional claim was first scientifically validated by the investigations carried out by Fernando *et. al* [17] which demonstrated the hypoglycaemic potential of the leaf extract. This preliminary work has been followed by many other studies which have provided insights into the efficacy, safety, mechanisms of action and the presence of other bioactivities of therapeutic potential in *A. heterophyllus* leaves. This chapter is based on the investigations carried out by Chackrewarthy *et al* [18] to evaluate the hypoglycaemic and hypolipidaemic potential of an ethylacetate fraction of *A. heterophyllus* leaves using a normal and streptozotocin induced diabetic rat models.

2. Phytochemical screening and standardized extraction

Plant extracts used in traditional medicine are chemically complex and may contain one or more structurally related active compounds that produce a combined effect. Standardization and phytochemical screening are essential measurements of ensuring quality control of herbal drugs.

Phytochemical screening of the aqueous extract of the leaves has revealed the presence of a range of polyphenols such as flavanoids, anthocyanins, tannins and polysaccharides as constituents [19]. In a more recent study of the aqueous extract of leaves, the presence of proteins, saponins, sterols, glycosides and lipids have been revealed in addition to the compounds mentioned [20]. A total ash value of 0.84%, acid insoluble ash value of 0.12% and water soluble ash value of 0.35% on dry weight basis have been reported for the aqueous extract of the leaves.

The purpose of standardized extraction procedures of plant crude extracts is to attain the therapeutically desired fractions and to eliminate unwanted material by treatment with selective solvents. In general, the solvent system used for the extraction plays a significant role in the solubility of the active principles of plant materials which in turn influence the bioactivities of the fractions [21].

Plant crude extracts usually contain large amounts of carbohydrates and/or lipoidal material and the concentration of the phenolics in the crude extract may be low [22]. To concentrate and obtain polyphenol rich fractions before analysis, strategies including sequential extraction is commonly used. Sequential extraction with solvents of increasing polarity; eg: hexane, dichloromethane (DCM), ethyl acetate, methanol and water leads to initial fractionation of constituents of plant materials based mainly on their nature of polarity and with minimal chemical damage [23]. Based on this procedure an initial fractionation of the constituents of *A. heterophyllus* leaves was carried out in the present study. Generally, waxy and lipoid substances are extracted into hexane and DCM and polyphenols are extracted into more polar solvents such as ethylacetate, methanol and water. In particular, methanol has been generally found to be more efficient in extraction of sugars, organic acids and lower molecular weight polyphenols while the higher molecular weight flavanols are better extracted with ethylacetate [24-27]. In recent studies, the phytochemical screening of the ethylactate fraction of A. heterophyllus leaves and bark has revealed the presence of flavanoids in high content. [28,29]. All fractions were evaporated to dryness and the residues stored at -4^{0}C until use.

3. Hypoglycaemic activity of *A.heterophyllus* leaves

3.1. Effects on fasting blood glucose levels

The hypoglycemic potential of fractions separated from *A. heterophyllus* leaves by sequential fractionation, were tested using a normoglycaemic rat model. Male Wistar rats were fasted overnight, devided into groups and each group was treated with a different fraction by oral administration at a dose equivalent to 50 mg/kg body weight. The ethylacetate (EA) fraction and the water fraction were found to exert the highest hypoglycemic effects compared to the controls treated with distilled water (Fig 2). The reduction in fasting blood glucose levels at +2 hr mediated by ethylacetate and water fractions were 42.5% and 28.7% respectively. This demonstrates that both these fractions contain the active principals mediating the hypoglycaemic effect in varying proportions. Methanol fraction also had significant activity similar to the aqueous fraction, but the initial hypoglycaemic effect (+1 hr) was more prominent in the aqueous fraction (30% vs 16%). In experiments carried out by Fernando *et al* [17] with the crude extract of *A. heterophyllus* leaves, the fasting blood glucose levels of normoglycaemic rats were reduced by 24% at +3hr. However, this reduction was obtained with a higher dose of 10g/kg body weight of *A. hetertophyllus* starting material. Further, purification and fractionation results in an enhancement of bioactivity by eliminating the unwanted material which could exert inhibitory effects on the bioactivity of interest. Since the ethylacetate fraction has been shown to contain a high content of flavanoids by phyotochemical screening [19,28,29], the hypoglycaemic activity of this fraction could be attributed to a high molecular weight flavanoid which has a higher solubility in ethylacetate than in water.

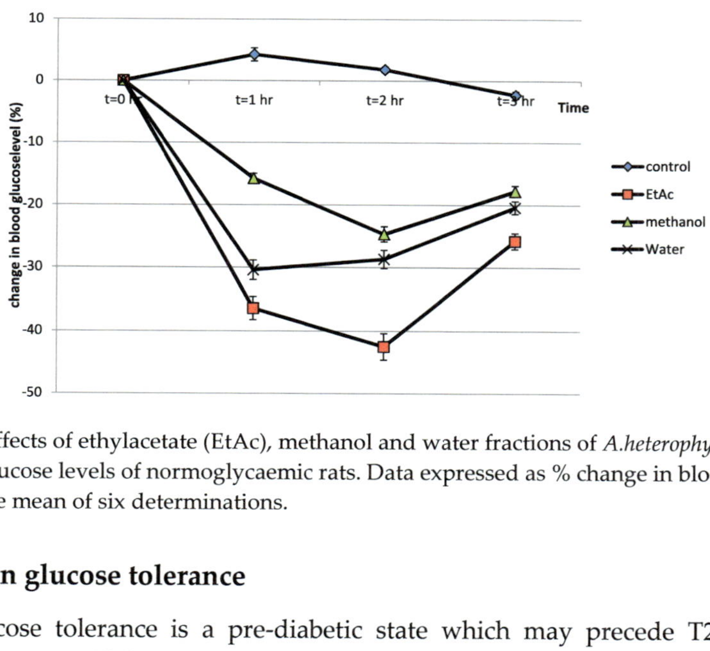

Figure 2. The effects of ethylacetate (EtAc), methanol and water fractions of *A.heterophyllus* leaves on fasting blood glucose levels of normoglycaemic rats. Data expressed as % change in blood glucose level. Each point is the mean of six determinations.

3.2. Effects on glucose tolerance

Impaired glucose tolerance is a pre-diabetic state which may precede T2DM. The oral glucose tolerance test (OGTT) was used as a screening method for acute antihyperglycemic activity since the results give the overall effect of the test material on the handling of an external glucose load [30].

Glucose tolerance studies with normoglycaemic rats, receiving the ethylacetate fraction showed a significant improvement in their ability to utilize the external glucose load compared to the control group (Fig. 3). This was dose dependant, and a dosage of 20mg/kg was found to be more effective than 10 mg/kg. Compared with the controls, the reduction in blood glucose concentration at 2 hr post glucose administration was 18.9% and 26.4% for dosages of 10 mg/kg and 20 mg/kg respectively (Table 1). Reductions in blood glucose levels were statistically significant between the control curve and test curves at all time intervals. In similar experiments a higher dose of 150mg/kg of the ethylacetate fraction had resulted in a 36.9% reduction in blood glucose at 2 hr post glucose administration [28].

Effects of the hot water extract of *A. heterophyllus* leaves on glucose tolerance of healthy individuals and maturity onset diabetic patients have been investigated by Fernando *et al* [31]. Oral administration of the hot water extract equivalent to a dose of 20g/kg starting material, one hour before the glucose load of 50 g, resulted in a significant improvement in the glucose tolerance of normal subjects and in the diabetic patients compared to the controls receiving distilled water. These data provide confirmatory evidence for the presence of antidiabetic principals in the leaf extract and validate its use in the treatment of diabetes by traditional medical practitioners.

	Mean serum glucose concentration (mg/dl)		% reduction in serum glucose compared to control
	Fasting	2 hrs post glucose	
Control	95.1 ± 4.4	169.5 ± 3.6	
EA fraction (10 mg/kg)	96.5 ± 2.3	137.3 ± 2.7	18.9*
EA fraction (20 mg/kg)	98.6 ± 3.5	124.8 ± 4.2	26.4*
Gibenclamide (0.6 mg/kg)	98.3 ± 1.9	108.5 ± 2.9	35.9*

*Significantly different (p<0.05) compared to control

Table 1. Effect of ethylacetate fraction on glucose tolerance

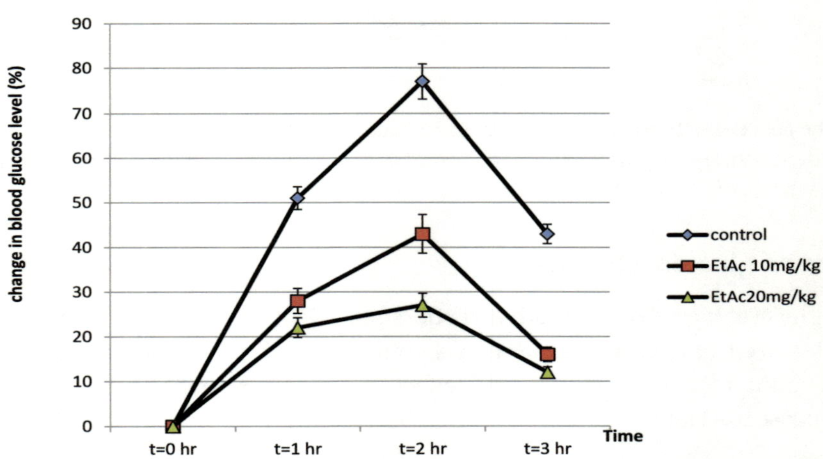

Figure 3. The effects of ethylacetate (EtAc) fraction of *A.heterophyllus* leaves at doses of 10 mg/kg and 20 mg/kg bodyweight, on glucose tolerance of normoglycaemic rats. Data expressed as % change in blood glucose level. Each point is the mean of six determinations.

3.3. Animal models of diabetes mellitus

Non-insulin-dependent forms of diabetes can be produced by administration of a low dose of Streptozotocin (STZ) or alloxan [32]. These kinds of models of diabetes are considered a screening step in the search for drugs for the treatment of diabetes [33].

Streptozotocin (STZ) is an antibiotic derived from *Streptomyces achromogenes* and structurally is a glucosamine derivative of nitrosourea. Its structural similarity to glucose allows it to enter the pancreatic beta-cell via a glucose transporter-GLUT-2 and causes alkylation of deoxyribonucleic acid (DNA). Furthermore, STZ induces activation of poly-adenosine diphosphate ribosylation and nitric oxide release. As a result of STZ action, pancreatic beta-cells are destroyed by necrosis [34]. The diabetes induced by STZ is associated with polydipsia and loss in body weight [35]. Although high-dose STZ severely impairs insulin secretion mimicking type 1 diabetes, low-dose STZ has been known to induce a mild impairment of insulin secretion which generate an impairment in glucose metabolism leading to glucose intolerance and mild, moderate or severe hyperglycaemia [36, 37]. Further, it also affects the lipid metabolism which leads to hyperlipidaemia which closely mimic the natural course of pathogenesis of T2DM [36-39]. The potential problem with STZ is that its toxic effects are not restricted to pancreatic beta-cells since it may cause renal injury [40], oxidative stress, inflammation and endothelial dysfunction [41]. Despite its widespread use, there is a wide variability in the extent of diabetes depending on species, strain and age limiting the predictability of its effects and precautions should be taken when trying to extrapolate the findings to the clinical practice [42,43].

3.4. Effect of chronic administration of ethylacetate extract on fasting blood glucose levels of sterptozotocin-induced diabetic rats

Diabetes was induced in male Wistar rats by a single intravenous injection of freshly prepared STZ solution (in 0.1 M citrate buffer pH = 4.5) at a dose of 60 mg/kg body weight. The efficacy of antidiabetic plant materials may vary with time and investigating the effects of sub chronic or chronic administration is a necessary requirement in evaluating the profile of long term effects of herbal extracts [44].

Chronic administration (Table 2) of the EA fraction to rats at dose of 20 mg/kg for five consecutive weeks caused a significant fall ($P < 0.05$) in the fasting blood sugar levels of diabetic rats when compared with diabetic controls which did not receive the ethylacetate fraction. This is evident in the second week itself and the reduction in the fasting blood sugar in the ethylacetate fraction treated rats (22.8%) was fairly comparable to that produced by the reference drug glibenclamide (32.2%) during the same time period. As in the glibenclamide-treated rats, in rats receiving the ethylacetate fraction also, the fall in the blood sugar level continued progressively till the end of the fifth week. A maximum fall of 39.1% and 55.7% were seen for for the ethylacetate fraction and glibenclamide respectively at the end of the fifth week. In a more recent study, chronic administration of the aqueous extract of *A. heterophyllus* leaves to streptozotocin induced diabetic rats has shown similar results [20]. There was a 51% decrease in fasting blood sugar level for a dose of 250 mg/kg in diabetic rats at the end of the first week when compared with diabetic controls. The fall in fasting blood sugar has continued progressively during the period of treatment with the extract. In another study conducted by Mohana Priya *et al* [29] using a similar protocol, chronic administration of an ethylacetate fraction of the *A. heterophyllus* bark extract has resulted in a maximum fall of fasting blood glucose level by 27.5% for a dose of 400mg/kg body weight.

Glibenclamide being a standard drug for the treatment of T2DM, stimulates insulin secretion from pancreatic β-cells.[45] Therefore, it may be suggested that stimulation of insulin release from the still functioning β-cells by active principles in ethylacetate fraction may be one of the mechanisms by which this fraction mediates its hypoglycemic effect, as proposed for some other plant extracts.[46,47] Further, components of the ethylacetate fraction as proposed by Gomes *et al*.[48] with reference to *Camellia sinensis* (black tea), may be able to generate β-cells of the pancreas or protect the intact β-cells from further deterioration so that they may remain active and continue to produce insulin. Histopathological analysis of pancreas of streptozotocin induced diabetic rats chronically treated with an ethylacetate fraction of *A. heterophyllus* bark extract has revealed initial stages of regenerating islet cells with loss of degenerative features when compared with diabetic controls in which progressive β cell vacuolation, occasional apoptotic cells with vascular congestion and fibrous tissue infilteration was observed in the pancreas. All the above findings provide the biochemical basis for the use of *A. heterophyllus* leaves in the management of patients with diabetes and confirms its role as a traditional antidiabetic remedy.

Groups	Post STZ	2 weeks	4 weeks	5 weeks
Normal control	98.4± 2.9	90.6± 5.7	91.6 ± 4.8	92.7 ± 6.6
Diabetic control	254.3± 2.5	245.5± 6.6[a]	250.0 ± 3.9[a]	253.4 ± 6.3[a]
Diabetic + EA fraction (20 mg kg^{-1} bw)	252.8±11.9	189.4± 5.1[b]	160.1±11.0[b]	154.2± 11.1[b]
Diabetic + Glibenclamide (0.6 mg kg^{-1} bw)	235.2 ± 8.3	166.4 ± 4.8[c]	126.6 ± 9.2[c]	112.3 ± 7.5[c]

Serum glucose levels in mg dl^{-1}. Significantly different ($p<0.05$) compared to normal controls[a], compared to diabetic controls[b], EA treated diabetic rats[c]

Table 2. Serum glucose levels in STZ-induced diabetic rats after prolonged treatment with ethylacetate fraction

4. Effect of chronic administration of ethylacetate extract on body weights and hyperlipidaemia associated with diabetes

Hyperlipidemia is a metabolic complication of both clinical and experimental diabetes.[49] Insulin plays a major role in lipid metabolism apart from its regulation of carbohydrate metabolism. Insulin increases the receptor mediated removal of LDL cholesterol and activates lipoprotein lipase for the hydrolysis of triacylglycerols in lipoproteins. Therefore, reduced activity if insulin in diabetes causes hypercholesterolaemia and hypertriglyceridaemia. This is cleary demonstrated in the diabetic controls of the present study by the increased levels of serum total cholesterol (TC) and triacylglycerols (TG) in diabetic rats when compared to normal control rats (Table 3).

Groups	Total Cholesterol(mg/dl)	Triglycerides (mg/dl)	Body weight (g)
Normal control	78.2 ± 3.8	102.2 ± 2.3	201.0 ± 8.5
Diabetic control	127.9 ± 3.2 [a]	199.8 ± 6.2 [a]	172.1± 5.5
Diabetic + EA fraction (20 mg kg^{-1} bw)	98.5 ± 4.3 [b]	119.0 ± 2.5 [b]	190.4 ± 1.2
Diabetic + Glibenclamide (0.6 mg kg^{-1} bw)	87.4 ± 3.2 [c]	116.8 ± 1.3 [c]	196.5 ± 3.3

Significantly different ($p<0.05$) compared to normal controls a ,compared to diabetic controls b ,EA treated diabetic rats[c]

Table 3. Serum total cholesterol, triglyceride levels and body weight in STZ-induced diabetic rats after five weeks of treatment with ethylacetate fraction

Alterations in the lipid profiles and body weights of STZ-induced diabetic rats are summarized in Table 3. Treatment of diabetic rats with the ethylacetate fraction resulted in a significant fall ($P < 0.05$) in the levels of both total cholesterol (TC) and TGs compared to diabetic controls. The fall in serum TG levels (40%) was more marked than that of cholesterol levels (23%). This effect on diabetic hypertriglyceridemia in ethylacetate fraction treated rats could be due to improved glycemic control. The improved glycemic control by sulfonylureas accompanied by decreased serum very low density lipoprotein (VLDL) and TG levels has already been reported.[50] The reduction in cholesterol levels in diabetic test rats could be due to an inhibitory effect of the active principles on enzymes of cholesterol biosynthesis[51,52] and/or due to the enhanced activity of enzymes involved in bile acid synthesis and its excretion [53]. Further, stimulation of insulin secretion in response to the treatment with the extract could increase the uptake of low density lipoprotein (LDL) cholesterol by extrahepatic tissues contributing to the cholesterol lowering effects of the ethylacetate fraction. However, to obtain confirmatory evidence of these views, further studies on the effects of the ethylacetate fraction on LDL and high density lipoprotein (HDL) cholesterol levels and their clearance need to be investigated. A high fat intake and increased levels of free fatty acids in circulation have been implicated in the development of insulin resistance.[54,55] Based on these observations, it could be speculated that the EA fraction mediated reduction in circulating levels of TGs may also help to ameliorate insulin resistance in diabetic rats and thereby stimulate glucose utilization by peripheral tissues.[56] In a more recent study the chronic administration of aqueous extract of *A. heterophyllus* leaves have been shown to reduce the serum total cholesterol level and improve the HDL levels and the body weight in streptozotocin induced diabetic rats [20]. Similar effects have been shown for the ethyacetate fraction of *A. heterophyllus* bark on diabetic rats [29].

Loss of body weight in diabetic rats is due to increased muscle wasting and loss of tissue proteins [57]. As evident from Table 3, the ethylacetate fraction had an improving effect on the BW (11%) of diabetic rats, which was restored to near normal levels. This may be a reflection of improved health resulting from the effects of the ethylacetate fraction on insulin release.

5. Toxicity

The use of herbal medicines for the treatment or prevention of a variety of diseases has increased markedly. Herbal medicines are believed to be benign and not cause severe toxicity. This coupled with lower costs compared with conventional medications is the major attraction to these treatments. The active ingredients of plant extracts are chemicals similar to those in purified medications, and they have the same potential to cause serious side effects. The usefulness of any drug depends not only on its therapeutic efficacy but also on its lack of toxicity or adverse side effects. Therefore, toxicological investigations have to be carried out before any drug can be considered as safe. This is specially important in the case of antidiabetic drugs, which have to be administered over a relatively long period of time to obtain their pharmacological potency.

Hot water extracts of *A. heterophyllus* leaves have been used from ancient times as a treatment for diabetes in traditional medicine in Sri Lanka and no evidence has been reported of any toxicity or adverse side effects. However, this requires scientific validation with toxicological studies. An in vivo study using Sprague Dawley rats carried out by Fernando and Thabrew [58] has demonstrated that an aqueous extract of mature leaves of *A. heterophyllus* exerted no adverse effects even after daily administration for 30 days, as assessed by effects on (a) liver function, (b) haematological parameters such as haemoglobin concentration, red blood cell count, white blood cell count and packed cell volume, (c) reproductive ability of experimental animals and (d) histology of body organs (heart, liver, lung,kidney, intestine and pancreas). Investigations carried out by Chandrika *et al* [28] also have revealed that the chronic administration of the ethylacetate fraction of *A. heterophyllus* leaves to normoglycaemic rats over a period of twelve weeks at a dose of 50 mg/kg body weight failed to bring any overt signs of toxicity such as salivation, diarrhea, lacrymation, postural abnormalities or behavioural changes. No significant differences had been observed in the liver function tests and the histology of various body organs between the test and the control groups. *A. heterophyllus* leaf extract can therefore be considered to be free of any major toxic compounds or adverse effects.

6. Mechanism of action

Antidiabetic activity of plant extracts is mainly due to their ability to restore the function of the pancreatic tissue by causing an increase in insulin secretion or inhibit the intestinal absorption of glucose or by facilitation of the insulin dependant process.

In investigations carried out by Fernando & Thabrew [59] to investigate the mechanism of action, the hypoglycaemic activity of the aqueous extract of *A. heterophyllus* leaves has been attributed to an extra pancreatic effect, resulting from the inhibition or destruction of insulinase by the constituents of the leaf extract. Improved glycaemic control is achieved by prolonging the half life of insulin. Further, no effects of the extract have been observed on the intestinal glucose absorption in experimental rats.

In vitro investigations carried out by Kotowaroo *et al* [60], on the mechanism of action have revealed that aqueous leaf extract of *A. heterophyllus* significantly ($p < 0.05$) inhibited α-amylase activity in rat plasma. Further, enzyme kinetic studies using the Michaelis-Menten and Lineweaver-Burk equations have established that the aqueous leaf extract of *A. heterophyllus* behaved as a competitive inhibitor. Results from this study indicated that *A. heterophyllus* could act as a 'starch blocker' thereby reducing post-prandial glucose peaks. However, this finding does not agree with the fact that the leaf extract significantly improves the glucose tolerance by improving the ability to handle an external glucose load, which has been consistently demonstrated in both animal and human studies conducted so far. However, the possibility exists, that the leaf extract could exert its hypoglycaemic effects through more than one mechanism.

Furthermore, avialable evidence indicates that the active principals mediating the antidiabetic effect in *A. heterophyllus* leaves to be flavanoids. There is evidence that flavonoids, can increase the viability of beta-cells exposed to STZ or other oxidative stress conditions and improve beta-cell function [61-64]. Increased oxidative stress due either to fasting or postprandial hyperglycemia is accepted as a participant in increased beta-cell damage contributing to the development and progression of diabetes [65]. There is also evidence that the antioxidant defense system is under-expressed in pancreatic cells [66] and flavonoid-rich extracts administration to diabetic animal models has been shown to increase expression of enzymes like catalase and superoxide dismutase as well as glutathione peroxidase system [67, 68]. Therefore, there is a strong possibility of a pancreatic mechanism either by induction of insulin secretion or by recovery of beta-cell mass through which the hypoglycaemic activity of the leaf extract could be exerted. However, further research is necessary to elucidate the mechanism(s) of action.

7. Conclusions

An ethylacetate fraction of *A. heterophyllus* leaf extract exerts stong hypoglycaemic activity in both normoglycaemic and diabetic rats. Chronic administration of the ethylacetate fraction to STZ-induced diabetic rats resulted in a significant improvement in the hyperlipidaemia associated with diabetes leading to a significant lowering of serum total cholesterol and triglycerides. The effects of the improved glycaemic control was evident in the improvement of body weights in diabetic rats under chronic treatment with the ethylacetate fraction. Isolation and characterization of the active principals in the ethylacetate fraction followed by further pharmacological and clinical studies would provide with a novel herbal drug for T2DM therapy.

Author details

Sureka Chackrewarthy
Department of Biochemistry and Clinical Chemistry, Faculty of Medicine, University of Kelaniya, Thalagolla Road, Ragama, Sri lanka

M.I. Thabrew
Institute of Biochemistry, Molecular Biology and Biotechnology, University of Colombo, Sri Lanka

8. References

[1] International Diabetes Federation. IDF Diabetes Atlas. Epidemiology and Mobidity. In: International Diabetes Federation. Available from http://www.idf.org/. Accessed on 1 March 2011

[2] Frank B Hu. Globalization of Diabetes. Diabetes Care 2011, 34(6): 1249-1257

[3] Farnsworth NR (1994) Ethnopharmacology and drug development. In: Chadwick DJ, Marsh J (eds) Ethnobotany and the search for new drugs Ciba Foundation Symposium185. JohnWiley and Sons, Chichester New York, pp 42–51

[4] A.Y.Oubre′ , T.J. Carlson, S.R. King, G.M.Reaven. From plant to patient: an ethnomedical approach to the identification of new drugs for the treatment of NIDDM. Diabetologia 1997, 40: 614–617

[5] Ivorra MD, Paya M, Villar A. A review of natural products and plants as potential antidiabetic drugs. Journal of Ethnopharmacology 1989, 27: 243–275

[6] Nilam, A. Sangal, In: P.D. Flaps, (Ed.), New Developments in Nutrition Research (Nova Science Publisher USA, 2006) 99-115

[7] Bailey, C.J. and Day, C. Traditional plant medicines as treatments for diabetes. *Diabetes Care* 1989, 12, 553–564

[8] F.J. Alarcon-Aguilara, R. Roman-Ramos, S. Perez-Gutierrez, A. Aguilar-Contreras, C.C.Contreras-Weber, J.L. Flores-Saenz. *J. Ethnopharmacol*, 1998, 61,101-110

[9] Chhetri, D.R., Parajuli, P., Subba, G.C. Antidiabetic plants used by Sikkim and Darjeeling Himalayantribes, India. Journal of Ethnopharmacology 2005, 99, 199–202

[10] Roman Ramos, R., Lara Lemus, A., Alarcon Aguilar, F., Flores Saenz, J.L. (1992) Hypoglycemic activity of some antidiabetic plants. Archives of Medical Research 1992, 23, 105–109

[11] World Health Organization, Expert Committee on Diabetes Mellitus: Second WHO Technical Report Series 646. Geneva: World Health Organization, 1980, 61

[12] Dey, L., Attele, A.S., Yuan, C.S. Alternative therapies for type 2 diabetes. Alternative Medicine Review 2002, 7, 45–58.

[13] Morton, J. 1987. Fruits of Warm Climates. Julia F. Morton, Miami, Florida. <http://www.hort.purdue.edu/newcrop/ morton/jackfruit_ars.html>.

[14] Khare C P; Indian medicinal plants: An Illustrated Dictionary. Springer: New York. 2007; 65-66.

[15] Tripathi B. Charak Samhinta, 5th ed., Vol. 2. Varanasi, India:Chaukhamba Surbharti Prakashan, 1998.

[16] Jayaweera DM . Medicinal plants used in Ceylon. Colombo: National Science Council of Sri Lanka; 1982. .4-89.

[17] Bever BO, Zahad GR. Plants with oral hypoglycemic action. Q J Crude Drug Res 1979;17:139-96.

[18] Fernando MR, Thabrew MI, Karunanayake EH. Hypoglycaemic activity of somemedicinal plants in Sri Lanka. Gen Pharmac 1990;21:779-82.

[19] Chackrewarthy S, Thabrew MI, Weerasuriya MKB, Jayasekera S. Evaluation of hypoglycaemic and hypolipidaemic effects of an ethylacetate fraction of *Artocarpus heterophyllus* leaves in STZ-induced diabetic rats. Phcog Mag, 2010; 6923): 186-190.

[20] Chandrika JG, Fernando WS, Wickremasinghe SMDN, Wedage WS. Effects of proanthocyanidine and flavanoid fractions of Artocarpus heterophyllus leaves on blood glucose levels in healthy amle Wistar rats. Journal of Gampaha Ayurveda Wickramarachchi Institute 2004; (2)1:26-29.

[21] Nazli S, Mohamed Ali. Pharmacognostical standardization and antidiabetic activity of *Artocarpus heterophyllus* leaves. Int Imperial J Phcog Natr Pdts. 2012: 2(1); 24-30.

[22] Nair R, Kalariya T, Chanda S. Antibacterial activity of some selected Indian medicinal flora. Turk J Biol. 2005; 29: 41- 47.

[23] Neergheen, V.S.; Soobrattee, M.A.; Bahorun, T.; Aruoma, O.I. Characterization of the phenolic constituents in Mauritian endemic plants as determinants of their antioxidant activities *in vitro*. *J. Plant Physiol.* 2006, *163*, 787-799

[24] Xu, B.J.; Chang, S.K. A comparative study on phenolic profiles and antioxidant activities of legumes as affected by extraction solvents. *J. Food Sci.* 2007, *72*, S159-166.

[25] Metivier, R.P.; Francis, F.J.; Clydesdale, F.M. Solvent extraction of anthocyanins from wine pomace. *J. Food Sci.* 1980, *45*, 1099-1100.

[26] Prior, R.L.; Lazarus, S.A.; Cao, G.; Muccitelli, H.; Hammerstone, J.F. Identification of procyanidins and anthocyanins in blueberries and cranberries (Vaccinium spp.) using highperformance liquid chromatography/mass spectrometry. *J. Agric. Food Chem.* 2001, *49*, 1270-1276.

[27] Guyot, S.; Marnet, N.; Drilleau, J. Thiolysis-HPLC characterization of apple procyanidins covering a large range of polymerization states. *J. Agric. Food Chem.* 2001, *49*, 14-20.

[28] Labarbe, B.; Cheynier, V.; Brossaud, F.; Souquet, J.M.; Moutounet, M. Quantitative fractionation of grape proanthocyanidins according to their degree of polymerization. *J. Agric. Food Chem.* 1999, *47*, 2719-2723.

[29] Chandrika UG, Wedage WS, Wickremasinghe SM, Fernando WS. Hypoglycaemic action of the flavonoid fraction of *Artocarpus heterophyllus* leaf. Afr J Trad CAM 2006;3:42-50.

[30] Mohana Priya E, Gothandam KM, Karthikeyan S. Antidiabetic activity of *Feronia limonia* and *Artocarpus heterophyllus* in STZ induced diabetic rats.. Am J food Tech 2012; 7(1); 43-49.

[31] Verspohl EJ. 2002. Recommended testing in diabetes research. Planta Med 68: 581–590.

[32] Fernando MR, Wickremasinghe SM, Thabrew MI, Ariyananda P, Karunanayake EH. Effect of *Artocarpus heterophyllus* and *Asteracanthus longifolia* on glucose tolerance in

normal human subjects and in maturity onset diabetic patients. J Ethanopharmacol 1991;31:277-82.

[33] Bailey CJ, Flatt PR. Animal syndromes resembling type II diabetes. In: Pickup JC, Williams G, editors Textbook for Diabetes. 3rd Ed. Oxford UK: Blackwell publishing company; 2003, p25.1-25.30.

[34] Kecshemeti V, Bagi Z, Pacher P, Posa I, Kocsics E, Koltai MZ. New Trends in development of antidiabetic drugs. Current Med Chem 2002; 9: 53-71.

[35] Mythili, M.D., R. Vyas, G. Akila and S. Gunasekaran, 2004. Effect of STZ on the ultrastructure of rat pancreatic islets. Microsc. Res. Tech., 63: 274-281

[36] Kim, J. D.; Kang, S. M.; Seo, B. I.; Choi, H. Y.; Choi, H. S. & Ku, S. K. Anti-diabetic activity of SMK001, a poly herbal formula in streptozotocin-induced diabetic rats: therapeutic study. *Biol. Pharm. Bull., 2006, 29(3)*:477-82.

[37] Srinivasan K, Viswanad B, Lydia Asrat, Kaul CL, Ramarao P. Combination of high-fat diet-fed and low-dose streptozotocin-treated rat: A model for type 2 diabetes and pharmacological screening. Pharmacological Research 52 (2005) 313–320

[38] Reed MJ, Meszaros K, Entes LJ, Claypool MD, Pinkett JG, Gadbois TM, et al. A new rat model of type 2 diabetes: the fat-fed, streptozotocin-treated rat. Metabolism 2000;49:1390–4.

[39] TheMing Zhang, Xiao-Yan Lv, Jing Li, Zhi-Gang Xu, and Li Chen. Characterization of High-Fat Diet and Multiple Low-Dose Streptozotocin Induced Type 2 Diabetes Rat Model. Experimental Diabetes Research Volume 2008 (2008), Article ID 704045, 9 pages

[40] K. Sahin, M. Onderci, M. Tuzcu, et al., "Effect of chromium on carbohydrate and lipid metabolism in a rat model of type 2 diabetes mellitus: the fat-fed, streptozotocin-treated rat," Metabolism, 2007, 56(9), pp. 1233–1240,

[41] Valentovic MA, Alejandra N, Carpenter AB, Brown PI, ramos K. Streptozotocin (STZ) diabetes enhances benzo(α)pyrene induced rena linjury in Sprague Dawley rats. Toxicology letters, 2006; 164: 214-220.

[42] Yu-Chen Lei, Jing-Shiang Hwang, Chang-Chuan Chan, Chung-Te L, Tsun-Jen Cheng. Enhanced oxidative stress and endothelial dysfunction in streptozotocin-diabetic rats exposed to fine particles. Environmental research 2005, 99(3), 335-343

[43] Arias-Dias, J. Balibrea, J. Modelos animals de intolerancia a la glucose y diabetes tipo 2. Nutricion Hospitalaria. 2007, 22(2): 160-168.

[44] Rodrigues, B., Poucheret, P., Battel, M.L., McNeill, J.H. 1999. Streptozotocin-induced diabetes: induction, mechanism(s) and dose dependency. In: McNeill, J.H. (Ed).Experimental Models of Diabetes, Boca Raton, FL, CRC. 3-19.

[45] Day, C., Bailey, C.J. 2006. Preclinical and clinical methods for evaluating antidiabetic activity of plants. In: Soumyanath, A. (Ed.), Traditional medicines for modern times: Antidiabetic plants. CRC Taylor and Francis.

[46] Tian YM, Johnson G, Ashcroft JH. Sulfonylureas enhance exocytosis from pancreatic β–cells by a mechanism that does not involve direct activation of proteinkinase C. Diabetes 1998;47:1722-6.

[47] Chakrabarti S, Bijwas TK, Rokeya B, Mosihuzzaman M, Ali L, Nahar N, Mukherjee B. Advanced studies in hypoglycaemic effect of *Caesalpinia bonducella* F. intype 1 and 2 diabetes in Lon-Evans rats. J Ethanopharmacol 2003;84:41-6.

[48] Bakirel T, Bakirel U, Keles OU, Ulgen SG, Yardibi H. *In vivo* assessment of antidyabetic and antioxidant activities of rosemary (*Rosemarinus officinale*) in alloxantreated diabetic rats. J Ethanopharmacol 2008;116:64-73.
[49] Gomes A, Vedasiromoni JR, Das M, Sharma RM, Ganguly DK. Antihyperglycaemic effect of black tea (*Camellia sinensis*) in rat. J Ethanopharmacol 2001;27:243-75.
[50] Bierman EL, Amaral JA, Balknap BH. Hyperlipidaemia and diabetes mellitus. Diabetes1975;25:509-15.
[51] Rao BK , Kesavulu RG, Rao CA . Antidiabetic and hypolipidaemic effects of *Momordica cymbalaria* hook fruit powder in alloxan diabetic rats. J Ethanopharmacol 1999;67:103-9.
[52] Sharma SB, Nasir A, Prabhu KM , Murthy PS, Dev G. Hypoglycaemic and Hypolipidaemic effect of ethanolic extract of seeds of *Eugeneia Jambolana* in alloxaninduced diabetic rats. J Ethanopharmacol 2003;85:201-6.
[53] Ju JB, Kim JS, Choi CW, Lee HK, Oh TK, Kim SC. Comparison between ethanolic and aqueous extract from Chinese *Juniper berries* for hypoglycaemic and hypolipidaemic effects in alloxan induced diabetic rats. J Ethanopharmacol 2008;115110-5.
[54] Sethupathy SC, Elanchezhiyan K, Vasudevan G, Rajgopal. Antiaterogenic effect in high fat fed rats. Indian J. Exp. Biol. 2002, 40: 1169.
[55] Manco M, Bertuzzi A, Salinari S, Scarfone A, Calvani M, Greco AV, *et al.* The ingestion of saturated fatty acid triglycerides acutely affects insulin secretion and insulinsensitivity in human subjects. Br J Nutr 2004;92:895-903.
[56] Manco M, Calvani A, Mingrone G. Effects of dietary fatty acids on insulin sensitivityand secretion. Diabetes, Obesity and Metabolism. 2004;6:402-13.
[57] Kamanyi, Njamen AD, Nikeh B. Hypoglycaemic properties of aqueous root extract of *Morinda lucida* studies in mouse. Phytotherapy Res1994;8:369-71.
[58] Chatterjee, M. N., Shinde, R. (2002) Metabolism of carbohydrates. In: Chatterjee, M. N., Shinde, R. (eds) Textbook of medical biochemistry. JayPee Publications, New Delhi, India, p. 317
[59] Fernando, M.R., Thabrew, M.I.. Studies on the possible toxicity of Artocarpus heterophyllus. Ceylon Journal of Medical Sciences, 1989, 32, 1 – 7.
[60] Fernando MR, Thabrew MI. Extra pancreatic effects contributing to the hypoglycaemic activity of Artocarpus herterophyllys. Cey J Med Sci 200;, 44: 1-10
[61] M. I. Kotowaroo, M. F. Mahomoodally, A. Gurib-Fakim, A. H. Subratty. Screening of Phytotherapy Research Volume 20, Issue 3, pages 228–231, March 2006
[62] Thomas, D.A., Stauffer, C., Zhao, K., Yang, H., Sharma, V.K., Szeto, H.H., Suthanthiran, M. Mitochondrial targeting with antioxidant peptide SS-31 prevents mitochondrial depolarization, reduces islet cell apoptosis, increases islet cell yield, and improvesposttransplantation function. Journal of the American Society of Nephrology 2007, 18: 213-222.
[63] Kamalakkannan, N., Prince, P.S.M. 2006. Antihyperglycemic and antioxidant effect o frutin, a polyphenolic flavonoid, in streptozotocin-induced diabetic wistar rats. Basic andClinical Pharmacology and Toxicology 98: 97-103
[64] Kim, E.K., Kwon, K.B., Song, M.Y., Han, M.J., Lee, J.H., Lee, Y.R. Lee, J.H., Ryu, D.G., Park, B.H., Park, J.W. Flavonoids protect against cytokine-induced pancreatic beta-cell

damage through suppression of nuclear factor kappa B activation. Pancreas 2007(b). 35(4): e1-e9.

[65] Lee, Y.J., Suh, K.S., Choi, M.C., Chon, S., Oh, S., Woo, J-T., Kim, S-W., Kim, J-W., Km, Y.S.. Kaempferol protects HIT-T15 pancreatic beta cells from 2-deoxy-D-riboseinduced oxidative damage. Phytotherapy research. 2010, 24: 419-423

[66] Bonora, E. Protection of pancreatic beta-cells: is it feasible? Nutrition, metabolism, and cardiovascular diseases. 2008, 18: 74-83.

[67] Hotta, M., Yamato, E., Miyazaki, J. 2000. Oxidative stress and pancreatic beta-cell destruction in insulin dependent diabetes mellitus. In: Packer, L., Rosen, P., Tritschler, H.J., Azzi, A. (Eds.) Antioxidants in diabetes management. Marcell Dekker, Inc. New York.

[68] Kim, M.J., Leem, K.A., Kim, H.K.. Hydrangea dulcis folium preserves beta-cell mass in diabetic db/db mice. Food and Chemical Toxicology. 2009, 47: 1685–1688.

[69] Bagri, P., Ali, M., Aeri, V., Bhowmik, M., Sultana, S. Antidiabetic effect of Punica granatum flowers: effect on hyperlipidemia, pancreatic cells lipid peroxidation and antioxidant enzymes in experimental diabetes. Food and Chemical Toxicology. 2009, 47(1): 50- 54.

Chapter 13

Non-Obese Type 2 Diabetes Animals Models

Yukihito Ishii, Takeshi Ohta and Tomohiko Sasase

Additional information is available at the end of the chapter

http://dx.doi.org/10.5772/52712

1. Introduction

Diabetes mellitus has become a global health problem, and the incidence of the disease is increasing rapidly in all regions of the world. Furthermore, the prevalence of diabetes is increasing worldwide at an alarming rate. For example, prevalence of diabetes across the world is forecast to increase from 171 million in 2000 to 366 million in 2030 [1].

Diabetes mellitus is classified into two categories, type 1 and type 2. Type 1 diabetes mellitus (T1D or IDDM; Insulin Dependent Diabetes Mellitus) is characterized by a loss of insulin secretion due to pancreatic β-cell degeneration, leading to autoimmune attack. Type 2 diabetes mellitus (T2D or NIDDM; Non Insulin Dependent Diabetes Mellitus) is metabolic disorder that is caused by insufficient insulin secretion and/or insulin resistance in peripheral and liver tissues. It is known that 90-95% of diabetes is diagnosed as T2D [2]. Development of T2D is usually caused by several factors, which are combined with lifestyle, genetic defects, virus infection, and drugs [3, 4]. Sustained hyperglycemia causes severe diabetic microvascular complications, such as retinopathy, peripheral neuropathy, and nephropathy. In the diabetic states, multiple mechanisms have been implicated in glucose-mediated vascular damage and contribute to diabetic microvascular complications. In addition, postprandial state is also an important factor in the development of macroangiopathy. In diabetes, the postprandial phase is characterized by an exaggerated rise in blood glucose levels. It has recently been shown that postprandial hyperglycemia is relevant to onset of cardiovascular complications. From this evidence, treatment of diabetes has become a part of the strategies for the prevention of diabetic vascular complications.

To help develop new diabetic treatments, it is important to reveal the complex mechanisms of diabetes. In particular, studies using diabetic animal models are essential to aid in clarification of the pathogenesis and progression in human disease course. Types of T2D animal models are classified into three groups, non-obese T2D, obese T2D, and new T2D models. In this chapter, we review these three types of T2D animal models with respect to characteristic features, including impaired glucose tolerance.

2. Non-obese type 2 diabetic animal models

Certain non-obese diabetic models are used in the investigation of T2D in humans. Spontaneous models are well known in this category, e.g., Goto-Kakizaki (GK) rats, Spontaneously Diabetic Torii (SDT) rats, Cohen diabetic rats, Wistar Bonn/Kobori (WBN/Kob) rats, Akita mice, Horino-Niki diabetic (HND) mice, Diabetes Mellitus Saitama (DMS) mice, and Chinese hamsters with spontaneous diabetes (CHAD). Chemically-induced diabetes models such as neonatally streptozotocin-induced (nSTZ) diabetic rats are also used.

2.1. Goto-Kakizaki (GK) rat

2.1.1. Background

Goto-Kakizaki (GK) rat is a non-obese animal with mild T2D [5, 6]. Glucose intolerance is developed early, at 2 weeks of age. Since the GK rat is generally considered as one of the best models of T2D, many researchers have used this animal model to study the physiology of diabetes and its complications, and to evaluate anti-diabetes drugs. In 1973, Goto and Kakizaki of Tohoku University (Japan) started selection of this substrain from Wistar rats by mating pairs with glucose intolerance. Since F8, sister-brother mating has been repeated, and were established as an SPF animal at F29. Today, many colonies of the GK rat exist and the rats are available for purchase from several breeders.

The major quantitative trait locus (QTL) for impaired glucose tolerance is *Niddm1*, identified in chromosome 1. Several loci linked to pathophysiologic characteristics was observed on chromosomes 2, 4, 5, 8, 10, and 17, indicating that the diabetic features in GK rats are inherited as polygenic traits and that GK rats would provide insights into genetics of human T2D [7].

2.1.2. Glucose tolerance and insulin sensitivity

Non-fasting blood insulin levels in GK rats are slightly higher than in age-matched Wistar rats. Impaired glucose-stimulated insulin secretion has been reported in GK rat *in vivo* [8], in the isolated pancreas [9], and in isolated pancreatic islets [10]. Perfusion experiments using isolated pancreas showed that the first phase of insulin secretion by glucose stimulation was impaired in GK rats, although the response to arginine was preserved [9].

"Starfish-shaped" islets are a morphological feature of GK rat. The number of enlarged islets with irregular shape, ill-defined borders, and fibrous strands of endocrine cells is increased in aged GK rats. These islets showed similar or moderately decreased insulin content compared with control rats. Pancreatic glucagon content is at almost the same level as in Wistar rats, and somatostatin content is slightly higher in GK rats [11]. The defective insulin response to glucose in β-cells is due to abnormalities in the function of K^{+}_{ATP} channels and L-type Ca^{2+} channels [12].

The GK rats show mild insulin resistance, mainly considered to be due to increased hepatic glucose production [8]. Decreased glycogen synthesis from glucose, and glucose uptake in skeletal muscle and adipose tissue are also observed in GK rat.

2.1.3. Drug treatment and diabetic complications

GK rats have been widely used for evaluating anti-diabetic drugs. Almost all types of such drugs have been tested with GK rats, including sulfonylureas [13], an α-glucosidase inhibitor [14], a thiazolidinedione derivative (troglitazone) [15], a biguanide (metformin) and a gluconeogenesis inhibitor [16], a GLP-1 analog and a dipeptidyl peptidase-4 inhibitor (DPPIV-i) [17], and an SGLT2 inhibitor [18].

In addition to its useful features as a T2D model, GK rat has been used as model of diabetic complications. Reduced motor nerve conduction velocity (MNCV) in the caudal nerve is reported in 2-month-old GK rats [19]. Increase of glomerular basal membrane was observed at 3 months [8]. Electroretinogram (ERG) showed functional abnormalities of photoreceptors in GK rats [20]. Aged GK rats at eight months showed higher endothelial/pericyte ratio than in normal rats, indicating retinopathy [21].

2.2. Neonatally streptozotocin-induced (nSTZ) diabetic rat

2.2.1. Background

Streptozotocin (STZ) is an antibiotic derived from *Streptomyces achromogenes* that has selective toxicity to pancreatic β-cells. STZ induces DNA strand breaks and a consequent excess activation of poly (ADP-ribose) synthetase, an enzyme that repairs DNA, depleting NAD in cells, which leads to energy depletion and finally causes β-cell death [22]. Therefore, STZ is widely used as an agent to induce IDDM (or T1D) experimentally: injection of a single high dose of STZ causes T1D in adult rats.

On the other hand, when the STZ is injected neonatally, rats develop T2D in adulthood. Neonatal rats treated with STZ at birth (nSTZ rat) revealed acute insulin deficient diabetes at 3-5 days after birth [23]. Their pancreatic insulin contents reduced to 7% that of normal rats, and showed hyperglycemia in this period. However, after this period, blood glucose and insulin levels in nSTZ rats were almost the same as in control rats at 3 weeks of age. At eight weeks of age, nSTZ rats showed mild hyperglycemia and impaired glucose tolerance with a 50% decrease in pancreatic insulin content [24].

Recently, Masiello et al. have reported a new method of inducing T2D in rat by administration of STZ combination with nicotinaminde (NA) [25]. Adult (3 months old) Wistar rats treated with NA intraperitoneally 15 min before STZ administration (STZ/NA rat) have shown moderate and stable hyperglycemia with 40% preservation of pancreatic insulin stores. When given a calorie-controlled high fat diet, hyperlipidemia and insulin resistance without obesity were observed [26]. These models of T2D similar to human T2D may provide a particularly advantageous tool for pharmacological investigations of new insulinotropic agents.

2.2.2. *Glucose tolerance*

The reduction of β-cell number and insulin content in the pancreas leads to defective insulin response *in vivo*. An isolated pancreas perfusion study using adult nSTZ rats showed lack of insulin response to glucose stimulation, indicating loss of β-cell function [27]. Both the first and the second phase of insulin response were severely impaired. Reduction of GLUT2 expression in β-cells may attribute to impaired glucose entry into β-cells and the following insulin secretion [28]. Reduced sensitivity of K_{ATP} channel to extracellular glucose has also been suggested by the patch-clamp technique [29]. Furthermore, an *in vivo* study has indicated that the hepatic glucose production (HGP) in the basal state is higher in adult nSTZ rats than in control animals [30]. From these observations, a lack of insulin response to glucose in pancreas and an increased insulin action upon HGP *in vivo* are major causes of mild basal hyperglycemia and impaired glucose tolerance in nSTZ rats.

2.2.3. *Drug treatment*

The features of nSTZ rats as a T2D model make this model valuable for evaluation of many hypoglycemic drugs, including a sulfonylurea [31], a thiazolidinedione (pioglitazone) [32], a biguanide (metformin) [33], a glucose sensor enhancer [34], a DPPIV-i [35], and an SGLT2 inhibitor [36]. nSTZ rats are also a useful model for assessment of therapeutic drugs that enhance β-cell regeneration. Tourrel et al. reported improved beneficial effects of GLP-1 and its analog exendin-4 on β-cell mass recovery and glucose homeostasis [37]. Ghrelin, the hunger-stimulating peptide produced in stomach, also promotes regeneration of β-cells in nSTZ rats. Treatment with ghrelin increased pancreatic expression of insulin and Pdx1 mRNA with a consequent improvement of hyperglycemia in nSTZ rats [38].

3. Obese type 2 diabetes animal models

Obesity is a well-established risk factor for many chronic disorders, such as T2D [39]. To understand the complicated features of the disease, spontaneously T2D models provide important knowledge. In particular, the development of diabetic animal models and pathophysiological analyses of the models are very important to aid in clarification of the pathogenesis and the patterns of progression in the human disease course. Genetic models of obesity and diabetes, such as *db/db* mice, *ob/ob* mice, Zucker diabetic fatty (ZDF) rats, Otsuka Long-Evans Tokushima Fatty (OLETF) rats, and Wistar fatty rats are most commonly used in such studies.

3.1. Zucker diabetic fatty (ZDF) rat

3.1.1. *Background*

Zucker diabetic fatty (ZDF) rat is an obese animal associated with hyperphagia, hyperglycemia, hyperinsulinemia, and hyperlipidemia. Insulin resistance is caused by age-dependent degeneration in pancreatic β-cells that trigger hyperglycemia. Thus, ZDF rat is a widely studied model of obesity and insulin resistance and is used for evaluation of anti-diabetic drugs. ZDF rat was discovered in a colony of outbred Zucker fatty (ZF) rat in the laboratory of Dr. Walter Shaw at Eli Lilly Research laboratories during the 1980's. ZF rat, discovered in crosses between Sherman and Merck stock M rats (13M strain) in 1961 [40], was identified as carrying a mutation in *fa* gene, and exhibits hyperphagia/obesity. Dr. Richard Peterson at Indiana University Medical School (IUMS) started selection of this rederivation, and established an inbred line of ZDF rat in 1985. It is well known that sexual differences exist in the incidence and progression of diabetes mellitus in ZDF rat [41]. Diabetes mellitus has developed in more 90% of the males, whereas the blood glucose level remains normal in most females. However, female ZDF rat became diabetic on high-fat diet, and it was shown that the dietary fat content affected development of diabetes in females [41]. Today, ZDF rat is available for purchase from Charles River.

3.1.2. Glucose tolerance and insulin sensitivity

Serum glucose levels in ZDF rat are usually elevated from 7-10 weeks of age. The increase was sustained until about 14 weeks of age. ZDF rats showed hyperinsulinemia from 6 to 12 weeks, but after about 14 weeks of age their insulin levels showed a tendency to decrease. Impaired glucose tolerance has been reported in ZDF rat at 5-7 weeks of age. Glucose intolerance at 12 weeks becomes more severe than that at 5-7 weeks of age [42, 43]. Age-dependent degenerative changes of pancreatic islets showed decreased production and secretion of insulin, and atrophy of islets. Early pathological changes of the pancreatic islets, such as hypertrophy, disarray of islet architecture, and irregular islet boundaries, were observed by 10-12 weeks of age [44, 45]. The specific factor that causes deterioration of pancreatic β-cells has not been identified, but changes in β-cell structure and function have been well studied. It was reported that lipotoxicity based on high plasma free fatty acid could attribute to β-cell dysfunction [46]. Reduction of islet mRNAs in β-cells, such as those for insulin, GLUT2, and glucokinase, contributes to the β-cell deterioration [42]. Furthermore, decrease in GLUT4 expression is also observed in skeletal muscle and adipose tissue of ZDF rat [47].

3.1.3. Drug treatment and diabetic complications

It is well known that ZDF rat is a useful model for evaluating anti-diabetic compounds. Some studies have shown that DPPIV-i improve the diabetic condition in ZDF rat. Other compounds also have been evaluated in ZDF rat, including a sulfonylurea [48], α-glucosidase inhibitors [49], a thiazolidinedione (pioglitazone) [50], a biguanide (metformin) [51], a GLP-1 analog [52], an SGLT2 inhibitor [53], a β3-andrenergic receptor agonist [54], and a variety of other compounds [55-58].

A number of studies demonstrated that ZDF rat can be used as model of diabetic complications. Blood urea nitrogen (BUN) levels and urinary protein excretion in ZDF rat were elevated from about 40-50 weeks of age. Renal morphologic changes were observed at 40 weeks of age [59]. It is shown that ZDF rat exhibits renal hypertrophy. Reduced MNCV in the sciatic nerve is observed from 12–14 weeks of age in ZDF rats, and endoneurial blood flow (EBF) in the sciatic nerve is also decreased after 24 weeks of age [60]. It is suggested that ZDF rat develops neural dysfunction. The degeneration and swelling of fibrae lentis, formation of Morgagnian globules, and stratification of epithelium lentis cells is observed in ZDF rat at 21 weeks of age [61, 62]. It is shown that diabetic cataract is observed in ZDF rat.

3.2. Otsuka-Long-Evans-Tokushima-Fatty (OLETF) rat

3.2.1. Background

Otsuka-Long-Evans-Tokushima-Fatty (OLETF) rat is a mildly obese animal associated with polydipsia, polyuria, polyphagia, hyperglycemia, and hyperlipidemia. The incidence of diabetes mellitus in this rat might be related to weakness of β-cells. OLETF rat is considered to be a suitable model for understanding the properties of T2D with mild obesity. The spontaneously obese rat with T2D was obtained from a colony of outbred Long-Evans rat, available for purchase from Charles River, in 1984 at laboratory of Otsuka pharmaceuticals, Tokushima [63]. A strain of this rat was established by sister-brother mating with obesity and glucose intolerance. According to the results of a study by Takiguchi [64, 65], a disrupted cholecystokinin-A (CCK-A) receptor gene in peripheral tissues and central nervous system is found in the OLETF rats [64]. The function of CCK-A in central nervous system is to regulate food intake directly [66]. Meanwhile, in peripheral tissues, CCK-A also controls satiety signals through the vagal afferent neurons [67]. Thus, dysfunctional signal of CCK may cause obese T2D, leading to hyperphagia in OLETF rats. Today, OLETF rats are available for purchase from Japan SLC, Inc., but this rat is limited in use to non-profit purposes.

3.2.2. Glucose tolerance and insulin sensitivity

Non-fasting plasma glucose levels in OLETF rats were elevated from 18 weeks of age, and the increase was sustained until 40 weeks of age. Diabetes mellitus developed in about 90% of OLETF rats at 30 weeks of age, whereas the plasma glucose level remained normal in most females at 24 weeks of age [63, 68]. Sexual differences exit in the incidence and progression of diabetes mellitus in OLETF rats [69]. In glucose tolerance test, marked elevation of plasma glucose and insulin level responses to glucose are observed at 24 weeks of age [63]. Impaired glucose tolerance becomes more severe after 24 weeks of age. Age-dependent degenerative changes of pancreatic islets are observed from 16 weeks of age [70]. The pathological changes of the pancreatic islets, such as hypertrophy, atrophy of insulin positive-β-cells, fibrosis, and indistinct, irregular islet boundaries, were observed by 30 weeks of age [71]. These dysfunctions of β-cells seem to cause the development of glucose intolerance in OLETF rats. Insulin resistance has been reported in OLETF rats at 16 weeks of age, as measured by hyperinsulinemic euglycemic clamp technique [70]. In adipocytes, the GLUT4 protein expression considerably decreased in OLETF rats at 30 weeks of age. The decrease in GLUT4 protein in muscles is also observed in OLETF rats at 30 weeks of age [72]. These abnormalities of GLUT4 protein expression lead to insulin resistance in the peripheral tissues of OLETF rats.

3.2.3. *Drug treatment and diabetic complications*

OLETF rats have been widely used for pharmacological evaluation while testing for many anti-diabetic drugs, including a Ca^{2+} antagonist [73], sulfonylureas [74], an α-glucosidase inhibitor [75], a thiazolidinedione [76], a biguanide (metformin) and a gluconeogenesis inhibitor [77], and a GLP-1 analog [78].

OLETF rats are also used as a model for assessment of diabetic complications. It was reported that histopathological changes in the kidney were observed after 23 weeks of age. OLETF rats at 55 weeks of age showed an expansion of the mesangial matrix and aneurismal dilatation of intraglomerular vessels [63]. Development of diabetic nephropathy was also observed in OLETF rats. It is known that lenticular sorbitol level increases in OLETF rats from 40 weeks of age [79]. OLETF rats show swelling and liquefaction of lens fibers in the subcapsular and supranuclear region at 60 weeks of age. It is suggested that diabetic cataract is observed in OLETF rats.

3.3. Wistar fatty rat

3.3.1. *Background*

Wistar fatty rat develops obesity with hyperphagia, hyperglycemia, hyperinsulinemia, hyperlipidemia, and glucose intolerance. Wistar fatty rat is a good model for studying obesity and insulin resistance, and for evaluation of anti-diabetic drugs. Wistar fatty rat was established as a congenic line of the insulin resistance of the Wistar Kyoto strain (WKY) rat by introducing the *fa* allele of the ZF rat for obesity into the WKY rat genome in the laboratory of Dr. Hitoshi Ikeda at Takeda Chemical Industries [80]. At 5th generation of backcrossing, male obese animals exhibit hyperglycemia, and were established as Wistar fatty rat at 10th generation. Sex differences in diabetes have been reported in Wistar fatty rat. The female Wistar fatty rat sustained the euglycemia until 22 weeks of age [81]. The molecular basis for this sex difference has not been identified.

3.3.2. *Glucose tolerance and insulin sensitivity*

Nonfasting plasma glucose levels in Wistar fatty rats were elevated until 8 weeks of age, and this level was sustained until 24 weeks of age. Wistar fatty rats also exhibited hyperinsulinemia and hypertriglyceridemia. Wistar fatty rat is a widely studied model used to investigate the pathogenesis of obesity and insulin resistance, and for evaluation of anti-diabetic drugs. In glucose tolerance test conducted at 12 weeks of age, Wistar fatty rat showed higher serum glucose and insulin levels after glucose loading compared with WKY rat, and glucose intolerance became more severe age-dependently. Pronounced glucose intolerance was observed in Wistar fatty rat. Hypertrophied pancreatic islets in Wistar fatty rat were increased in pancreas compared with WKY rat [80]. Insulin resistance has been reported in Wistar fatty rats, confirmed by glucose clamp technique [82]. Decreased insulin-stimulated glycogen synthesis and glycolysis in the isolated soleus muscles, and insulin-stimulated glucose oxidation and lipogenesis in adipocytes were observed in Wistar fatty rats [83]. It is considered that these abnormalities in the peripheral tissues lead to insulin resistance in Wistar fatty rats.

3.3.3. Drug treatment and diabetic complications

Wistar fatty rats have been used as a good model for evaluation of a number of anti-diabetic drugs, including a biguanide [84], an α-glucosidase inhibitor [75], a thiazolidinedione [85], and an DPPIV-i [86].

Wistar fatty rats are also used as a model of diabetic complications. It was reported that age-related increases in urinary NAG (N-acetyl-beta-D-glucosaminidase) and urinary protein and albumin excretion in Wistar fatty rat were elevated from 5-11 weeks of age. Wistar fatty rats at 26 weeks of age showed an expansion of the glomerular mesangial matrix and local formation of a nodular-like lesion. The development of diabetic nephropathy was observed in Wistar fatty rats [87]. Reduced MNCV in the fibula nerve and histopathological changes, such as demyelination and axonal degeneration, were observed in Wistar fatty rats [88]. It is suggested that Wistar fatty rat develops neural dysfunction.

4. New type 2 diabetes animal models

4.1. Spontaneously Diabetic Torii (SDT) rat

4.1.1. Background

The Spontaneously Diabetic Torii (SDT) rat is a new inbred strain of Sprague-Dawley (SD) rat established as a non-obese model of type 2 diabetes mellitus. Glucosuria appeared at approximately 20 weeks in male SDT rats. The cumulative incidence of diabetes was 100% by 32 weeks in male SDT rats, while it was only 33% in females even at 65 weeks. A clear sex difference is observed in the onset of diabetes in SDT rats. Male SDT rats showed high plasma glucose levels (over 700 mg/dL) by 20 weeks [89]. As a result of chronic severe hyperglycemia, the SDT rats developed severe complications in eyes, peripheral nerves, and kidneys. Especially, ocular complications including the diabetic retinopathy in SDT rats is noteworthy [90]. Of many diabetic ocular complications, cataract, retinopathy, and neovascular glaucoma (hemorrhagic glaucoma) are the most important clinically. SDT rats are the first diabetic model with all of these complications [89, 90].

4.1.2. Glucose tolerance and insulin sensitivity

In SDT rats, development of hyperglycemia may be more dependent on decreased insulin secretion than insulin resistance, as shown by the fact that the blood insulin concentration tended to be lower than in normal SD rats even before the onset of diabetes, and marked hypoinsulinemia developed after the onset of hyperglycemia [91-93], indicating that this strain of rat is a model of non-obese T2D associated with impaired insulin secretion. It is clinically known that glucose tolerance decreases before the onset of T2D. In oral glucose tolerance test in SDT rats, glucose tolerance markedly decreased at least 3 months before manifestation of hyperglycemia (around 16 weeks old), and the rate of rise in blood glucose level after glucose-loading increased with age. We examined the glucose tolerance periodically at 5, 9, and 13 weeks of age in SDT rats (Figure 1.).

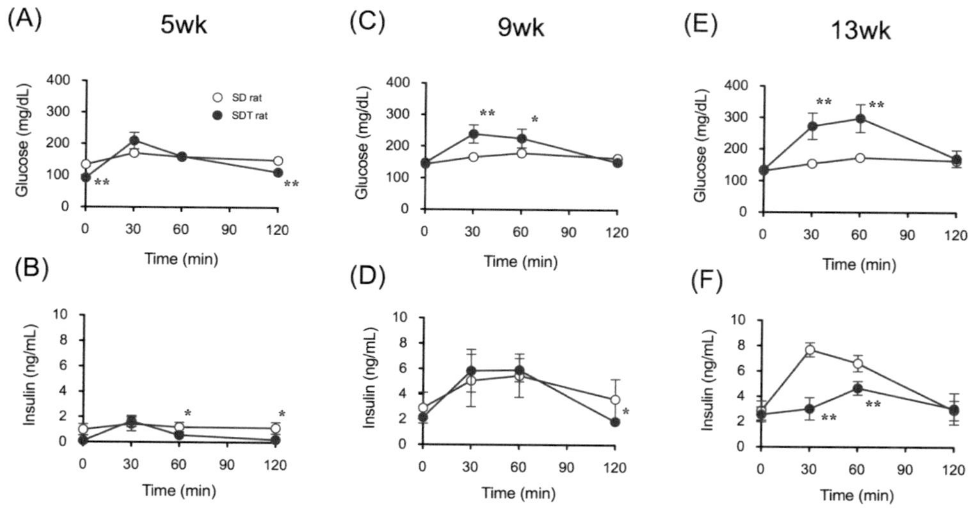

Figure 1. Glucose tolerance test (GTT) at 5, 9, and 13 weeks of age in SD rats and SDT rats. Glucose solution (2g glucose/kg) were administered to SD rats and SDT rats. The glucose and the insulin levels were examined at immediately before glucose-loading, 30, 60, and 120 min after glucose-loading. (A), (B) 5 weeks of age, (C), (D) 9 weeks of age, (E), (F) 13 weeks of age. The data are shown as the mean ± standard deviation (n=4-6). * $P<0.05$, ** $P<0.01$ significantly different from SD rats.

At 5 weeks of age, blood glucose level at 30 min after glucose-loading in SDT rats tended to increase as compared with that in SD rats (Figure 1A.). The blood glucose level before glucose-loading and the level at 120 min after glucose-loading in SDT rats significantly decreased as compared with those in SD rats. The blood insulin level at 30 min after glucose-loading was not different from that in SD rats, but the insulin levels at the other points significantly decreased as compared with those in SD rats (Figure 1B.). Also, the insulinogenic index at 5 weeks of age in SDT rats was comparable with that in SD rats (Figure 2.).

At 9 weeks of age, the blood glucose levels after glucose-loading in SDT rats were more elevated as compared with those in the rats at 5 weeks of age, suggesting that the glucose tolerance was deteriorated with age (Figure 1C.). The insulin levels at points except for 120 min after glucose-loading in SDT rats was comparable with those in SD rats (Figure 1D.), but the insulinogenic index showed a lower level than SD rats (Figure. 2). At 13 weeks of age, the impaired glucose tolerance (IGT) in SDT rats was accelerated and a peak value in the blood glucose level reached to about 300 mg/dl (Figure 1E.). The insulin level at 30 min after glucose-loading did not increase in SDT rats (Figure 1F.), suggesting that the glucose stimulated insulin secretion (GSIS) was almost deleted in the rats at 13 weeks of age (Figure 2.). In male rats, the severity of impaired glucose tolerance before the onset of diabetes was closely correlated with the age. Impaired glucose tolerance was related to decreased insulin secretory response after glucose-loading, and decrease in the fasting plasma insulin concentration (lower than 1 ng/ml) and loss of insulin secretory response after glucose-loading were also observed after the onset of diabetes (Figure 3.).

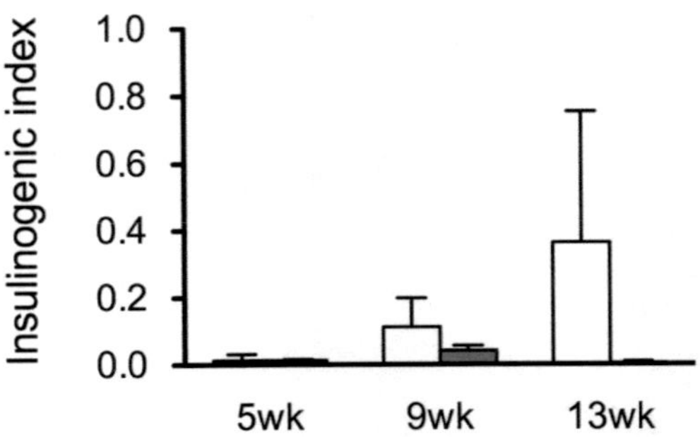

Figure 2. Insulinogenic index at 5, 9, and 13 weeks of age in SD rats and SDT rats. Insulinogenic index (ΔInsulin/ΔGlucose) was calculated using incremental blood insulin and glucose levels for 0 to 30 min after glucose-loading. The data are shown as the mean ± standard deviation (n=4-6).

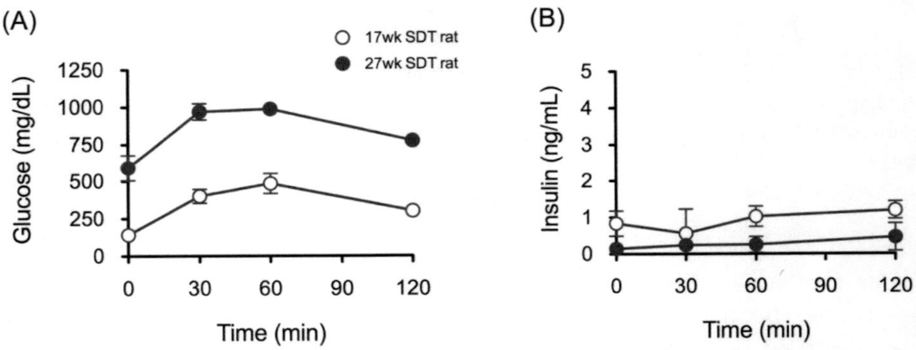

Figure 3. Glucose tolerance test (GTT) at 17 and 27 weeks of age in SDT rats. Glucose solution (2g glucose/kg) were administered to SDT rats. The glucose (A) and the insulin (B) levels were examined at immediately before glucose-loading, 30, 60, and 120 min after glucose-loading. The data are shown as the mean ± standard deviation (n=5).

In addition, the insulin secretion level in pancreatic islets of Langerhans from SDT rats after glucose treatment markedly decreased at 12 weeks of age and thereafter compared with normal SD rats. Likewise, the mRNA expression levels for GLUT2 and glucokinase (GK) in the isolated pancreatic islets of Langerhans markedly decreased at 12 weeks and thereafter in SDT rats [94]. In female rats, glucose tolerance also decreased, at 25 weeks and thereafter, but insulin was secreted after glucose-loading, indicating that some factors cause insulin resistance or insulin requirement in the females, unlike in the males [95].

It is reported that the pancreatic insulin content in SDT rats at 7 weeks of age decreased as compared with that in SD rats [96]. In human, β cell mass in impaired fasting glucose (IFG) subjects significantly decreased as compared with that in nondiabetic subjects [97]. In further study, the change of β-cell mass in pre-diabetic SDT rats should be elucidated.

Other non-obese type 2 diabetic models, such as GK rats and the nSTZ rats, did not show a pre-diabetic state. Since the SDT rat shows a pre-diabetic state for a long term, the rat is valuable as IGT model as well as a type 2 diabetic model.

4.1.3. Drug treatment

In previous study, α-glucosidase inhibitor voglibose was administered to male SDT rats in a pre-diabetic stage, and the effects of voglibose on the glucose intolerance and the development of diabetes were investigated [98]. In SDT rats at 10 weeks of age, a single dose of voglibose (0.03, 0.1, 0.3 mg/kg) improved the glucose tolerance dose-dependently. Moreover, voglibose was administered as a dietary mixture to SDT rats from 10 to 20 weeks of age. As a result, voglibose suppressed the incidence of diabetes in SDT rats. In clinical study, α-glucosidase inhibitor, such as voglibose and acarbose, showed a prevention of type 2 diabetes mellitus [99, 100]. The pharmacological intervention delayed progression of IGT to diabetes. The results showed that pharmacological intervention with voglibose in SDT rats with IGT can delay progression to T2D. SDT rat is considered to be useful for development of a preventive drug on T2D. SDT rat is available for purchace from CLEA Japan.

4.2. Spontaneously Diabetic Torii *Leprfa* (SDT fatty) rat

4.2.1. Background

Type 2 diabetes mellitus is a polygenic disorder that is caused by a metabolic and/or hormonal imbalance between insulin secretion from β cells and insulin sensitivity in peripheral tissues, both of which might be modified by genetic and environmental factors [101]. The decreased sensitivity to insulin leads to an increased requirement for insulin, and is often associated with obesity in which metabolic disturbances are marked in insulin-target organs, such as the liver, muscle and adipose tissues [102]. Obesity plays key roles in the pathophysiology of several metabolic diseases and is a risk factor for diabetes mellitus and dyslipidemia. Based on the above concept, a novel model of obesity-related diabetes was established by Masuyama *et al.* [103]. They established a congenic line of the Spontaneously Diabetic Torii (SDT) rat by introducing the *fa* allele of the ZF rat into the SDT rat genome via the Speed Congenic Method using a PCR technique with DNA markers. This congenic strain has been maintained by inter-crossing between *fa*-heterozygous littermates.

4.2.2. Glucose tolerance, insulin sensitivity and drug treatment

Metabolic disorder in SDT fatty rats was obviously promoted as compared with SDT rats [104, 105]. Serum glucose levels in SDT fatty rats of both sexes were elevated from 6 weeks, and lipid parameters such as serum triglyceride and total cholesterol levels in the rats were elevated from 4 weeks of age. The hyperglycemia and hyperlipidemia were sustained for a long time afterwards. With early incidence of diabetes mellitus, diabetes-associated complications in SDT fatty rats were seen at younger ages than those in the SDT rats. SDT fatty rats did not almost show a pre-diabetic state, since the rats showed a hyperglycemia from a young age. However, the glucose intolerance in SDT fatty rats is considered to exist with the progression of diabetes mellitus.

We evaluated the pharmacological effects of an anti-diabetic drug, DPPIV-i on SDT fatty rats. Male SDT fatty rats at 9 weeks of age were used after overnight fasting. The effect of drug on blood glucose and insulin levels in glucose-loaded animals was examined by means of an oral glucose tolerance test (1g glucose/kg) 30 min after single oral administration of DPPIV-i. When DPPIV-i was administered at doses of 1 and 10 mg/kg, the impaired glucose tolerance was improved dose dependently and insulin secretion was enhanced (Figure 4.).

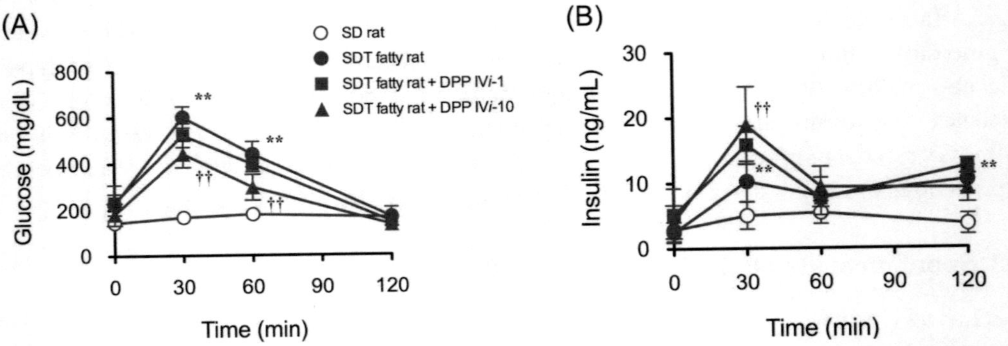

Figure 4. Effect of DPPIV-i on blood glucose (A) and insulin (B) levels in glucose-loaded SDT fatty rats. DPPIV-i was administered orally 30 min before glucose-loading (1g glucose/kg). The data are shown as the mean ± standard deviation (n=5). * P<0.05, ** P<0.01 significantly different from the control. #P<0.05, ## P<0.01 significantly different from SD rat.

Furthermore, we investigated the chronic effect of DPPIV-i in male SDT fatty rats. DPPIV-i (1, 10 mg/kg) was given as a dietary admixture in the powder diet for 4 weeks. Non-fasted blood glucose levels decreased dose-dependently after 3 weeks of administration with DPPIV-i, and the hemoglobin A1c (HbA1c) levels at 4 weeks after the administration tended to decrease (HbA1c level, control: 7.31 ± 0.22%, DPPIV-i 1 mg/kg: 6.99 ± 0.24%, DPPIV-i 10 mg/kg: 7.03 ± 0.17%). There was no change in body weights during the experimental period. DPPIV-i is expected to control postprandial hyperglycemia in patients with type 2 diabetes mellitus without increasing body weight. SDT fatty rats at 9 weeks of age showed a prominent hyperglycemia after glucose-loading (Figure 4A.). The glucose levels at 30 and 60 min after glucose-loading in the SDT fatty rats significantly increased as compared with those in SD rats. Moreover, the insulin levels at 30 and 120 min after glucose-loading in the SDT fatty rats increased as compared with those in SD rats (Figure 4B.). The GSIS in SDT fatty rats was accelerated as compared with SD rats, suggesting that hyperinsulinemia (insulin resistance) exists in the SDT fatty rats at 9 weeks of age. In the other hand, the insulinogenic index in SDT fatty rats was lower than that in SD rats (SDT fatty rat, 0.021 ± 0.010, and SD rat, 0.112 ± 0.087, respectively). Glucose intolerance in SDT fatty rats is considered to be related with both the insulin resistance and the impaired insulin secretion. SDT fatty rat is available for purchace from CLEA Japan.

	Non-obesity			Obesity			
	GK	nSTZ	SDT	ZDF	OLETF	Wistar fatty	SDT fatty
Sexual dimorphism	No	No	Yes (Male>Female)	Yes	Yes (Male)	Yes	No
Obesity	No	No	No	Yes	Yes	Yes	Yes
Hyperphagia	No	No	No	Yes	Yes	Yes	Yes
Pancreatic islet	Degeneration	Degeneration	Degeneration	Hypertrophy → Degeneration	Hypertrophy	Hypertrophy	Hypertrophy → Degeneration
β cell number	Decrease	Decrease	Decrease	Increase → Decrease	Increase → Decrease	Increase	Increase → Decrease?
Impaired insulin secretion	Yes	Yes	Yes	Yes (Hypersecretion)	Yes	Yes? (Hypersecretion)	Yes (Hypersecretion)
Onset of diabetes	8wk	8wk	20wk	7wk	18wk	8wk	5wk
Insulin resistance	Yes	–	?	Yes	Yes	Yes	Yes
Diabetic complications	Nephropathy (Mild) Retinopathy Neuropathy		Nephropathy Retinopathy Cataract	Nephropathy Neuropathy Cataract	Nephropathy Cataract	Nephropathy Neuropathy	Nephropathy Retinopathy /Uveitis Neuropathy Cataract Osteoporosis

Table 1. Characteristic of type 2 diabetes models.

5. Conclusion

There are many type 2 diabetic animal models, and they can be classified into the following three groups: non-obese T2D, obese T2D, and new type 2 diabetic models.

Each of these models has different features as described above (Table 1.), and each model acts as an important tool for revealing the complex mechanisms of diabetes and developing new anti-diabetic drugs. Studies using diabetic animal models are especially essential to aid in clarification of the pathogenetic development in human T2D. On the other hand, these animal models do not exhibit the human characteristics perfectly. New T2D animal models that more closely resemble the human conditions are required for further investigation of the disease mechanisms in the future.

Author details

Yukihito Ishii*, Takeshi Ohta and Tomohiko Sasase
Japan Tobacco Inc., Central Pharmaceutical Research Institute, Murasaki-cho, Takatsuki, Osaka, Japan

6. References

[1] Wild S, Roglic G, Green A, Sicree R, King H. Global prevalence of diabetes: estimates for the year 2000 and projections for 2030. Diabetes Care 2004;27(5):1047-53.
[2] Inzucchi SE, Sherwin RS. The prevention of type 2 diabetes mellitus. Endocrinol Metab Clin North Am 2005;34(1):199-219, viii.
[3] Zimmet P, Alberti KG, Shaw J. Global and societal implications of the diabetes epidemic. Nature 2001;414(6865):782-7.
[4] Miyake K, Yang W, Hara K, Yasuda K, Horikawa Y, Osawa H, et al. Construction of a prediction model for type 2 diabetes mellitus in the Japanese population based on 11 genes with strong evidence of the association. J Hum Genet 2009;54(4):236-41.
[5] Goto Y, Suzuki K-I, Sasaki M, Ono T, Abe S. GK rats as amodel of nonobese, noninsulin-dependent diabetes. Selective breeding over 35 generations. In: Shafrir E, Renold AE, editors. Lessons from Animal Diabetes II. London: John Libbey; 1988. p. 301-3.
[6] Goto Y, Kakizaki M, Masaki N. Spontaneous diabetes produced by selective breeding of normal Wistar rats. Proc Jpn Acad 1975;51:80-5.
[7] Granhall C, Park HB, Fakhrai-Rad H, Luthman H. High-resolution quantitative trait locus analysis reveals multiple diabetes susceptibility loci mapped to intervals<800 kb in the species-conserved Niddm1i of the GK rat. Genetics 2006;174(3):1565-72.
[8] Suzuki K-I, Goto Y, Toyota T. Spontaneously diabetic GK (Goto-Kakizaki) rats. In: Shafrir E, editor. Lessons from Animal Diabetes IV. London: Smith-Gordon; 1992. p. 107-16.
[9] Kimura K, Toyota T, Kakizaki M, Kudo M, Takebe K, Goto Y. Impaired insulin secretion in the spontaneous diabetes rats. Tohoku J Exp Med 1982;137(4):453-9.
[10] Ostenson CG, Khan A, Abdel-Halim SM, Guenifi A, Suzuki K, Goto Y, et al. Abnormal insulin secretion and glucose metabolism in pancreatic islets from the spontaneously diabetic GK rat. Diabetologia 1993;36(1):3-8.

---

* Corresponding Author

[11] Abdel-Halim SM, Guenifi A, Efendic S, Ostenson CG. Both somatostatin and insulin responses to glucose are impaired in the perfused pancreas of the spontaneously noninsulin-dependent diabetic GK (Goto-Kakizaki) rats. Acta Physiol Scand 1993;148(2):219-26.

[12] Tsuura Y, Ishida H, Okamoto Y, Kato S, Sakamoto K, Horie M, et al. Glucose sensitivity of ATP-sensitive K+ channels is impaired in beta-cells of the GK rat. A new genetic model of NIDDM. Diabetes 1993;42(10):1446-53.

[13] Ladriere L, Malaisse-Lagae F, Fuhlendorff J, Malaisse WJ. Effect of antidiabetic agents on the increase in glycemia and insulinemia caused by refeeding in hereditarily diabetic rats. Res Commun Mol Pathol Pharmacol 1997;97(1):53-9.

[14] Koyama M, Wada R, Mizukami H, Sakuraba H, Odaka H, Ikeda H, et al. Inhibition of progressive reduction of islet beta-cell mass in spontaneously diabetic Goto-Kakizaki rats by alpha-glucosidase inhibitor. Metabolism 2000;49(3):347-52.

[15] O'Rourke CM, Davis JA, Saltiel AR, Cornicelli JA. Metabolic effects of troglitazone in the Goto-Kakizaki rat, a non-obese and normolipidemic rodent model of non-insulin-dependent diabetes mellitus. Metabolism 1997;46(2):192-8.

[16] Yoshida T, Okuno A, Tanaka J, Takahashi K, Nakashima R, Kanda S, et al. Metformin primarily decreases plasma glucose not by gluconeogenesis suppression but by activating glucose utilization in a non-obese type 2 diabetes Goto-Kakizaki rats. Eur J Pharmacol 2009;623(1-3):141-7.

[17] Simonsen L, Pilgaard S, Orskov C, Rosenkilde MM, Hartmann B, Holst JJ, et al. Exendin-4, but not dipeptidyl peptidase IV inhibition, increases small intestinal mass in GK rats. Am J Physiol Gastrointest Liver Physiol 2007;293(1):G288-95.

[18] Ueta K, Ishihara T, Matsumoto Y, Oku A, Nawano M, Fujita T, et al. Long-term treatment with the Na+-glucose cotransporter inhibitor T-1095 causes sustained improvement in hyperglycemia and prevents diabetic neuropathy in Goto-Kakizaki Rats. Life Sci 2005;76(23):2655-68.

[19] Goto Y, Kakizaki M, Yagihashi S. Neurological findings in spontaneously diabetic rats. Excerpta Medica ICS 1982;581:26-38.

[20] Matsubara H, Kuze M, Sasoh M, Ma N, Furuta M, Uji Y. Time-dependent course of electroretinograms in the spontaneous diabetic Goto-Kakizaki rat. Jpn J Ophthalmol 2006;50(3):211-6.

[21] Agardh CD, Agardh E, Zhang H, Ostenson CG. Altered endothelial/pericyte ratio in Goto-Kakizaki rat retina. J Diabetes Complications 1997;11(3):158-62.

[22] Yamamoto H, Uchigata Y, Okamoto H. Streptozotocin and alloxan induce DNA strand breaks and poly(ADP-ribose) synthetase in pancreatic islets. Nature 1981;294(5838):284-6.

[23] Portha B, Levacher C, Picon L, Rosselin G. Diabetogenic effect of streptozotocin in the rat during the perinatal period. Diabetes 1974;23(11):889-95.

[24] Portha B, Picon L, Rosselin G. Chemical diabetes in the adult rat as the spontaneous evolution of neonatal diabetes. etologia 1979;17(6):371-7.

[25] Masiello P, Broca C, Gross R, Roye M, Manteghetti M, Hillaire-Buys D, et al. Experimental NIDDM: development of a new model in adult rats administered streptozotocin and nicotinamide. Diabetes 1998;47(2):224-9.

[26] Nakamura T, Terajima T, Ogata T, Ueno K, Hashimoto N, Ono K, et al. Establishment and pathophysiological characterization of type 2 diabetic mouse model produced by streptozotocin and nicotinamide. Biol Pharm Bull 2006;29(6):1167-74.

[27] Giroix MH, Portha B, Kergoat M, Bailbe D, Picon L. Glucose insensitivity and amino-acid hypersensitivity of insulin release in rats with non-insulin-dependent diabetes. A study with the perfused pancreas. Diabetes 1983;32(5):445-51.

[28] Thorens B, Weir GC, Leahy JL, Lodish HF, Bonner-Weir S. Reduced expression of the liver/beta-cell glucose transporter isoform in glucose-insensitive pancreatic beta cells of diabetic rats. Proc Natl Acad Sci U S A 1990;87(17):6492-6.

[29] Tsuura Y, Ishida H, Okamoto Y, Tsuji K, Kurose T, Horie M, et al. Impaired glucose sensitivity of ATP-sensitive K+ channels in pancreatic beta-cells in streptozotocin-induced NIDDM rats. Diabetes 1992;41(7):861-5.

[30] Kergoat M, Portha B. In vivo hepatic and peripheral insulin sensitivity in rats with non-insulin-dependent diabetes induced by streptozocin. Assessment with the insulin-glucose clamp technique. Diabetes 1985;34(11):1120-6.

[31] Serradas P, Bailbe D, Portha B. Long-term gliclazide treatment improves the in vitro glucose-induced insulin release in rats with type 2 (non-insulin-dependent) diabetes induced by neonatal streptozotocin. Diabetologia 1989;32(8):577-84.

[32] Takada J, Fonseca-Alaniz MH, de Campos TB, Andreotti S, Campana AB, Okamoto M, et al. Metabolic recovery of adipose tissue is associated with improvement in insulin resistance in a model of experimental diabetes. J Endocrinol 2008;198(1):51-60.

[33] Rossetti L, DeFronzo RA, Gherzi R, Stein P, Andraghetti G, Falzetti G, et al. Effect of metformin treatment on insulin action in diabetic rats: in vivo and in vitro correlations. Metabolism 1990;39(4):425-35.

[34] Ohta T, Furukawa N, Yonemori F, Wakitani K. JTT-608 controls blood glucose by enhancement of glucose-stimulated insulin secretion in normal and diabetes mellitus rats. Eur J Pharmacol 1999;367(1):91-9.

[35] Sangle GV, Lauffer LM, Grieco A, Trivedi S, Iakoubov R, Brubaker PL. Novel biological action of the dipeptidylpeptidase-IV inhibitor, sitagliptin, as a glucagon-like peptide-1 secretagogue. Endocrinology 2012;153(2):564-73.

[36] Fujimori Y, Katsuno K, Ojima K, Nakashima I, Nakano S, Ishikawa-Takemura Y, et al. Sergliflozin etabonate, a selective SGLT2 inhibitor, improves glycemic control in streptozotocin-induced diabetic rats and Zucker fatty rats. Eur J Pharmacol 2009;609(1-3):148-54.

[37] Tourrel C, Bailbe D, Meile MJ, Kergoat M, Portha B. Glucagon-like peptide-1 and exendin-4 stimulate beta-cell neogenesis in streptozotocin-treated newborn rats resulting in persistently improved glucose homeostasis at adult age. Diabetes 2001;50(7):1562-70.

[38] Irako T, Akamizu T, Hosoda H, Iwakura H, Ariyasu H, Tojo K, et al. Ghrelin prevents development of diabetes at adult age in streptozotocin-treated newborn rats. Diabetologia 2006;49(6):1264-73.

[39] Bjorntorp P. Metabolic implications of body fat distribution. Diabetes Care 1991;14(12):1132-43.

[40] Zucker LM, Zucker TF. Fatty, a new mutation in the rat. J Hered 1961;52(6):275-8.

[41] Corsetti JP, Sparks JD, Peterson RG, Smith RL, Sparks CE. Effect of dietary fat on the development of non-insulin dependent diabetes mellitus in obese Zucker diabetic fatty male and female rats. Atherosclerosis 2000;148(2):231-41.
[42] Tokuyama Y, Sturis J, DePaoli AM, Takeda J, Stoffel M, Tang J, et al. Evolution of beta-cell dysfunction in the male Zucker diabetic fatty rat. Diabetes 1995;44(12):1447-57.
[43] Ohneda M, Inman LR, Unger RH. Caloric restriction in obese pre-diabetic rats prevents beta-cell depletion, loss of beta-cell GLUT 2 and glucose incompetence. Diabetologia 1995;38(2):173-9.
[44] Pick A, Clark J, Kubstrup C, Levisetti M, Pugh W, Bonner-Weir S, et al. Role of apoptosis in failure of beta-cell mass compensation for insulin resistance and beta-cell defects in the male Zucker diabetic fatty rat. Diabetes 1998;47(3):358-64.
[45] Unger RH, Orci L. Diseases of liporegulation: new perspective on obesity and related disorders. Faseb J 2001;15(2):312-21.
[46] Lee Y, Hirose H, Ohneda M, Johnson JH, McGarry JD, Unger RH. Beta-cell lipotoxicity in the pathogenesis of non-insulin-dependent diabetes mellitus of obese rats: impairment in adipocyte-beta-cell relationships. Proc Natl Acad Sci U S A 1994;91(23):10878-82.
[47] Slieker LJ, Sundell KL, Heath WF, Osborne HE, Bue J, Manetta J, et al. Glucose transporter levels in tissues of spontaneously diabetic Zucker fa/fa rat (ZDF/drt) and viable yellow mouse (Avy/a). Diabetes 1992;41(2):187-93.
[48] Mine T, Miura K, Kitahara Y, Okano A, Kawamori R. Nateglinide suppresses postprandial hypertriglyceridemia in Zucker fatty rats and Goto-Kakizaki rats: comparison with voglibose and glibenclamide. Biol Pharm Bull 2002;25(11):1412-6.
[49] Peterson RG. alpha-Glucosidase inhibitors in diabetes: lessons from animal studies. Eur J Clin Invest 1994;24 Suppl 3:11-8.
[50] Hirasawa Y, Matsui Y, Yamane K, Yabuki SY, Kawasaki Y, Toyoshi T, et al. Pioglitazone improves obesity type diabetic nephropathy: relation to the mitigation of renal oxidative reaction. Exp Anim 2008;57(5):423-32.
[51] Han SJ, Choi SE, Kang Y, Jung JG, Yi SA, Kim HJ, et al. Effect of sitagliptin plus metformin on beta-cell function, islet integrity and islet gene expression in Zucker diabetic fatty rats. Diabetes Res Clin Pract 2011;92(2):213-22.
[52] Larsen PJ, Wulff EM, Gotfredsen CF, Brand CL, Sturis J, Vrang N, et al. Combination of the insulin sensitizer, pioglitazone, and the long-acting GLP-1 human analog, liraglutide, exerts potent synergistic glucose-lowering efficacy in severely diabetic ZDF rats. Diabetes Obes Metab 2008;10(4):301-11.
[53] Han S, Hagan DL, Taylor JR, Xin L, Meng W, Biller SA, et al. Dapagliflozin, a selective SGLT2 inhibitor, improves glucose homeostasis in normal and diabetic rats. Diabetes 2008;57(6):1723-9.
[54] Blachere JC, Perusse F, Bukowiecki LJ. Lowering plasma free fatty acids with Acipimox mimics the antidiabetic effects of the beta 3-adrenergic agonist CL-316243 in obese Zucker diabetic fatty rats. Metabolism 2001;50(8):945-51.
[55] Ishikawa Y, Saito MN, Ikemoto T, Takeno H, Watanabe K, Tani T. Actions of the novel oral antidiabetic agent HQL-975 in insulin-resistant non-insulin-dependent diabetes mellitus model animals. Diabetes Res Clin Pract 1998;41(2):101-11.

[56] Schafer HL, Linz W, Falk E, Glien M, Glombik H, Korn M, et al. AVE8134, a novel potent PPARalpha agonist, improves lipid profile and glucose metabolism in dyslipidemic mice and type 2 diabetic rats. Acta Pharmacol Sin;33(1):82-90.

[57] Schreibelt G, Klinkenberg LJ, Cruz LJ, Tacken PJ, Tel J, Kreutz M, et al. The C-type lectin receptor CLEC9A mediates antigen uptake and (cross-)presentation by human blood BDCA3+ myeloid dendritic cells. Blood;119(10):2284-92.

[58] Chen L, Yao X, Young A, McNulty J, Anderson D, Liu Y, et al. Inhibition of apical sodium-dependent bile acid transporter as a novel treatment for diabetes. Am J Physiol Endocrinol Metab;302(1):E68-76.

[59] Vora JP, Zimsen SM, Houghton DC, Anderson S. Evolution of metabolic and renal changes in the ZDF/Drt-fa rat model of type II diabetes. J Am Soc Nephrol 1996;7(1):113-7.

[60] Oltman CL, Coppey LJ, Gellett JS, Davidson EP, Lund DD, Yorek MA. Progression of vascular and neural dysfunction in sciatic nerves of Zucker diabetic fatty and Zucker rats. Am J Physiol Endocrinol Metab 2005;289(1):E113-22.

[61] Shibata T, Takeuchi S, Yokota S, Kakimoto K, Yonemori F, Wakitani K. Effects of peroxisome proliferator-activated receptor-alpha and -gamma agonist, JTT-501, on diabetic complications in Zucker diabetic fatty rats. Br J Pharmacol 2000;130(3):495-504.

[62] Kim J, Kim CS, Sohn E, Kim H, Jeong IH, Kim JS. Lens epithelial cell apoptosis initiates diabetic cataractogenesis in the Zucker diabetic fatty rat. Graefes Arch Clin Exp Ophthalmol 2010;248(6):811-8.

[63] Kawano K, Hirashima T, Mori S, Saitoh Y, Kurosumi M, Natori T. Spontaneous long-term hyperglycemic rat with diabetic complications. Otsuka Long-Evans Tokushima Fatty (OLETF) strain. Diabetes 1992;41(11):1422-8.

[64] Takiguchi S, Takata Y, Funakoshi A, Miyasaka K, Kataoka K, Fujimura Y, et al. Disrupted cholecystokinin type-A receptor (CCKAR) gene in OLETF rats. Gene 1997;197(1-2):169-75.

[65] Takiguchi S, Takata Y, Takahashi N, Kataoka K, Hirashima T, Kawano K, et al. A disrupted cholecystokinin A receptor gene induces diabetes in obese rats synergistically with ODB1 gene. Am J Physiol 1998;274(2 Pt 1):E265-70.

[66] Mori T, Nagai K, Nakagawa H, Yanaihara N. Intracranial infusion of CCK-8 derivatives suppresses food intake in rats. Am J Physiol 1986;251(4 Pt 2):R718-23.

[67] Lorenz DN, Goldman SA. Vagal mediation of the cholecystokinin satiety effect in rats. Physiol Behav 1982;29(4):599-604.

[68] Kawano K, Hirashima T, Mori S, Natori T. OLETF (Otsuka Long-Evans Tokushima Fatty) rat: a new NIDDM rat strain. Diabetes Res Clin Pract 1994;24 Suppl:S317-20.

[69] Shi K, Mizuno A, Sano T, Ishida K, Shima K. Sexual difference in the incidence of diabetes mellitus in Otsuka-Long-Evans-Tokushima-Fatty rats: effects of castration and sex hormone replacement on its incidence. Metabolism 1994;43(10):1214-20.

[70] Ishida K, Mizuno A, Min Z, Sano T, Shima K. Which is the primary etiologic event in Otsuka Long-Evans Tokushima Fatty rats, a model of spontaneous non-insulin-dependent diabetes mellitus, insulin resistance, or impaired insulin secretion? Metabolism 1995;44(7):940-5.

[71] Lee E, Ryu GR, Ko SH, Ahn YB, Yoon KH, Ha H, et al. Antioxidant treatment may protect pancreatic beta cells through the attenuation of islet fibrosis in an animal model of type 2 diabetes. Biochem Biophys Res Commun 2011;414(2):397-402.

[72] Toide K, Man ZW, Asahi Y, Sato T, Nakayama N, Noma Y, et al. Glucose transporter levels in a male spontaneous non-insulin-dependent diabetes mellitus rat of the Otsuka Long-Evans Tokushima Fatty strain. Diabetes Res Clin Pract 1997;38(3):151-60.

[73] Harada N, Ohnaka M, Sakamoto S, Niwa Y, Nakaya Y. Cilnidipine improves insulin sensitivity in the Otsuka Long-Evans Tokushima fatty rat, a model of spontaneous NIDDM. Cardiovasc Drugs Ther 1999;13(6):519-23.

[74] Mori Y, Komiya H, Kurokawa N, Tajima N. Comparison of the effects of glimepiride and glibenclamide on adipose tissue tumour necrosis factor-alpha mRNA expression and cellularity. Diabetes Obes Metab 2004;6(1):28-34.

[75] Yamamoto M, Otsuki M. Effect of inhibition of alpha-glucosidase on age-related glucose intolerance and pancreatic atrophy in rats. Metabolism 2006;55(4):533-40.

[76] Nakagawa T, Goto H, Hussein G, Hikiami H, Shibahara N, Shimada Y. Keishibukuryogan ameliorates glucose intolerance and hyperlipidemia in Otsuka Long-Evans Tokushima Fatty (OLETF) rats. Diabetes Res Clin Pract 2008;80(1):40-7.

[77] Kosegawa I, Katayama S, Kikuchi C, Kashiwabara H, Negishi K, Ishii J, et al. Metformin decreases blood pressure and obesity in OLETF rats via improvement of insulin resistance. Hypertens Res 1996;19(1):37-41.

[78] Wang Y, Guo XH. [Effects of GLP-1 treatment on protection of B cells in Otsuka Long-Evans Tokushima fatty rats]. Beijing Da Xue Xue Bao 2006;38(4):375-80.

[79] Kubo E, Maekawa K, Tanimoto T, Fujisawa S, Akagi Y. Biochemical and morphological changes during development of sugar cataract in Otsuka Long-Evans Tokushima fatty (OLETF) rat. Exp Eye Res 2001;73(3):375-81.

[80] Ikeda H, Shino A, Matsuo T, Iwatsuka H, Suzuoki Z. A new genetically obese-hyperglycemic rat (Wistar fatty). Diabetes 1981;30(12):1045-50.

[81] Kava RA, West DB, Lukasik VA, Greenwood MR. Sexual dimorphism of hyperglycemia and glucose tolerance in Wistar fatty rats. Diabetes 1989;38(2):159-63.

[82] Tominaga M, Kimura M, Igarashi M, Eguchi H, Igarashi K, Abe T, et al. Slight but significant improvement of insulin resistance of Wistar fatty rats by treatment with a disaccharidase inhibitor, AO-128. Tohoku J Exp Med 1997;181(3):353-60.

[83] Sugiyama Y, Taketomi S, Shimura Y, Ikeda H, Fujita T. Effects of pioglitazone on glucose and lipid metabolism in Wistar fatty rats. Arzneimittelforschung 1990;40(3):263-7.

[84] Suzuki M, Odaka H, Suzuki N, Sugiyama Y, Ikeda H. Effects of combined pioglitazone and metformin on diabetes and obesity in Wistar fatty rats. Clin Exp Pharmacol Physiol 2002;29(4):269-74.

[85] Ikeda H, Sugiyama Y. [Insulin resistance-reducing effect of a new thiazolidinedione derivative, pioglitazone]. Nihon Yakurigaku Zasshi 2001;117(5):335-42.

[86] Feng J, Zhang Z, Wallace MB, Stafford JA, Kaldor SW, Kassel DB, et al. Discovery of alogliptin: a potent, selective, bioavailable, and efficacious inhibitor of dipeptidyl peptidase IV. J Med Chem 2007;50(10):2297-300.

[87] Suzuki M, Yamada Y, Yamasaki H, Anayama H, Sasaki S, Odaka H, et al. Nephropathy in Genetically Obese - Diabetic Wistar Fatty Rats -Characterization and Prevention-. Jpn Pharmacol Ther 1997;25(2):363-71.

[88] Berti-Mattera LN, Lowery J, Day SF, Peterson RG, Eichberg J. Alteration of phosphoinositide metabolism, protein phosphorylation, and carbohydrate levels in sciatic nerve from Wistar fatty diabetic rats. Diabetes 1989;38(3):373-8.

[89] Shinohara M, Masuyama T, Shoda T, Takahashi T, Katsuda Y, Komeda K, et al. A new spontaneously diabetic non-obese Torii rat strain with severe ocular complications. Int J Exp Diabetes Res 2000;1(2):89-100.
[90] Sasase T, Ohta T, Ogawa N, Miyajima K, Ito M, Yamamoto H, et al. Preventive effects of glycaemic control on ocular complications of Spontaneously Diabetic Torii rat. Diabetes Obes Metab 2006;8(5):501-7.
[91] Masuyama T, Komeda K, Hara A, Noda M, Shinohara M, Oikawa T, et al. Chronological characterization of diabetes development in male Spontaneously Diabetic Torii rats. Biochem Biophys Res Commun 2004;314(3):870-7.
[92] Ohta T, Matsui K, Miyajima K, Sasase T, Masuyama T, Shoda T, et al. Effect of insulin therapy on renal changes in spontaneously diabetic Torii rats. Exp Anim 2007;56(5):355-62.
[93] Ohta T, Miyajima K, Yamada T. Pathophysiological changes in pre-diabetic stage of Spontaneously Diabetic Torii (SDT) rats. J Anim Vet Adv 2011;10(7):813-17.
[94] Matsui K, Oda T, Nishizawa E, Sano R, Yamamoto H, Fukuda S, et al. Pancreatic function of spontaneously diabetic torii rats in pre-diabetic stage. Exp Anim 2009;58(4):363-74.
[95] Shinohara M, Oikawa T, Sato K, Kanazawa Y. Glucose intolerance and hyperlipidemia prior to diabetes onset in female Spontaneously Diabetic Torii (SDT) rats. Exp Diabesity Res 2004;5(4):253-6.
[96] Ohta T, Shinohara M, Miyajima K, Yamada T. Pancreatic abnormalities at a young age in pre-diabetic stage of Spontaneously Diabetic Torii (SDT) rats. J Anim Vet Adv 2012;11(9):1322-6.
[97] Butler AE, Janson J, Bonner-Weir S, Ritzel R, Rizza RA, Butler PC. Beta-cell deficit and increased beta-cell apoptosis in humans with type 2 diabetes. Diabetes 2003;52(1):102-10.
[98] Ohta T, Miyajima K, Shinohara M, Yamamoto T, Yamada T. Inhibition of postprandial hyperglycemia prevents the incidence of diabetes in pre-diabetic stage of Spontaneously Diabetic Torii (SDT) rats. J Anim Vet Adv 2012;11(10):1583-7.
[99] Chiasson JL, Josse RG, Gomis R, Hanefeld M, Karasik A, Laakso M. Acarbose for prevention of type 2 diabetes mellitus: the STOP-NIDDM randomised trial. Lancet 2002;359(9323):2072-7.
[100] Kawamori R, Tajima N, Iwamoto Y, Kashiwagi A, Shimamoto K, Kaku K. Voglibose for prevention of type 2 diabetes mellitus: a randomised, double-blind trial in Japanese individuals with impaired glucose tolerance. Lancet 2009;373(9675):1607-14.
[101] Report of the Expert Committee on the Diagnosis and Classification of Diabetes Mellitus. Diabetes Care 1997;20(7):1183-97.
[102] Cavaghan MK, Ehrmann DA, Polonsky KS. Interactions between insulin resistance and insulin secretion in the development of glucose intolerance. J Clin Invest 2000;106(3):329-33.
[103] Masuyama T, Katsuda Y, Shinohara M. A novel model of obesity-related diabetes: introgression of the Lepr(fa) allele of the Zucker fatty rat into nonobese Spontaneously Diabetic Torii (SDT) rats. Exp Anim 2005;54(1):13-20.
[104] Ishii Y, Ohta T, Sasase T, Morinaga H, Ueda N, Hata T, et al. Pathophysiological analysis of female Spontaneously Diabetic Torii fatty rats. Exp Anim 2010;59(1):73-84.
[105] Matsui K, Ohta T, Oda T, Sasase T, Ueda N, Miyajima K, et al. Diabetes-associated complications in Spontaneously Diabetic Torii fatty rats. Exp Anim 2008;57(2):111-21.